The NEW Carbohydrate, Fat, Protein & Calories Counter

DR. HATEM MAHER

Table of Contents

NTRODUCTION

Making healthy food choices isn't always easy. Whether you want to lose weight, gain muscle mass, manage diabetes or hypertension, prevent health issues, or simply provide healthy meals for you and your family, this book is for you.

you know dozens of people on the ketogenic diet, Atkins diet, Paleo diet, low-carb diets, low glycemic iets, there's a good reason: These diets really promote weight-loss, prevent weight gain, reverse some 1ronic disease, maintain health condition and improve blood markers. That's why more and more people ave turned to them as their primary diets to reach their weight management or health goals.

lowever, all dieters will struggle to keep their macronutrients and nutrients counts within the strict limits ecommended by their diets without having a reliable and complete food counter.

his simple-to-understand, well-organized, easy-to-use, comprehensive guidebook provides all the iformation you need, whether your goal is to lose weight, gain muscle mass, prevent chronic disease, or imply want to eat healthy foods.

y providing extensive nutritional information for more than 6500 foods as well as optimized dietary uidelines, and glycemic index tables, this book has everything you need to know to count 1acronutrients, nutrients or glycemic index and glycemic load in your diet, and reach your goals, whether our objective is to lose weight, gain mass muscles, improve blood markers, prevent weight gain, maintain ealth condition, reverse diabetes, manage hypertension or simply eat healthy food.

he 2019 Complete Guide provides the following for more than 6500 foods commonly eaten:

- Calorie counts
- Carbohydrate grams
- Net Carbohydrates grams
- Protein grams
- Fiber grams
- Fat grams
- Cholesterol milligrams
- Sodium milligrams

n addition to comprehensive tables of Glycemic index and glycemic load. Foods are divided into three ategories according to their glycemic index:

- Low glycemic index food
- Moderate glycemic index food
- High glycemic index food

500 popular foods are divided into eighteen categories, including:

- Cereal Grains,
- Breakfast Cereals
- Condiments
- Dairy & Eggs
- Beverages

- Fast food
- Fats and Oils
- Restaurant Foods
- Backed Product
- Fruits and Juices
- Vegetables and Vegetable Products
- Herbs & Spices
- Nuts and Seeds
- Pork Products
- Poultry Products

What can you expect by using this book?

This book will give you an extensive and authoritative collection of accurate data essential to reach your weight management or health goals. You will be able to keep your daily carbohydrates intakes within the strict limits recommended by the diet you follow.

The first part provides general dietary guidelines that will allow you to understand the importance of the quality of macronutrients and gives you recommendation on how to choose healthy foods.

In the second part, you will find the carb grams, protein grams, fat grams, calories, fiber grams, sodium milligrams of 6,500 foods commonly eaten divided into eighteen categories including Dairy and Eggs Products, Beverages, Baked Products, Cereal Grains and Pasta, Fruits and Fruit Juices, Meals, Entrees, and Side Dishes; Nut and Seed Products, Vegetables...

The third part is divided into three chapters. The first chapter provides an exhaustive table that lists foods that meet the criteria of the low glycemic index (LGI). LGI foods are presented and sorted alphabetically. The second chapter provides a table of moderate glycemic index food with the glycemic index and glycemic load values. The third chapter provides a listing of foods that must be avoided due to their high glycemic index values.

All the data provided in this book come from the most authoritative organizations in the field. Those data are essential for you in order to succeed in your diet journey (ketogenic diet, the Atkins diet, low-carb, diabetes management or prevention), and achieve a long-term and lasting results (weight loss, weight gain prevention, diabetes control plan...)

PART I: General Dietary Guidelines

Chapter 1: Choose the good Carbohydrates

Insulin, cortisol, leptin, ghrelin and peptides YY are hormones that play key roles for successful and long-lasting weight loss diets. The choice of high-quality macronutrient — carbohydrates, fats and protein— is then crucial and will ensure long-term results, blood markers improvements and general health condition maintenance.

How to make the hormones work for you to beat obesity and overweight?

Before going deeper in the choice of healthy carbohydrates, we have to notice that we must achieve the following "Hormones regulation concepts":

Getting and maintaining the insulin down, this will allow to increase your body insulin sensitivity and reduce any form of insulin resistance.

Avoiding spikes in insulin level, which is harmful for the pancreas and may induce insulin resistance, and induce increase of cortisol levels —*the hormone of stress*— when the blood sugar decrease abruptly.

Avoiding ultra-processed and high-processed foods that compromise the integrity of the guts and inhibits or reduce the release of leptin —*the hormone of satiety.*—

Reduce the release of ghrelin — *the hormone of hunger*— by eating some nutrients that slowdown the ghrelin release in the bloodstream.

Carbohydrates in low-glycemic diet

Carbohydrate is one of the main three macronutrients found in food. On a ketogenic diet, Carbohydrates is drastically restricted to enable the body to enter the ketosis stage with a lot of side effect especially for women associated to the drastic carbohydrates reduction and increase of cortisol level. Conversely, in **low-GI diet, the daily intake of carbohydrates is 40% mainly complex carbohydrates**.

Regardless of the diet, complex carbs have several positive benefits particularly for men's and women's health. Thus, optimizing the choice of your dietary carbohydrates is a mandatory step to achieve long-term weight loss, weight gain prevention, insulin resistance reversal, diabetes control and prevention.
It is essential that you understand vital information provided in this chapter and gain insights and general knowledge that will guide you throughout your diet journey.

Types of Carbohydrate in Your Diet
The main function of carbohydrates is to provide energy through a known mechanism. Dietary carbohydrates can be divided into three major categories:
- Sugars: Short-chain carbs found in foods such as fructose, glucose, sucrose and galactose.
- Starches: Long-chain of glucose molecules, which get transformed into glucose during digestion.
- Fibers: are divided into soluble and insoluble.

Carbohydrates can also be divided according to their chemical composition into simple and complex carbs.

- Complex carbohydrates are formed by sugar molecules that are linked together in complex and long chains. Complex carbs are found in foods such as vegetables, fruits, peas, beans, and whole grains and contain natural fiber. These types of food are healthy.

- Simple carbohydrates are transformed quickly by the body and induce an increased sugar blood level. Simple carbs are found in foods such as milk, milk products and some fruits. They are found in high amount in processed foods and refined sugars. The consumption of this type of carbs is associated with health problems like type 2 diabetes, obesity, metabolism problem. Simple carbs foods are also deprived of essential nutrients and vitamins.

Choosing the best carbohydrates

For a lasting weight loss and prevention of weight gain, you have to remember always that the main concept is to adapt your diet to make the five hormones of weight gain working for you.
Thus, the *quality* of the carbohydrates you eat is crucial in adjusting the hormones level as stated in the beginning of this chapter.
For instance, low-quality carbs are quickly digested and lead to blood sugar spikes, which will play against you and cause weight gain, obesity, insulin resistance and increased level of cortisol. Conversely, the soluble and insoluble fibers in whole foods are known to offset the glucose conversion of glucose, preventing higher insulin supplies, and avoiding irregular variation of blood sugar that induce excess of cortisol.

In low-glycemic diet, we recommend shifting to eat according to the glycemic index and glycemic load which include whole grains, nuts and seeds, vegetables, fruits, and dairy. We also recommend shifting away from refined carbohydrates, added sugars in beverages, ultra-processed and high-processed meals.

Added sugar, the hidden enemy
The quality of carbohydrates is so crucial for the success of the "hormones revolution concepts" that drive weight loss, prevent weight gain, reduce insulin resistance and improve critical metabolic functions.

So you have To improve the quality of carbohydrates in your diet, by choosing more whole grains and avoiding foods that have added sugars. This can be achieved partly, by cooking low-glycemic-index food at home and eating whole foods according to their glycemic index value and glycemic load, rather than processed ones, or those with high glycemic index or high glycemic load.

Processed and refined carbohydrates like grains, starches, and sugars must be avoided. In your low-glycemic diet start by removing these foods from your pantry. And, replace them with high-quality carbohydrates sources like fruits, vegetables, nuts, seeds, raw honey and maple syrup.

The consumption of sugar, refined grains, and other nutrient-poor foods lead to high blood sugar levels; with sharp peaks of insulin secretion. Which is harmful to your health and pancreas.
Added sugar is obviously in fruit drinks, soda, sweets, snacks, and in general in foods that are not naturally sweets. However, it's also in significant quantities in foods that aren't considered sweets, including yogurt, bread, pasta, breakfast cereals, salad dressings, sauces, processed meats, and processed foods.

We recommend that women following the low-glycemic index limit added sugar intake to 16 grams (the equivalent of 4 teaspoons) per day and to 20 grams (the equivalent of 5 teaspoons) for man.

Net Carb concept

The concept of net carbs is based on the principle that not all carbohydrates affect the body in the same manner.

Some carbs, like refined or simple starches and sugars, are metabolized rapidly and have a high glycemic index meaning they cause high spikes of blood sugar in the bloodstream after eating. The Excess of simple and refined carbohydrates are stored in your body as fat.

Other carbohydrates, have different metabolism action such as dietary fibers (soluble and insoluble) found in whole grains, vegetables and fruits, are metabolized slowly which raises the blood sugar in a balanced and which raises the blood sugar in a regulated, balanced way. Dietary fibers are safe and must not be counted in the Net Carb formula.

Sugar alcohols is another type of carbohydrates that is metabolized slowly, but must be included in the Net Carbs calculation. Unlike food companies that didn't count sugar alcohols in Net Crab formula. There is a consensus between researchers that Sugar alcohols must be must be count in the Net Carb formula. There are sugar alcohols that can raise blood sugar quickly, and have a higher glycemic index, and must be counted as carbohydrates.

We estimate that 50% of sugar alcohols must be counted in the Net Carb formula.

Chapter 2: Choose the good fats

After carbohydrates, it is essential to optimize the choice of your dietary fat.
Fat is one of the three macronutrients found in food. On a ketogenic diet for example, fat is the primary energy source, however, as you may have noticed in our approach, you should optimize the choice of your dietary fat, by choosing the healthy types and eating the just right amount recommended by your diet, in addition, to the proper supply of high-quality carbs and proteins.
So, it is essential that you gain insights that will guide you throughout your diet journey.

What is fat, and why it is essential for your health?

Dietary fats are found in both animals and vegetables and are essential for your living since they provide your body energy and support cell growth.
Fats also provide some valuable benefits and play essential roles, including:

- Help your body absorb some nutrients such as vitamins A, D, E, and K.

- Help your body produce necessary hormones.

- Regulate inflammation and immunity issues.

- Maintain the health of your cells (skin, hair cells)

How many different fats are there?

There are four major fats in food, based on their chemical structures and physical properties:

- Saturated fat (bad fat): is a kind of fat in which the fatty acid chain of carbon atoms holds as many hydrogen atoms as possible (saturated with hydrogens). This form of saturated fat is associated with various negative health effects while recent studies moderate the common belief, and question about how bad they impact the health.
- Trans fat (bad fat): (trans-unsaturated fatty acids or trans fatty acids) are a form of unsaturated fat associated with various adverse health effects.
- Monounsaturated fats (healthy fat): are a type of unsaturated fat, but have only one double bond. These fats are associated with positive health effect and may replace the bad fats. Monounsaturated fats are found in olive oil, avocados and some nuts).
- Polyunsaturated fat (healthy fat): The two major classes of polyunsaturated fats are omega-3 and omega-6 fatty acids

What is cholesterol?

Cholesterol is a waxy, fat-like substance found in all the cells in your body. Plus, your body needs some cholesterol to produce steroid hormones, vitamin D, and bile acid that helps you digest fats. Contrary to the common belief, your body produces all the cholesterol it needs in the liver. Cholesterol is supplied in small quantities (less than 15%) by plant and animals foods.

In fact, more than 85% of the cholesterol in your bloodstream comes from your liver rather than from the food you eat. Dietary cholesterol has a little impact on raising blood cholesterol levels, which is valuable information from a diet perspective.

While a high level of cholesterol in the blood can be dangerous, maintaining the right balance of cholesterol in the blood is essential for your health.

What types of fat should you eat?

We recommend that you consume fats found naturally in food and not being processed.
Several healthy sources of fat exist such as:

- Butter and ghee (clarified butter)
- Cream
- Coconut oil
- Cheese
- Lard and tallow
- Avocado (the fruit and/or avocado oil)
- Coconut (meat, cream, oil, milk, butter)
- Cacao butter
- Tallow
- Duck fat
- Medium-chained triglyceride (MCT) oil
- Pepperoni/salami/prosciutto
- Bacon fat/lard/beef
- Sardines, anchovies
- Salmon
- Olives and olive oil
- Avocados and avocado oil
- Macadamias and macadamia oil
- Almonds, Brazil nuts, hazelnuts, pecans
- Polyunsaturated fat sources

What Are Fatty Acids?

Fatty acids are a form of hydrocarbon chains with carboxyl at one end and methyl at the other. The biological activity of fatty acids is determined by the length of their carbon chain and by the number and position of their double bonds.

While saturated fatty acids do not contain double bonds within the acyl chain, unsaturated fatty acids include at least one double bond.

When two or more double bonds are present in their chain, unsaturated fatty acids are referred to as Dietary polyunsaturated fatty acids (PUFAs) and have been associated with cholesterol-lowering properties. The two families of PUFA are omega-3 and omega-6.

What Are Omega-3 Fatty Acids?

Omega-3 fatty acids are a type of polyunsaturated fats. Since your body can't produce omega-3s, this kind of fats is classified as "essential fats," implying that you have to get them from your diet.

There are various types of omega-3 fats, which differ by their chemical structure. The three most common types of omega-3 are:

- Eicosapentaenoic acid (EPA)
- Docosahexaenoic acid (DHA)
- Alpha-linolenic acid (ALA)

Omega-3 fats play a crucial role in your body, including:

- Improves heart health
- Supports mental health
- Reduces weight and waist size
- Decreases liver fat
- Supports infant brain development
- Fights inflammation
- Prevents dementia
- Promotes bone health

Omega-3 are essential fats that you must integrate into low carb or GI diet. They have significant benefits for your heart, brain and metabolism.

What are Omega-6 Fatty Acids?

Like omega-3, omega-6 fatty acids are polyunsaturated fatty acids. Omega-6 fatty acids are primarily used for energy, so you need to get them from your diet in the right quantities.
Following different studies and guidelines, we recommend a ratio of 4/1 omega-6 to omega-3 or less.
Which mean that for 400 milligrams of omega-6 you have to consume 100 milligram of omega-3.
This ratio is very important, when we know that western diets have very high ratio between 10/1 and 50/1.

Why and how is the excess of omega-6 harmful?
A high amount of omega-6 polyunsaturated fatty acids associated with a very high ratio omega-6/omega-3 is a constant in a majority of Western diets including the keto-basic diet. That increase the pathogenesis of several diseases, such as cancer, cardiovascular disease, autoimmune and inflammatory diseases.
Conversely high levels of omega-3 associated with a low ratio of omega-6/omega-3 induce health benefits. For example, a ratio omega-6/omega-3 of 4/1 was correlated to a 70% reduction in mortality.
The lower omega-6/omega-3 ratio in women suffering from breast cancer was connected to decreased risk. This explains why the notion of omega-6 / omega-3 ratio is essential in weight loss and health.

As for high-quality carbs, the low-glycemic index diet will provide you with the right fatty acids in proper proportion to benefit from sustainable weight loss and health.

A traditional low-glycemic diet for example may be low in omega-3 fatty acids but rich in omega-6 and saturated fatty acids, and induced health concerns, increase the risk of insulin resistance, prediabetes, weight gain.

Thus, achieving a balance of omega-6 and omega-3 is a decisive element of your low carb or GI diet. Unlike the ketogenic -basic diet, or Atkins diet in which fats are prescribed in general, we recommend the right ratios for long-term results, including the omega-6: omega-3 ratio.
A low carb, low GI diet is based on a ratio of omega-6 to omega-3 essential fatty acids of approximately 1.5 to 2.5. Consuming fatty fish twice a week, eating whole foods, choosing dairy products and meat from grass-fed animals, can help you improve your omega-6: omega-3 ratio.

Chapter 3: Choose the right proteins

Protein is one of the three macronutrients found in food. On a low-glycemic diet, protein is consumed in a moderate amount to enable the body to have the necessary amount of this essential macronutrient.

Eating an adequate amount of protein is extremely important for women's and men's health. Protein is an essential component of every cell in your body. Protein plays a crucial role in vital processes and metabolism of your body such as building and repairing tissues, building muscles, blood, hair, and skin and producing hormones, enzymes, and other body chemicals.

Unlike carbohydrates and fat, your body does not store protein, and you need to eat the necessary amount to keep the right hormonal balance and a healthy body.

Plus, eating protein reduces levels of the ghrelin (the hunger hormone) and stimulates the production of the satiety hormones (PYY and GLP-1)
When you eat protein, it's transformed into amino acids, which help your body with various processes such as building muscle and regulating immune function

Guidelines for individualized protein intake

The RDA (international Recommended Dietary Allowance) for protein is 0.8 g per kg of body weight, regardless of age. This recommendation is derived as the minimum amount to maintain nitrogen balance; however, it is not optimized for women and men needs nor for physical activity level.

Taking into account different parameters, we recommend a protein intake of 1.4-1.8 grams per kg of your body weight. Going to 1.9 grams per kg of the body weight for woman in the premenstrual phase may be the right choice if she suffers from troubles associated with period approaches.

Protein Quality

The optimal source of protein is based on the calculation of the PDCAA (Protein Digestibility Corrected Amino Acid) Score, or the DIAA (Digestibility Indispensable Amino Acid) Score.

Following these quality parameters, animal-based foods are identified as a superior source of protein because they offer a complete composition of essential amino acids, with higher bioavailability and digestibility (>90%).

Collagen, an essential ingredient in low carb and GI diet:

Consuming a right amount of collagen, is an essential element in your diet.

The most abundant type of protein in your body is collagen. Ligaments, tendons, skin, hair, nails, discs, and bones are made up of collagen.

During the normal aging process, your body begins to experience a decline in the synthesis of collagen proteins. According to studies, this decline in collagen production starts around the age of 30, at a rate of 1% per year. At the age of fifty, the rate jump to up to 3%, causing health issues: :

- muscle stiffness,
- aching joints,
- wrinkles and fine lines,
- lack of tone,
- sagging skin,
- healing of wounds slower,
- frequent fatigue.

In low-glycemic diet, consuming more collagen will boost your body collagen protection (particularly for women). So we recommend that daily intake of collagen represent 25 to 35% of protein.

The beneficial effects are:
- Promote intestinal health
- Reduce articular pain
- Decrease hair loss
- Better skin
- Increase muscle mass

Better foods rich in collagen

Here are some of the best collagen-rich foods you can add to your diet:

Bone broth
Made by simmering bones, tendons, ligaments and skin of beef, bone broth is an excellent source of collagen, as well as several essential amino acids. Bone broth also available in powder, bar or even capsule for a collagen food supplement that is easy to add to your routine.

Spirulina
This type of seaweed is an excellent source of plant-based amino acids, which are a key component of collagen. Spirulina can be found in dried form at most health food stores.

Codfish
Codfish, like most other types of white fish, is a good source of collagen in addition to selenium, vitamin B6 and phosphorus.

Eggs
Eggs are a good source of collagen, including glycine and proline.

Gelatin
Gelatin is one of the best collagen-rich foods available. This is why it is advised to include it in your Low carb or GI diet.

Chapter 4: Weight Loss and Insulin Hormone

Insulin is a polypeptide hormone that regulates the absorption of sugar by body cells and maintains the level of sugar present in the blood at a healthy level.. This hormone is produced by the β cells of the pancreas. When we eat, food travels to our stomach and intestines where it is broken down into micronutrients.

These micronutrients are absorbed and transported by our bloodstream. The pancreas, which is the main regulator of our blood sugar, produces the insulin hormone, and releases it into the bloodstream when we eat.

Insulin is a hormone that controls the level of glucose in the blood by controlling its production by the liver and its use by the muscle. Its primary function is to allow body cells, including muscles and other cells to absorb and transform sugar (glucose) into energy throughout the body.

Insulin sends also signals to liver, muscle, and adipocytes (fat cells) to store the excess of glucose for further use. Excess sugar is stored in 3 ways:
* In muscle tissues in the form of glycogen.
* In the liver in the form of glycogen.
* In adipose tissue (fat reserves of the body) in the form of triglycerides which are fat molecules that store energy

Weight gain and insulin

Weight gain is explained by the secretion of insulin. Insulin is the hormone responsible for weight gain secreted by the pancreas. If you do not secrete pancreas insulin, you do not gain weight.

Hyperglycemia is the abnormally high blood sugar level. Hyperglycemia is felt like a rush of adrenaline, a gain of energy, making us feel extremely good.
However, hyperglycemia lasts only a short time because when the blood sugar level is too high, the pancreas will secrete insulin to release the sugar in the blood and pass it to the cells.

As seen earlier, excess of sugar is stored in 3 ways, including in adipose tissue (fat reserves of the body) in the form of triglycerides which are fat molecules that store energy.
Refined sugar and starches consumption have also been associated with a higher risk of obesity, insulin resistance, fatty liver, metabolic syndrome, and a higher risk of chronic disease.

Insulin Resistance

Insulin resistance is a serious and silent health condition that occurs when cells in your muscles, liver and body fat start ignoring the signal that insulin hormone is sending out in order to transfer sugar (glucose) out of the bloodstream and put it into your body cells.
As insulin resistance develops, the body reacts by producing more and more insulin to lower the blood sugar. Over time (months or years depending on the severity of the metabolic disfunction), the β cells in the pancreas that are working hard to make a higher supply of insulin, can no longer keep working to provide more and more insulin. Consequently, your blood sugar may reflect the pancreas failure to maintain the level in the healthy range, and your blood sugar begins to rise, indicating pre-diabetes or at worst diabetes type 2.

Symptoms of insulin resistance

Insulin resistance is silent and presents no symptoms in the first stage of its development. The symptoms start to appear later when the condition worsens, and the pancreas fails to produce enough amount of insulin to keep your blood sugar within the normal ranges. When this occurs, the symptoms may include:
- Excessive hunger
- Lethargy or tiredness
- Difficulty concentrating
- Brain fog
- Waist weight gain
- High blood pressure

Can insulin resistance be reduced or reversed?

Fortunately, It is possible to reduce the effects of insulin resistance and boost your insulin sensitivity by following a number of effective methods, including:

- Low glycemic diets

- Low carbohydrate diets

- Low carbohydrate and high-fat diet (ketogenic diets)

- Low-calorie diets

- Weight loss surgery

- Regular exercise in combination with healthy diets

These methods have a similar way of working in that they all reduce the daily glucose intake drastically, lower the body's need for insulin, reduce insulin spike in the bloodstream, promote weight loss and prevent weight gain.

How to make insulin working for you:
1. Get the insulin down, to reduce your body fat

2. Get the insulin down, by following a low glycemic index diet

3. Get the insulin down, by following a low carb diet

4. Avoid eating refined sugars, and added sugar meals

5. Avoid sweetened beverages and including fruit juices, soda,

6. Avoid processed meals and boxed foods

7. Limit your daily intake of carbohydrates to complex carbohydrates

Chapter 5: Weight Loss and Cortisol Hormone

Cortisol is the stress hormone, produced by the adrenal gland when the body is in stressful situations. The hypothalamus, via the pituitary gland, sends a chemical signal to the adrenal glands to produce and release both adrenaline and cortisol.

Cortisol is naturally released every day in small and regular quantities. However, like adrenaline, cortisol can also be secreted and released in reaction to physical and emotional stress and triggers the body's fight-or-flight response.

These two stress hormones work simultaneously: adrenaline produces a significant increase in strength, performance, awareness, and increases metabolism. It also let fat cells to release additional energy. Cortisol helps the body produce glucose from proteins, and increase the body's energy in times of stress quickly.

However, cortisol is also involved in a variety of essential function for your health. Most of the body cells have cortisol receptors to use this steroid hormone for a variety of critical functions, including:
- blood sugar regulation
- metabolism regulation
- inflammation reduction
- memory formulation

Cortisol is important for your health, but an excess of cortisol can harm your body and induce a variety of unwanted symptoms.

What cause high cortisol levels?
A high cortisol level can be caused by several things. High cortisol is known as Cushing syndrome. This health condition results from your body secreting and releasing too much cortisol.

Cushing syndrome causes many unwanted symptoms, including:
- obesity
- weight gain
- fatty deposits, especially in the face, midsection, and between the shoulders
- purple stretch marks on the arms, breasts, thighs, and abdomen
- thinning skin
- slow-healing injuries

Being under stress, induce a constant state of excess cortisol production. And, as seen above, this cortisol drives excess glucose production in a non-fight-or-flight situation.

This excess glucose is converted into fat and stored by the body. Thus, high levels of produced cortisol increase the risk of obesity highly, induce abdominal obesity, and increased the amount of fat storage.

Other factors that cause peaks in cortisol production are carbohydrates deprivation (in low carb diet, for example) and overconsumption of simple carbohydrates.

In both cases, when blood sugar levels fall, this induces a surge of stress hormones, including cortisol and adrenaline.

Stress hormones and their role in the body

Stress hormones are released in reply to body stressors. Hormonal responses of the woman body to stress are essential provided they occur in less frequently. They may become damaging and unhealthy when they happen too often. Prolonged exposure to porn induce severe damages to the brain and presents evidence that porn is not a healthy stressor.

Stress is habitually accompanied by high energy demand. Consequently, a severe stress situation induces a fast glucose release into the blood, which provides the required energy to deal with the stressful situation.

The principal players in the stress mechanism are:
- The adreno-corticotropic hormone (ACTH),
- The glucocorticoids such as cortisol, adrenaline
- and noradrenaline.

When this happens, blood glucose levels rise, concurrently with heart rate and blood pressure.

So at its simplest, stress leads to an increase in blood glucose, heart rate, and blood pressure, which induces an increased insulin release.

How to make cortisol working for you:
1. Get the cortisol down, to reduce your body fat

2. Get the cortisol down, by following a low glycemic index diet

3. Get the cortisol down, by eating healthy fats and keeping your ratio omega 6/ omega 3 inferior to 3.

4. Avoid eating refined sugars, and added sugar meals

5. Avoid sweetened beverages and including fruit juices, soda,

6. Avoid processed meals and boxed foods

7. Limit your daily intake of carbohydrates to complex carbohydrates (low GI foods)

PART II: Carbohydrates, Fat, Protein, Calories & Sodium Counts

BACKED PRODUCTS

Food Name ---> per 100 g	Protein (g)	Fat (g)	Carb (g)	Calories	Fiber (g)	Sodium (mg)	Cholesterol (mg)	Net Carb (g)
Bagels, plain, enriched, with calcium propionate (includes onion, poppy, sesame)	10.56	1.32	52.38	264	1.6	422	0	50.78
Bagels, plain (includes onion, poppy, sesame), toasted	11.14	1.43	57.39	287	1.8	457	0	55.59
Bagels, egg	10.6	2.1	53	278	2.3	505	24	50.7
Bagels, cinnamon-raisin	9.8	1.7	55.2	274	2.3	344	0	52.9
Bagels, cinnamon-raisin, toasted	10.6	1.8	59.3	294	2.5	370	0	56.8
Bagels, oat bran	10.7	1.2	53.3	255	3.6	590	0	49.7
Biscuits, plain or buttermilk, frozen, baked	6.2	11.03	53.87	338	1.3	942	1	52.57
Biscuits, plain or buttermilk, dry mix	8	15.4	63.4	428	2.1	1276	2	61.3
Biscuits, plain or buttermilk, dry mix, prepared	7.3	12.1	48.4	335	1.8	955	4	46.6
Biscuits, plain or buttermilk, refrigerated dough, lower fat	6.7	7.83	43.7	270	2	828	0	41.7
Biscuits, plain or buttermilk, refrigerated dough, lower fat, baked	7.8	9.1	51.6	319	2.3	962	0	49.3
Biscuits, plain or buttermilk, refrigerated dough, higher fat	6.66	10.58	46.32	307	0.7	977	1	45.62
Biscuits, plain or buttermilk, refrigerated dough, higher fat, baked	6.79	11.22	49.05	324	2.8	1002	0	46.25
Biscuits, plain or buttermilk, prepared from recipe	7	16.3	44.6	353	1.5	580	3	43.1
Biscuits, mixed grain, refrigerated dough	6.1	5.6	47.4	263	0	670	0	47.4
Bread, banana, prepared from recipe, made with margarine	4.3	10.5	54.6	326	1.1	302	43	53.5
Bread, boston brown, canned	5.2	1.5	43.3	195	4.7	631	1	38.6
Bread, cornbread, dry mix, enriched (includes corn muffin mix)	7	12.2	69.5	418	6.5	817	2	63
Bread, cornbread, dry mix, prepared with 2% milk, 80% margarine, and eggs	6.59	9.58	54.46	330	2.3	599	57	52.16
Bread, cornbread, prepared from recipe, made with low fat (2%) milk	6.7	7.1	43.5	266	0	658	40	43.5
Bread, cracked-wheat	8.7	3.9	49.5	260	5.5	538	0	44
Bread, egg	9.5	6	47.8	287	2.3	380	51	45.5
Bread, egg, toasted	10.5	6.6	52.6	315	2.5	417	56	50.1
Bread, french or vienna (includes sourdough)	10.75	2.42	51.88	272	2.2	602	0	49.68
Bread, french or vienna, toasted (includes sourdough)	13	2.14	61.93	319	3.1	720	0	58.83
Bread, irish soda, prepared from recipe	6.6	5	56	290	2.6	398	18	53.4
Bread, italian	8.8	3.5	50.1	271	3.2	550	0	46.9
Bread, multi-grain, toasted (includes whole-grain)	14.52	4.6	47.11	288	8.1	414	0	39.01
Bread, oat bran	10.4	4.4	39.8	236	4.5	353	0	35.3
Bread, oat bran, toasted	11.4	4.8	43.7	259	4.9	387	0	38.8
Bread, oatmeal	8.4	4.4	48.5	269	4	447	0	44.5
Bread, oatmeal, toasted	9.2	4.8	52.7	292	4.3	486	0	48.4
Bread, pita, white, enriched	9.1	1.2	55.7	275	2.2	536	0	53.5
Bread, pita, whole-wheat	9.8	1.71	55.89	262	6.1	527	0	49.79
Bread, protein (includes gluten)	12.1	2.2	43.8	245	3	404	0	40.8
Bread, pumpernickel	8.7	3.1	47.5	250	6.5	596	0	41
Bread, pumpernickel, toasted	9.5	3.4	52.2	275	7.1	655	0	45.1
Bread, raisin, enriched	7.9	4.4	52.3	274	4.3	347	0	48

Food Name ---> per 100 g	Protein (g)	Fat (g)	Carb (g)	Calories	Fiber (g)	Sodium (mg)	Cholesterol (mg)	Net Carb (g)
Bread, raisin, enriched, toasted	8.6	4.8	56.9	297	4.7	377	0	52.2
Bread, reduced-calorie, oat bran	8	3.2	41.3	201	12	459	0	29.3
Bread, reduced-calorie, oat bran, toasted	9.5	3.8	49.2	239	14.3	547	0	34.9
Bread, reduced-calorie, oatmeal	7.6	3.5	43.3	210	0	388	0	43.3
Bread, reduced-calorie, rye	9.1	2.9	40.5	203	12	513	0	28.5
Bread, reduced-calorie, wheat	13.32	2.92	42.47	217	11.1	332	0	31.37
Bread, reduced-calorie, white	8.7	2.5	44.3	207	9.7	479	0	34.6
Bread, rice bran	8.9	4.6	43.5	243	4.9	269	0	38.6
Bread, rye	8.5	3.3	48.3	259	5.8	603	0	42.5
Bread, rye, toasted	9.4	3.6	53.1	284	6.4	664	0	46.7
Bread, wheat	10.72	3.24	48.68	267	4	508	0	44.68
Bread, wheat, toasted	12.96	4.27	55.77	313	4.7	601	0	51.07
Bread, wheat bran	8.8	3.4	47.8	248	4	486	0	43.8
Bread, white, commercially prepared (includes soft bread crumbs)	8.85	3.33	49.42	266	2.7	490	0	46.72
Bread, white, commercially prepared, toasted	9	4	54.5	290	2.9	537	1	51.6
Bread, white, prepared from recipe, made with nonfat dry milk	7.7	2.6	53.6	274	2	336	0	51.6
Bread, white, prepared from recipe, made with low fat (2%) milk	7.9	5.7	49.6	285	2	359	3	47.6
Bread, whole-wheat, commercially prepared	12.45	3.5	42.71	252	6	455	0	36.71
Bread, whole-wheat, commercially prepared, toasted	16.27	4.07	51.16	306	7.5	565	0	43.66
Bread, whole-wheat, prepared from recipe	8.4	5.4	51.4	278	6	346	0	45.4
Bread, whole-wheat, prepared from recipe, toasted	9.2	5.9	56.4	305	6.7	381	0	49.7
Bread crumbs, dry, grated, plain	13.35	5.3	71.98	395	4.5	732	0	67.48
Bread sticks, plain	12	9.5	68.4	412	3	713	0	65.4
Bread stuffing, bread, dry mix	11	3.4	76.2	386	3.2	1405	1	73
Bread stuffing, bread, dry mix, prepared	2.73	12.05	18.84	195	0.8	479	0	18.04
Bread stuffing, cornbread, dry mix	10	4.2	76.7	389	14.3	1429	0	62.4
Bread stuffing, cornbread, dry mix, prepared	2.9	8.8	21.9	179	2.9	526	0	19
Cake, angelfood, commercially prepared	5.9	0.8	57.8	258	1.5	749	0	56.3
Cake, angelfood, dry mix	6.4	0.27	86.13	366	0.5	822	0	85.63
Cake, angelfood, dry mix, prepared	6.1	0.3	58.7	257	0.2	511	0	58.5
Cake, boston cream pie, commercially prepared	2.4	8.5	42.9	252	1.4	254	37	41.5
Cake, pudding-type, carrot, dry mix	5.1	9.8	79.2	415	0	567	0	79.2
Cake, cherry fudge with chocolate frosting	2.4	12.5	38	264	0.5	164	42	37.5
Cake, chocolate, commercially prepared with chocolate frosting, in-store bakery	3.48	20.05	52.84	389	2.2	348	22	50.64
Cake, pudding-type, chocolate, dry mix	4.6	8.14	80.16	391	2.3	767	0	77.86
Cake, chocolate, prepared from recipe without frosting	5.3	15.1	53.4	371	1.6	315	58	51.8
Cake, white, prepared from recipe with coconut frosting	4.4	10.3	63.2	356	1	284	1	62.2
Coffeecake, cheese	7	15.2	44.3	339	1	339	85	43.3
Coffeecake, cinnamon with crumb topping, commercially prepared, enriched	6.8	23.3	46.7	418	2	351	32	44.7
Coffeecake, creme-filled with chocolate frosting	5	10.8	53.8	331	2	323	69	51.8
Coffeecake, fruit	5.2	10.2	51.5	311	2.5	385	7	49
Coffeecake, cinnamon with crumb topping, dry mix	4.8	12	77.7	436	1.8	596	0	75.9
Coffeecake, cinnamon with crumb topping, dry mix, prepared	5.5	9.6	52.8	318	1.2	421	49	51.6

Food Name ---> per 100 g	Protein (g)	Fat (g)	Carb (g)	Calories	Fiber (g)	Sodium (mg)	Cholesterol (mg)	Net Carb (g)
Cake, fruitcake, commercially prepared	2.9	9.1	61.6	324	3.7	101	5	57.9
Cake, pudding-type, german chocolate, dry mix	4.17	3.24	81.25	350	2.1	841	0	79.15
Cake, gingerbread, dry mix	4.4	13.8	74.6	437	1.7	657	0	72.9
Cake, gingerbread, prepared from recipe	3.9	16.4	49.2	356	0	327	32	49.2
Cake, pudding-type, marble, dry mix	3.4	11.7	79.5	416	2.9	519	0	76.6
Cake, pineapple upside-down, prepared from recipe	3.5	12.1	50.5	319	0.8	319	22	49.7
Cake, pound, commercially prepared, butter (includes fresh and frozen)	5	13.96	53.64	353	0.6	377	66	53.04
Cake, pound, commercially prepared, other than all butter, enriched	5.2	17.9	52.5	389	1	400	58	51.5
Cake, shortcake, biscuit-type, prepared from recipe	6.1	14.2	48.5	346	0	506	3	48.5
Cake, snack cakes, creme-filled, chocolate with frosting	3.63	15.93	60.31	399	3.2	332	0	57.11
Cake, snack cakes, creme-filled, sponge	3.47	11.54	64.03	374	1	470	41	63.03
Cake, white, dry mix, special dietary (includes lemon-flavored)	3	8.4	79.6	397	0	260	0	79.6
Cake, sponge, commercially prepared	5.4	2.7	61	290	0.5	623	102	60.5
Cake, sponge, prepared from recipe	7.3	4.3	57.7	297	0	228	170	57.7
Cake, pudding-type, white, enriched, dry mix	3.9	9.5	80.9	423	0.7	665	0	80.2
Cake, white, prepared from recipe without frosting	5.4	12.4	57.2	357	0.8	327	2	56.4
Cake, yellow, commercially prepared, with chocolate frosting, in-store bakery	3.16	17.75	55.36	379	1.5	310	16	53.86
Cake, yellow, commercially prepared, with vanilla frosting	2.99	17.91	56.2	391	0.3	269	75	55.9
Cake, pudding-type, yellow, dry mix	4	9.8	80	423	0.7	860	0	79.3
Cake, yellow, enriched, dry mix	3.7	3.5	81.92	374	1.2	728	0	80.72
Cake, yellow, prepared from recipe without frosting	5.3	14.6	53	361	0.7	343	54	52.3
Cheesecake commercially prepared	5.5	22.5	25.5	321	0.4	438	55	25.1
Cheesecake prepared from mix, no-bake type	5.5	12.7	35.5	274	1.9	380	29	33.6
Cookies, brownies, commercially prepared	4.8	16.3	63.9	405	2.1	286	17	61.8
Cookies, brownies, dry mix, regular	4	14.9	76.6	434	0	303	0	76.6
Cookies, brownies, prepared from recipe	6.2	29.1	50.2	466	0	343	73	50.2
Cookies, butter, commercially prepared, enriched	6.1	18.8	68.9	467	0.8	282	117	68.1
Cookies, fudge, cake-type (includes trolley cakes)	5	3.7	78.3	349	2.8	192	0	75.5
Cookies, chocolate wafers	6.6	14.2	72.7	433	3.4	580	2	69.3
Cookies, chocolate chip, commercially prepared, regular, lower fat	5.97	17.91	67.49	451	3	418	0	64.49
Cookies, chocolate chip, commercially prepared, regular, higher fat, enriched	5.1	24.72	65.36	492	2	311	0	63.36
Cookies, chocolate chip, commercially prepared, soft-type	3.63	19.77	65.75	444	1.8	276	0	63.95
Cookies, chocolate chip, dry mix	4.6	25.2	66.1	497	0	290	0	66.1
Cookies, chocolate chip, refrigerated dough	3.98	21.33	61.02	451	1.5	321	7	59.52
Cookies, chocolate chip, refrigerated dough, baked	4.9	22.6	68.2	492	1.7	232	27	66.5
Cookies, chocolate chip, prepared from recipe, made with margarine	5.7	28.3	58.4	488	2.8	361	32	55.6
Cookies, chocolate sandwich, with creme filling, regular	5.21	19.14	71	464	2.9	388	0	68.1
Cookies, chocolate sandwich, with creme filling, regular, chocolate-coated	3.6	26.4	66.4	481	5.2	326	0	61.2
Cookies, chocolate sandwich, with extra creme filling	4.33	24.52	68.2	497	2.7	351	0	65.5

23

Food Name ---> per 100 g	Protein (g)	Fat (g)	Carb (g)	Calories	Fiber (g)	Sodium (mg)	Cholesterol (mg)	Net Carb (g)
Cookies, fig bars	3.7	7.3	70.9	348	4.6	350	0	66.3
Cookies, fortune	4.2	2.7	84	378	1.6	31	2	82.4
Cookies, gingersnaps	5.6	9.8	76.9	416	2.2	501	0	74.7
Cookies, graham crackers, plain or honey (includes cinnamon)	6.69	10.6	77.66	430	3.4	459	0	74.26
Cookies, graham crackers, chocolate-coated	4	25.8	66.78	500	2.2	265	1	64.58
Cookies, ladyfingers, with lemon juice and rind	10.6	9.1	59.7	365	1	147	221	58.7
Cookies, marshmallow, chocolate-coated (includes marshmallow pies)	4	16.9	67.7	421	2	188	0	65.7
Cookies, molasses	5.6	12.8	73.8	430	1	459	0	72.8
Cookies, oatmeal, commercially prepared, regular	6.2	18.1	68.7	450	2.8	383	0	65.9
Cookies, oatmeal, commercially prepared, soft-type	6.1	14.7	65.7	409	2.7	349	5	63
Cookies, oatmeal, dry mix	6.5	19.2	67.3	462	0	473	0	67.3
Cookies, oatmeal, refrigerated dough	5.4	18.9	59.1	424	2.5	294	24	56.6
Cookies, oatmeal, refrigerated dough, baked	6	21	65.7	471	2.8	327	26	62.9
Cookies, oatmeal, prepared from recipe, with raisins	6.5	16.2	68.4	435	0	538	33	68.4
Cookies, peanut butter, commercially prepared, regular	8.92	23.82	58.15	473	2.1	463	27	56.05
Cookies, peanut butter, commercially prepared, soft-type	5.3	24.4	57.7	457	1.7	336	0	56
Cookies, peanut butter, refrigerated dough	8.2	25	52.1	458	1.1	397	27	51
Cookies, peanut butter, refrigerated dough, baked	9.1	27.5	57.3	503	1.2	436	30	56.1
Cookies, peanut butter, prepared from recipe	9	23.8	58.9	475	0	518	31	58.9
Cookies, peanut butter sandwich, regular	8.8	21.1	65.6	478	1.9	368	0	63.7
Cookies, raisin, soft-type	4.1	13.6	68	401	1.2	418	2	66.8
Cookies, shortbread, commercially prepared, plain	5.37	26.22	63.78	514	1.3	353	0	62.48
Cookies, shortbread, commercially prepared, pecan	4.9	32.5	58.3	542	1.8	281	33	56.5
Cookies, brownies, dry mix, sugar free	2.9	12.5	80.4	426	4.2	83	0	76.2
Cookies, chocolate chip, commercially prepared, special dietary	3.9	16.8	73.4	450	1.6	244	0	71.8
Cookies, chocolate sandwich, with creme filling, special dietary	4.5	22.1	68	461	4.1	342	0	63.9
Cookies, oatmeal, commercially prepared, special dietary	4.8	18	69.9	449	2.9	273	0	67
Cookies, peanut butter sandwich, special dietary	10	34	50.8	535	0	412	0	50.8
Cookies, sugar wafer, with creme filling, sugar free	3.57	28.57	66.26	531	14.3	71	0	51.96
Cookies, sugar, commercially prepared, regular (includes vanilla)	5.35	19.55	67.34	464	1.3	385	12	66.04
Cookies, sugar, refrigerated dough	4	19.48	61.22	436	0.9	328	11	60.32
Cookies, sugar, refrigerated dough, baked	4.7	23.1	65.6	489	0.9	362	32	64.7
Cookies, sugar, prepared from recipe, made with margarine	5.9	23.4	60	472	1.2	491	26	58.8
Cookies, sugar wafers with creme filling, regular	3.84	23.24	70.64	502	1.6	103	0	69.04
Cookies, vanilla sandwich with creme filling	4.5	20	72.1	483	1.5	349	0	70.6
Puff pastry, frozen, ready-to-bake, baked	7.4	38.5	45.7	558	1.5	253	0	44.2
Cookies, vanilla wafers, lower fat	5	15.2	73.6	441	1.9	388	51	71.7
Cookies, vanilla wafers, higher fat	4.9	16.41	72.6	455	1.6	325	9	71
Crackers, cheese, regular	10.93	22.74	59.42	489	2.3	973	3	57.12
Crackers, cheese, sandwich-type with peanut butter filling	12.41	25.12	56.74	496	3.4	829	0	53.34
Crackers, crispbread, rye	7.9	1.3	82.2	366	16.5	410	0	65.7
Crackers, matzo, plain	10	1.4	83.7	395	3	0	0	80.7

Food Name ---> per 100 g	Protein (g)	Fat (g)	Carb (g)	Calories	Fiber (g)	Sodium (mg)	Cholesterol (mg)	Net Carb (g)
Crackers, matzo, egg	12.3	2.1	78.6	391	2.8	21	83	75.8
Crackers, matzo, whole-wheat	13.1	1.5	78.9	351	11.8	2	0	67.1
Crackers, melba toast, plain	12.1	3.2	76.6	390	6.3	598	0	70.3
Crackers, melba toast, rye (includes pumpernickel)	11.6	3.4	77.3	389	8	899	0	69.3
Crackers, melba toast, wheat	12.9	2.3	76.4	374	7.4	837	0	69
Crackers, milk	7.6	13.77	71.73	446	3.4	687	11	68.33
Crackers, rusk toast	13.5	7.2	72.3	407	0	253	78	72.3
Crackers, rye, sandwich-type with cheese filling	9.2	22.3	60.8	481	3.6	1044	9	57.2
Crackers, rye, wafers, plain	9.6	0.9	80.4	334	22.9	557	0	57.5
Crackers, rye, wafers, seasoned	9	9.2	73.8	381	20.9	887	0	52.9
Crackers, saltines (includes oyster, soda, soup)	9.46	8.64	74.05	418	2.8	941	0	71.25
Crackers, standard snack-type, regular	6.64	26.43	61.3	510	2.3	726	0	59
Crackers, standard snack-type, sandwich, with cheese filling	9.3	21.1	61.7	477	1.9	978	2	59.8
Crackers, standard snack-type, sandwich, with peanut butter filling	11.47	24.54	58.38	494	2.3	801	0	56.08
Crackers, wheat, regular	7.3	16.4	70.73	455	6.9	699	0	63.83
Crackers, wheat, sandwich, with cheese filling	9.8	25	58.2	497	3.1	839	7	55.1
Crackers, wheat, sandwich, with peanut butter filling	13.5	26.7	53.8	495	4.4	807	0	49.4
Crackers, whole-wheat	10.58	14.13	69.55	427	10.3	704	0	59.25
Cracker meal	9.3	1.7	80.9	383	2.6	16	0	78.3
Cream puff shell, prepared from recipe	9	25.9	22.8	360	0.8	483	171	22
Croissants, butter	8.2	21	45.8	406	2.6	467	67	43.2
Croissants, apple	7.4	8.7	37.1	254	2.5	274	31	34.6
Croissants, cheese	9.2	20.9	47	414	2.6	361	57	44.4
Croutons, plain	11.9	6.6	73.5	407	5.1	698	0	68.4
Croutons, seasoned	10.8	18.3	63.5	465	5	1089	7	58.5
Danish pastry, cinnamon, enriched	7	22.4	44.6	403	1.3	414	21	43.3
Danish pastry, cheese	8	21.9	37.2	374	1	417	23	36.2
Danish pastry, fruit, enriched (includes apple, cinnamon, raisin, lemon, raspberry, strawberry)	5.4	18.5	47.8	371	1.9	445	114	45.9
Danish pastry, nut (includes almond, raisin nut, cinnamon nut)	7.1	25.2	45.7	430	2	298	46	43.7
Doughnuts, cake-type, plain (includes unsugared, old-fashioned)	5.31	24.93	47.06	434	1.7	477	10	45.36
Doughnuts, cake-type, plain, chocolate-coated or frosted	4.93	25.25	51.33	452	1.9	326	19	49.43
Doughnuts, cake-type, plain, sugared or glazed	5.2	22.9	50.8	426	1.5	402	32	49.3
Doughnuts, cake-type, chocolate, sugared or glazed	4.5	19.9	57.4	417	2.2	215	57	55.2
Doughnuts, french crullers, glazed	3.1	18.3	59.5	412	1.2	345	11	58.3
Doughnuts, yeast-leavened, with creme filling	6.4	24.5	30	361	0.8	309	24	29.2
Doughnuts, yeast-leavened, glazed, enriched (includes honey buns)	6.14	22.7	47.93	421	2.1	316	30	45.83
Doughnuts, yeast-leavened, with jelly filling	5.9	18.7	39	340	0.9	455	26	38.1
English muffins, plain, enriched, with ca prop (includes sourdough)	8.87	1.69	44.17	227	3.5	425	0	40.67
English muffins, plain, toasted, enriched, with calcium propionate (includes sourdough)	10.32	2.02	52.65	270	2.8	477	0	49.85
English muffins, mixed-grain (includes granola)	9.1	1.8	46.3	235	2.8	298	0	43.5
English muffins, mixed-grain, toasted (includes granola)	9.9	1.9	50.3	255	3	324	0	47.3
English muffins, raisin-cinnamon (includes apple-cinnamon)	7.91	1.8	48.1	240	2.6	299	0	45.5

Food Name ---> per 100 g	Protein (g)	Fat (g)	Carb (g)	Calories	Fiber (g)	Sodium (mg)	Cholesterol (mg)	Net Carb (g)
English muffins, raisin-cinnamon, toasted (includes apple-cinnamon)	8.87	2.21	55.04	276	3	342	0	52.04
English muffins, wheat	8.7	2	44.8	223	4.6	353	0	40.2
English muffins, wheat, toasted	9.4	2.1	48.7	243	5	384	0	43.7
English muffins, whole-wheat	8.8	2.1	40.4	203	6.7	364	0	33.7
English muffins, whole-wheat, toasted	9.6	2.3	44.1	221	7.3	396	0	36.8
French toast, frozen, ready-to-heat	7.4	6.1	32.1	213	1.1	495	82	31
French toast, prepared from recipe, made with low fat (2%) milk	7.7	10.8	25	229	0	479	116	25
Hush puppies, prepared from recipe	7.7	13.5	46	337	2.8	668	45	43.2
Ice cream cones, cake or wafer-type	8.1	6.9	79	417	3	256	0	76
Ice cream cones, sugar, rolled-type	7.9	3.8	84.1	402	1.7	298	0	82.4
Muffins, plain, prepared from recipe, made with low fat (2%) milk	6.9	11.4	41.4	296	2.7	467	39	38.7
Muffins, blueberry, commercially prepared (Includes mini-muffins)	4.49	16.07	53	375	1.1	336	30	51.9
Muffins, blueberry, dry mix	3.48	3.25	61	293	1.4	479	0	59.6
Muffins, blueberry, toaster-type	4.6	9.5	53.3	313	1.8	417	6	51.5
Muffins, blueberry, prepared from recipe, made with low fat (2%) milk	6.5	10.8	40.7	285	0	441	37	40.7
Muffins, corn, commercially prepared	5.9	8.4	51	305	3.4	467	26	47.6
Muffins, corn, dry mix, prepared	7.4	10.2	49.1	321	2.4	795	62	46.7
Muffins, corn, toaster-type	5.3	11.3	57.9	346	1.6	430	13	56.3
Muffins, corn, prepared from recipe, made with low fat (2%) milk	7.1	12.3	44.2	316	0	585	42	44.2
Muffins, oat bran	7	7.4	48.3	270	4.6	393	0	43.7
Muffins, wheat bran, dry mix	7.1	12	73	396	0	700	0	73
Pancakes plain, frozen, ready-to-heat (includes buttermilk)	5.23	6.83	37.75	233	1	461	18	36.75
Pancakes, plain, dry mix, complete (includes buttermilk)	9.77	3.1	73.65	368	2.9	1082	2	70.75
Pancakes, plain, dry mix, complete, prepared	5.2	2.5	36.7	194	1.3	628	12	35.4
Pancakes, plain, dry mix, incomplete (includes buttermilk)	10	1.7	73.6	355	5.4	1496	0	68.2
Pancakes, plain, dry mix, incomplete, prepared	7.8	7.7	28.9	218	1.9	505	71	27
Pancakes, plain, prepared from recipe	6.4	9.7	28.3	227	0	439	59	28.3
Pancakes, blueberry, prepared from recipe	6.1	9.2	29	222	0	412	56	29
Pancakes, buckwheat, dry mix, incomplete	10.9	2.7	71.3	340	8.5	684	0	62.8
Pancakes, special dietary, dry mix	8.9	1.4	73.9	349	0	456	0	73.9
Pancakes, whole-wheat, dry mix, incomplete	12.8	1.5	71	344	0	1419	0	71
Pancakes, whole-wheat, dry mix, incomplete, prepared	8.5	6.5	29.4	208	2.8	572	61	26.6
Pie, apple, commercially prepared, enriched flour	1.9	11	34	237	1.6	201	0	32.4
Pie, apple, prepared from recipe	2.4	12.5	37.1	265	0	211	0	37.1
Pie, banana cream, prepared from mix, no-bake type	3.4	12.9	31.6	251	0.6	290	29	31
Pie, banana cream, prepared from recipe	4.4	13.6	32.9	269	0.7	240	51	32.2
Pie, blueberry, commercially prepared	1.8	10	34.9	232	1	287	0	33.9
Pie, blueberry, prepared from recipe	2.7	11.9	33.5	245	0	185	0	33.5
Pie, cherry, commercially prepared	2	11	39.8	260	0.8	246	0	39
Pie, cherry, prepared from recipe	2.8	12.2	38.5	270	0	191	0	38.5
Pie, chocolate creme, commercially prepared	4.15	22.41	38.44	353	0.8	266	12	37.64
Pie, chocolate mousse, prepared from mix, no-bake type	3.5	15.4	29.6	260	0	460	35	29.6

Food Name ---> per 100 g	Protein (g)	Fat (g)	Carb (g)	Calories	Fiber (g)	Sodium (mg)	Cholesterol (mg)	Net Carb (g)
Pie, coconut creme, commercially prepared	2.1	16.6	37.3	298	1.3	204	0	36
Pie, coconut cream, prepared from mix, no-bake type	2.8	17.6	28.5	276	0.5	329	23	28
Pie, coconut custard, commercially prepared	5.9	13.2	30.2	260	1.8	335	35	28.4
Pie, egg custard, commercially prepared	5.5	11.6	20.8	210	1.6	275	33	19.2
Pie, fried pies, fruit	3	16.1	42.6	316	2.6	333	0	40
Pie, lemon meringue, commercially prepared	1.5	8.7	47.2	268	1.2	172	45	46
Pie, lemon meringue, prepared from recipe	3.8	12.9	39.1	285	0	242	53	39.1
Pie, mince, prepared from recipe	2.6	10.8	48	289	2.6	254	0	45.4
Pie, peach	1.9	10	32.9	224	0.8	217	0	32.1
Pie, pecan, commercially prepared	4.5	16.69	59.61	407	2.1	275	42	57.51
Pie, pecan, prepared from recipe	4.9	22.2	52.2	412	0	262	87	52.2
Pie, pumpkin, commercially prepared	3.9	9.75	34.83	243	1.8	239	26	33.03
Pie, pumpkin, prepared from recipe	4.5	9.3	26.4	204	0	225	42	26.4
Pie, vanilla cream, prepared from recipe	4.8	14.4	32.6	278	0.6	260	62	32
Pie crust, standard-type, dry mix	6.9	31.4	52.1	518	0	753	0	52.1
Pie crust, standard-type, dry mix, prepared, baked	6.7	30.4	50.4	501	1.8	729	0	48.6
Pie crust, standard-type, frozen, ready-to-bake, enriched	6.16	26.07	48.62	457	2.5	409	0	46.12
Pie crust, standard-type, frozen, ready-to-bake, enriched, baked	6.5	28.59	56.24	508	3.3	467	0	52.94
Pie crust, standard-type, prepared from recipe, baked	6.4	34.6	47.5	527	1.7	542	0	45.8
Puff pastry, frozen, ready-to-bake	7.3	38.1	45.1	551	1.5	249	0	43.6
Phyllo dough	7.1	6	52.6	299	1.9	483	0	50.7
Popovers, dry mix, enriched	10.4	4.3	71	371	0	906	0	71
Rolls, dinner, plain, commercially prepared (includes brown-and-serve)	10.86	6.47	52.04	310	2	467	4	50.04
Rolls, dinner, egg	9.5	6.4	52	307	3.7	566	50	48.3
Rolls, dinner, oat bran	9.5	4.6	40.2	236	4.1	413	0	36.1
Rolls, dinner, rye	10.3	3.4	53.1	286	4.9	650	0	48.2
Rolls, dinner, wheat	8.6	6.3	46	273	3.8	524	0	42.2
Rolls, dinner, whole-wheat	8.7	4.7	51.1	266	7.5	521	0	43.6
Rolls, french	8.6	4.3	50.2	277	3.2	574	0	47
Rolls, hamburger or hotdog, plain	9.77	3.91	50.12	279	1.8	494	0	48.32
Rolls, hamburger or hotdog, mixed-grain	9.6	6	44.6	263	3.8	458	0	40.8
Rolls, hamburger or hotdog, reduced-calorie	8.3	2	42.1	196	6.2	410	0	35.9
Rolls, hard (includes kaiser)	9.9	4.3	52.7	293	2.3	544	0	50.4
Strudel, apple	3.3	11.2	41.1	274	2.2	135	6	38.9
Sweet rolls, cheese	7.1	18.3	43.7	360	1.2	357	76	42.5
Sweet rolls, cinnamon, commercially prepared with raisins	6.2	16.4	50.9	372	2.4	304	66	48.5
Sweet rolls, cinnamon, refrigerated dough with frosting	5	12.2	51.6	333	0	765	0	51.6
Sweet rolls, cinnamon, refrigerated dough with frosting, baked	5.4	13.2	56.1	362	0	832	0	56.1
Taco shells, baked	6.41	21.79	63.49	476	6.7	324	0	56.79
Toaster pastries, brown-sugar-cinnamon	4.06	7.98	72.64	370	2.3	361	0	70.34
Toaster pastries, fruit (includes apple, blueberry, cherry, strawberry)	4.2	9.95	70.32	388	1	334	0	69.32
Tortillas, ready-to-bake or -fry, corn	5.7	2.85	44.64	218	6.3	45	0	38.34
Tortillas, ready-to-bake or -fry, flour, refrigerated	8.2	7.99	49.38	306	3.5	736	0	45.88
Waffles, plain, frozen, ready-to-heat	6.47	9.7	42.98	285	2.2	638	14	40.78

Food Name ---> per 100 g	Protein (g)	Fat (g)	Carb (g)	Calories	Fiber (g)	Sodium (mg)	Cholesterol (mg)	Net Carb (g)
Waffles, plain, prepared from recipe	7.9	14.1	32.9	291	0	511	69	32.9
Wonton wrappers (includes egg roll wrappers)	9.8	1.5	57.9	291	1.8	572	9	56.1
Leavening agents, baking powder, double-acting, sodium aluminum sulfate	0	0	27.7	53	0.2	10600	0	27.5
Leavening agents, baking powder, double-acting, straight phosphate	0.1	0	24.1	51	0.2	7893	0	23.9
Leavening agents, baking powder, low-sodium	0.1	0.4	46.9	97	2.2	90	0	44.7
Leavening agents, baking soda	0	0	0	0	0	27360	0	0
Leavening agents, cream of tartar	0	0	61.5	258	0.2	52	0	61.3
Leavening agents, yeast, baker's, compressed	8.4	1.9	18.1	105	8.1	30	0	10
Leavening agents, yeast, baker's, active dry	40.44	7.61	41.22	325	26.9	51	0	14.32
Bread crumbs, dry, grated, seasoned	14.13	5.48	68.49	383	4.9	1336	1	63.59
Cookies, oatmeal, prepared from recipe, without raisins	6.8	17.9	66.4	447	0	598	36	66.4
Cookies, chocolate chip, prepared from recipe, made with butter	5.7	28.4	58.2	488	0	341	70	58.2
Bread, protein, (includes gluten), toasted	13.2	2.4	48.1	270	3.3	444	0	44.8
Bread, rice bran, toasted	9.7	5	47.3	264	5.3	292	0	42
Bread, wheat germ, toasted	10.7	3.3	54.3	293	2.3	621	1	52
Muffins, blueberry, toaster-type, toasted	4.9	10.1	56.7	333	1.9	444	5	54.8
Muffins, wheat bran, toaster-type with raisins, toasted	5.5	9.4	55.5	313	8.2	527	9	47.3
Pancakes, buttermilk, prepared from recipe	6.8	9.3	28.7	227	0	522	58	28.7
Rolls, dinner, plain, prepared from recipe, made with low fat (2%) milk	8.5	7.3	53.4	316	1.9	415	35	51.5
Pie crust, cookie-type, prepared from recipe, graham cracker, chilled	4.1	24.4	63.9	484	1.5	560	0	62.4
Crackers, matzo, egg and onion	10	3.9	77.1	391	5	285	45	72.1
Pie crust, cookie-type, prepared from recipe, vanilla wafer, chilled	3.7	36.2	50.2	531	0.1	515	39	50.1
Pie crust, standard-type, prepared from recipe, unbaked	5.7	30.8	42.3	469	3.4	482	0	38.9
Waffles, plain, frozen, ready -to-heat, toasted	7.19	9.61	49.29	312	2.4	730	15	46.89
Bagels, plain, enriched, without calcium propionate (includes onion, poppy, sesame)	10.5	1.6	53.4	275	2.3	534	0	51.1
Bagels, plain, unenriched, with calcium propionate (includes onion, poppy, sesame)	10.5	1.6	53.4	275	2.3	534	0	51.1
Bagels, plain, unenriched, without calcium propionate(includes onion, poppy, sesame)	10.5	1.6	53.4	275	2.3	534	0	51.1
Bread, cornbread, dry mix, unenriched (includes corn muffin mix)	7	12.2	69.5	418	6.5	1111	2	63
Bread, pita, white, unenriched	9.1	1.2	55.7	275	2.2	536	0	53.5
Bread, raisin, unenriched	7.9	4.4	52.3	274	4.3	390	0	48
Bread, white, commercially prepared, low sodium, no salt	8.2	3.6	49.6	267	2.3	298	1	47.3
Coffeecake, cinnamon with crumb topping, commercially prepared, unenriched	6.8	23.3	46.7	418	2	351	32	44.7
Cake, pound, commercially prepared, other than all butter, unenriched	5.2	17.9	52.5	389	1	400	58	51.5
Cake, pudding-type, white, unenriched, dry mix	3.9	9.5	81	423	0.7	665	0	80.3
Cake, yellow, unenriched, dry mix	4.4	11.6	78.1	432	1.1	657	2	77
Cookies, butter, commercially prepared, unenriched	6.1	18.8	68.9	467	0.8	351	117	68.1
Cookies, chocolate chip, commercially prepared,	5.4	22.6	66.8	481	2.5	315	0	64.3

Food Name ---> per 100 g	Protein (g)	Fat (g)	Carb (g)	Calories	Fiber (g)	Sodium (mg)	Cholesterol (mg)	Net Carb (g)
regular, higher fat, unenriched								
Cookies, ladyfingers, without lemon juice and rind	10.6	9.1	59.7	363	1	147	221	58.7
Crackers, melba toast, plain, without salt	12.1	3.2	76.6	390	6.3	19	0	70.3
Crackers, saltines, low salt (includes oyster, soda, soup)	9.5	8.85	74.34	421	2.9	198	0	71.44
Crackers, saltines, unsalted tops (includes oyster, soda, soup)	9.2	11.8	71.5	434	3	766	0	68.5
Crackers, standard snack-type, regular, low salt	7.4	25.3	61	502	1.6	216	0	59.4
Crackers, wheat, low salt	8.6	20.6	64.9	473	4.5	190	0	60.4
Crackers, whole-wheat, low salt	8.8	17.2	68.6	443	10.5	186	0	58.1
Danish pastry, cinnamon, unenriched	7	22.4	44.6	403	1.2	371	21	43.4
Danish pastry, fruit, unenriched (includes apple, cinnamon, raisin, strawberry)	5.4	18.5	47.8	371	1.9	354	40	45.9
Bread, white, commercially prepared, toasted, low sodium no salt	9	4	54.4	293	0	376	1	54.4
Danish pastry, lemon, unenriched	5.4	18.5	47.8	371	1.9	354	40	45.9
Crackers, cheese, low sodium	10.1	25.3	58.2	503	2.4	458	13	55.8
Danish pastry, raspberry, unenriched	5.4	18.5	47.8	371	1.9	354	40	45.9
Doughnuts, yeast-leavened, glazed, unenriched (includes honey buns)	6.4	22.8	44.3	403	1.2	342	6	43.1
English muffins, plain, enriched, without calcium propionate(includes sourdough)	7.7	1.8	46	235	2.7	464	0	43.3
English muffins, plain, unenriched, with calcium propionate (includes sourdough)	7.7	1.8	46	235	2.7	464	0	43.3
English muffins, plain, unenriched, without calcium propionate (includes sourdough)	7.7	1.8	46	235	2.7	464	0	43.3
Pie, apple, commercially prepared, unenriched flour	1.9	11	34	237	1.6	266	0	32.4
Pie, fried pies, cherry	3	16.1	42.6	316	2.6	374	0	40
Pie, fried pies, lemon	3	16.1	42.6	316	2.6	374	0	40
Pie crust, standard-type, frozen, ready-to-bake, unenriched	3.9	29.2	44.1	457	0.9	576	0	43.2
Popovers, dry mix, unenriched	10.4	4.3	71	371	0	906	0	71
Taco shells, baked, without added salt	7.2	22.6	62.4	468	7.5	15	0	54.9
Tortillas, ready-to-bake or -fry, corn, without added salt	5.7	2.5	46.6	222	5.2	11	0	41.4
Tortillas, ready-to-bake or -fry, flour, without added calcium	8.7	7.1	55.6	325	3.3	478	0	52.3
Cake, pound, commercially prepared, fat-free	5.4	1.2	61	283	1.1	341	0	59.9
Cake, yellow, light, dry mix	4.7	5.5	84.1	404	1.3	604	0	82.8
Crackers, saltines, fat-free, low-sodium	10.5	1.6	82.3	393	2.7	849	0	79.6
Breakfast tart, low fat	3.99	5.99	76.8	372	1.5	361	0	75.3
Toaster Pastries, KELLOGG, KELLOGG'S POP TARTS, Blueberry	4.6	13.3	68.41	412	1.1	398	0	67.31
Toaster Pastries, KELLOGG, KELLOGG'S POP TARTS, Frosted blueberry	4.6	10	71.77	391	1.1	320	0	70.67
Toaster Pastries, KELLOGG, KELLOGG'S POP TARTS, Brown sugar cinnamon	5.4	18.4	64.4	438	1.5	380	0	62.9
Toaster Pastries, KELLOGG, KELLOGG'S POP TARTS, Frosted brown sugar cinnamon	4.6	13.8	69	417	1.4	343	0	67.6
Toaster Pastries, KELLOGG, KELLOGG'S POP TARTS, Frosted cherry	4.2	10.2	72	397	1	320	0	71
Toaster Pastries, KELLOGG, KELLOGG'S POP TARTS, Frosted chocolate fudge	4.9	9.3	70.4	384	2.1	437	0	68.3
Toaster Pastries, KELLOGG, KELLOGG'S POP TARTS, Frosted	4.2	10.6	71.62	399	1	320	0	70.62

Food Name ---> per 100 g	Protein (g)	Fat (g)	Carb (g)	Calories	Fiber (g)	Sodium (mg)	Cholesterol (mg)	Net Carb (g)
TARTS, Frosted raspberry								
Toaster Pastries, KELLOGG, KELLOGG'S POP TARTS, S'mores	6.2	10.5	69.6	392	1.4	410	0	68.2
Toaster Pastries, KELLOGG, KELLOGG'S POP TARTS, Strawberry	4.7	10.5	71.1	398	1.1	355	0	70
Toaster Pastries, KELLOGG, KELLOGG'S POP TARTS, Frosted strawberry	4.1	9.8	71.7	390	1.3	331	0	70.4
Toaster Pastries, KELLOGG, KELLOGG'S POP TARTS, Frosted wild berry	4	9.5	72.4	390	1.3	315	0	71.1
Toaster Pastries, KELLOGG, KELLOGG'S LOW FAT POP TARTS, Frosted brown sugar cinnamon	4.7	5.9	73.7	366	5.5	379	0	68.2
Toaster Pastries, KELLOGG, KELLOGG'S LOW FAT POP TARTS, Frosted strawberry	4.2	5.4	74.4	363	5.6	357	0	68.8
KELLOGG, KELLOGG'S EGGO, Buttermilk Pancake	5.3	8	38.6	245	1	508	11	37.6
KELLOGG, KELLOG'S NUTRI-GRAIN CEREAL BARS, Mixed Berry	4.3	7.6	72.8	370	1.9	284	0	70.9
KELLOGG'S, EGGO, Waffles, Homestyle, Low Fat	6.3	3.5	44.9	229	1.3	393	23	43.6
KELLOGG'S, EGGO, NUTRI-GRAIN, Waffles, Low Fat	6.5	3.5	39	201	4	559	0	35
KELLOGG'S EGGO Lowfat Blueberry Nutri-Grain Waffles	5.95	2.83	42.71	208	3.5	591	0	39.21
ARCHWAY Home Style Cookies, Sugar Free Oatmeal	5.54	20.92	67.2	442	1.9	308	0	65.3
ARCHWAY Home Style Cookies, Chocolate Chip Ice Box	4.28	24.4	65.02	497	2	270	13	63.02
ARCHWAY Home Style Cookies, Coconut Macaroon	3.02	22.55	61.23	460	5.1	200	0	56.13
ARCHWAY Home Style Cookies, Date Filled Oatmeal	4.67	12.05	68.16	400	2.1	331	6	66.06
ARCHWAY Home Style Cookies, Dutch Cocoa	4.5	14.99	69.44	431	2.6	384	7	66.84
ARCHWAY Home Style Cookies, Frosty Lemon	4.41	17.11	64.78	430	0.7	449	0	64.08
ARCHWAY Home Style Cookies, Iced Molasses	3.5	14.43	69.12	420	1	605	12	68.12
ARCHWAY Home Style Cookies, Iced Oatmeal	4.89	16.53	66.76	435	2	377	8	64.76
ARCHWAY Home Style Cookies, Molasses	4.25	12.06	69.41	403	1.2	577	25	68.21
ARCHWAY Home Style Cookies, Oatmeal	5.48	14.08	68.17	421	2.9	394	10	65.27
ARCHWAY Home Style Cookies, Oatmeal Raisin	5.17	12.08	69.27	406	2.7	339	8	66.57
ARCHWAY Home Style Cookies, Old Fashioned Molasses	4.27	11.83	70.55	406	1.1	561	25	69.45
ARCHWAY Home Style Cookies, Old Fashioned Windmill Cookies	5.17	17.55	72.23	468	1.8	471	1	70.43
ARCHWAY Home Style Cookies, Peanut Butter	9	24.28	58.48	480	2.8	404	37	55.68
ARCHWAY Home Style Cookies, Raspberry Filled	4.35	13.26	65.92	400	2.2	334	6	63.72
ARCHWAY Home Style Cookies, Strawberry Filled	4.35	13.26	65.92	400	2.2	377	6	63.72
ARCHWAY Home Style Cookies, Reduced Fat Ginger Snaps	4.67	11.14	76.23	424	1.1	406	1	75.13
Artificial Blueberry Muffin Mix, dry	4.7	8.7	77.45	407	0	760	0	77.45
KRAFT, STOVE TOP Stuffing Mix Chicken Flavor	12.6	4.1	73.1	381	2.5	1532	4	70.6
GEORGE WESTON BAKERIES, Brownberry Sage and Onion Stuffing Mix, dry	13.3	5.1	72.7	390	5.4	1680	0	67.3
KEEBLER, KEEBLER Chocolate Graham SELECTS	7.1	16.6	71.8	465	0	357	0	71.8

Food Name ---> per 100 g	Protein (g)	Fat (g)	Carb (g)	Calories	Fiber (g)	Sodium (mg)	Cholesterol (mg)	Net Carb (g)
KEEBLER, Vanilla Wafers	4	17.4	73.1	462	1.4	402	1	71.7
CONTINENTAL MILLS, KRUSTEAZ Almond Poppyseed Muffin Mix, Artificially Flavored, dry	5.6	10.3	75.6	418	1.7	590	0	73.9
MCKEE BAKING, LITTLE DEBBIE NUTTY BARS, Wafers with Peanut Butter, Chocolate Covered	8	32.8	55.2	548	0	223	0	55.2
MARTHA WHITE FOODS, Martha White's Chewy Fudge Brownie Mix, dry	4.42	6.16	83.58	407	2.9	457	0	80.68
MARTHA WHITE FOODS, Martha White's Buttermilk Biscuit Mix, dry	7.81	13.23	59.41	388	1.5	1295	3	57.91
MISSION FOODS, MISSION Flour Tortillas, Soft Taco, 8 inch	8.7	6	49.6	287	0	898	0	49.6
NABISCO, NABISCO GRAHAMS Crackers	6.99	10	76.2	424	3.4	659	0	72.8
NABISCO, NABISCO OREO CRUNCHIES, Cookie Crumb Topping	4.78	21.5	70.23	476	3.2	528	0	67.03
NABISCO, NABISCO RITZ Crackers	7.23	23.21	63.51	492	2.3	882	0	61.21
PILLSBURY, Buttermilk Biscuits, Artificial Flavor, refrigerated dough	6.4	2.79	47.07	236	1.6	854	0	45.47
PILLSBURY, Chocolate Chip Cookies, refrigerated dough	3.82	21.26	60.75	450	1.7	326	6	59.05
PILLSBURY, Crusty French Loaf, refrigerated dough	8.59	2.88	46.35	243	2.6	575	0	43.75
PILLSBURY, Traditional Fudge Brownie Mix, dry	4.8	12.1	78.3	441	0	292	0	78.3
PILLSBURY GRANDS, Buttermilk Biscuits, refrigerated dough	6.16	11.34	42.41	293	1.5	1066	0	40.91
PILLSBURY Golden Layer Buttermilk Biscuits, Artificial Flavor, refrigerated dough	5.88	13.24	41.18	307	1.2	1059	0	39.98
PILLSBURY, Cinnamon Rolls with Icing, refrigerated dough	4.34	11.27	53.42	330	1.4	780	0	52.02
KRAFT FOODS, SHAKE 'N' BAKE ORIGINAL RECIPE, Coating for Pork, dry	6.1	3.7	79.8	377	0	2182	0	79.8
GEORGE WESTON BAKERIES, Thomas English Muffins	8	1.8	46	232	0	345	0	46
HEINZ, WEIGHT WATCHER, Chocolate Eclair, frozen	4.4	6.9	40.3	241	2.1	300	47	38.2
INTERSTATE BRANDS CORP, WONDER Hamburger Rolls	8.07	4.15	50.84	273	2.6	488	0	48.24
GENERAL MILLS, BETTY CROCKER SUPERMOIST Yellow Cake Mix, dry	3.8	8.1	81.3	413	0	672	0	81.3
NABISCO, NABISCO SNACKWELL'S Fat Free Devil's Food Cookie Cakes	5	1.09	74.25	305	1.6	174	0	72.65
Crackers, cheese, sandwich-type with cheese filling	8.92	24.41	58.76	490	1.9	878	6	56.86
USDA Commodity, Bakery, Flour Mix	8.47	12.9	62.53	400	7.1	1410	0	55.43
USDA Commodity, Bakery, Flour Mix Low-fat	9.07	4.7	70.59	361	3.5	1360	0	67.09
Waffles, buttermilk, frozen, ready-to-heat	6.58	9.22	41.05	273	2.2	621	15	38.85
Waffle, buttermilk, frozen, ready-to-heat, toasted	7.42	9.49	48.39	309	2.6	710	13	45.79
Waffle, buttermilk, frozen, ready-to-heat, microwaved	6.92	9.4	44.16	289	2.4	663	16	41.76
Waffle, plain, frozen, ready-to-heat, microwave	6.71	9.91	45.41	298	2.4	682	16	43.01
Pancakes, plain, frozen, ready-to-heat, microwave (includes buttermilk)	5.88	4.73	43.33	239	2.5	566	0	40.83
Toaster Pastries, fruit, frosted (include apples, blueberry, cherry, strawberry)	4.01	9.02	71.83	385	1.8	311	0	70.03
Toaster pastries, fruit, toasted (include apple, blueberry, cherry, strawberry)	4.7	11.03	72.7	409	1	354	0	71.7

Food Name ---> per 100 g	Protein (g)	Fat (g)	Carb (g)	Calories	Fiber (g)	Sodium (mg)	Cholesterol (mg)	Net Carb (g)
Muffin, blueberry, commercially prepared, low-fat	4.23	4.22	50.05	255	4.2	413	28	45.85
Pie Crust, Cookie-type, Graham Cracker, Ready Crust	5.1	24.83	64.3	501	1.9	471	0	62.4
Pie Crust, Cookie-type, Chocolate, Ready Crust	6.08	22.42	64.48	484	2.7	503	0	61.78
Pie, Dutch Apple, Commercially Prepared	2.17	11.5	44.54	290	1.6	200	0	42.94
Pie crust, deep dish, frozen, unbaked, made with enriched flour	5.52	28.74	46.79	468	1.4	353	0	45.39
Pie crust, refrigerated, regular, baked	3.41	28.69	58.52	506	1.4	472	0	57.12
Pie crust, deep dish, frozen, baked, made with enriched flour	6.1	31.84	52.47	521	2.3	393	0	50.17
Pie crust, refrigerated, regular, unbaked	2.97	25.46	51.11	445	1.8	409	0	49.31
Crackers, whole-wheat, reduced fat	11.34	7.59	75.52	416	10.9	745	0	64.62
Crackers, wheat, reduced fat	9.34	13.37	71.52	444	3.4	776	0	68.12
Waffles, chocolate chip, frozen, ready-to-heat	5.8	10.1	45.68	297	1.5	529	21	44.18
Tostada shells, corn	6.15	23.38	64.43	474	5.8	657	0	58.63
Bread, salvadoran sweet cheese (quesadilla salvadorena)	7.12	17.12	47.84	374	0.7	510	59	47.14
Bread, pound cake type, pan de torta salvadoran	7.06	17.45	51.29	390	1.7	390	0	49.59
Bread, pan dulce, sweet yeast bread	9.42	11.58	56.38	367	2.3	228	30	54.08
Keikitos (muffins), Latino bakery item	6.81	25.24	53.16	467	1.2	515	0	51.96
Cake, pound, BIMBO Bakeries USA, Panque Casero, home baked style	6.62	21.7	48.94	418	1	357	0	47.94
Pan Dulce, LA RICURA, Salpora de Arroz con Azucar, cookie-like, contains wheat flour and rice flour	8.81	16.11	66.28	445	1.2	445	0	65.08
Pastry, Pastelitos de Guava (guava pastries)	5.48	18.5	47.76	379	2.2	231	10	45.56
Crackers, snack, GOYA CRACKERS	14.25	13.35	64.35	433	3.8	665	0	60.55
Crackers, cream, GAMESA SABROSAS	7.01	20.37	64.55	484	2.4	1148	0	62.15
Crackers, cream, LA MODERNA RIKIS CREAM CRACKERS	7.19	19.5	64.88	464	2.4	752	0	62.48
Garlic bread, frozen	8.36	16.61	41.72	350	2.5	544	0	39.22
Cinnamon buns, frosted (includes honey buns)	4.45	26.61	48.6	452	1.2	305	5	47.4
Crackers, cheese, reduced fat	10	11.67	68.19	418	3.3	1167	0	64.89
Crackers, saltines, whole wheat (includes multi-grain)	7.14	10.71	68.25	398	6.7	1214	0	61.55
Bread, white wheat	10.66	2.15	43.91	238	9.2	478	0	34.71
Bagels, wheat	10.2	1.53	48.89	250	4.1	439	0	44.79
Cream puff, eclair, custard or cream filled, iced	4.41	18.52	37.43	334	0.9	265	66	36.53
Tortillas, ready-to-bake or -fry, flour, shelf stable	8.01	7.58	49.27	297	2.4	742	0	46.87
Bread, potato	12.5	3.13	47.07	266	6.3	375	0	40.77
Bread, cheese	10.42	20.83	44.83	408	2.1	750	10	42.73
Focaccia, Italian flatbread, plain	8.77	7.89	35.82	249	1.8	561	0	34.02
KASHI, TLC, Honey Sesame Crackers	8.7	10.4	72.2	398	5.8	471	0	66.4
KASHI, TLC, Original 7-Grain Crackers	13.9	11.9	63.2	385	9	530	0	54.2
KASHI, TLC, Country Cheddar Crackers	9.8	15.5	68	445	2.5	724	5	65.5
KASHI, TLC, Toasted Asiago Crackers	12.7	13.8	66.4	420	9.6	659	5	56.8
KASHI, Blueberry Waffle	5.7	7.1	34.6	192	9	476	0	25.6
KASHI, H2H Woven Wheat Cracker, Original	10.6	11.6	73.4	396	12.2	283	0	61.2
KASHI, Original Waffle	6	7.4	35.4	197	9.3	479	0	26.1
KASHI, TLC, Fire Roasted Vegetable Crackers	12	12.2	64.6	389	8.7	664	0	55.9
KASHI, H2H Woven Wheat Cracker, Roasted Garlic	10.5	11.7	73.2	440	12.2	240	0	61
AUSTIN, Cheddar Cheese on Wheat Crackers,	7.9	24.5	61.4	495	1.8	839	3	59.6

Food Name ---> per 100 g	Protein (g)	Fat (g)	Carb (g)	Calories	Fiber (g)	Sodium (mg)	Cholesterol (mg)	Net Carb (g)
sandwich-type								
AUSTIN, Cheddar Cheese on Cheese Crackers, sandwich-type	7.5	24.9	60	494	1.3	900	3	58.7
AUSTIN, Chocolatey Peanut Butter Crackers, sandwich-type	7.7	20.8	66.2	479	2	584	0	64.2
AUSTIN, Grilled Cheese on Wafer Crackers, sandwich-type	7.9	23.8	62	493	1.3	910	3	60.7
AUSTIN, Cheddar Cheese on Cheese Crackers, sandwich-type, reduced fat	7.8	17.5	68	461	1.4	884	3	66.6
AUSTIN, Peanut Butter on Cheese Crackers, sandwich-type, reduced fat	9.7	17.9	66.3	461	2.7	726	0	63.6
AUSTIN, Peanut Butter on Toasty Crackers, sandwich-type, reduced fat	9.5	18	67.2	463	2.7	648	0	64.5
AUSTIN, PB & J Crackers, sandwich-type	7.6	21.7	65.7	484	2	582	0	63.7
BARBARA DEE, Winter Mints Cookies	3.9	26	67.1	515	2	290	0	65.1
KELLOGG'S, BEANATURAL, Original 3-Bean Chips	22.9	25.3	46.5	487	14.2	794	0	32.3
BEAR NAKED, Double Chocolate Cookies	6.6	16.9	66.9	423	7	200	0	59.9
BEAR NAKED, Fruit & Nut Cookies	7.5	21.4	61.6	443	7.1	133	0	54.5
KELLOGG'S, EGGO, Biscuit Scramblers, Bacon, Egg & Cheese	8.8	7.9	38.3	258	2.1	610	27	36.2
KELLOGG'S, EGGO, Biscuit Scramblers, Egg & Cheese	8.8	7.6	38.3	254	2.3	583	28	36
KELLOGG'S, EGGO, French Toaster Sticks, Cinnamon	4.8	6.9	42.6	250	1	550	24	41.6
KELLOGG'S, EGGO, French Toaster Sticks, Original	5.3	7	39.4	239	0.9	598	26	38.5
KELLOGG'S, EGGO, Mini Muffin Tops, Blueberry	5	10.2	45.8	293	1	586	28	44.8
Rolls, pumpernickel	10.8	2.8	51.87	276	5.4	492	0	46.47

Beverages

Food Name ---> per 100 g	Protein (g)	Fat (g)	Carb (g)	Calories	Fiber (g)	Sodium (mg)	Cholesterol (mg)	Net Carb (g)
Alcoholic beverage, beer, regular, all	0.46	0	3.55	43	0	4	0	3.55
Alcoholic beverage, beer, regular, BUDWEISER	0.36	0	2.97	41	0	3	0	2.97
Alcoholic beverage, beer, light, BUDWEISER SELECT	0.2	0	0.87	28	0	3	0	0.87
Alcoholic beverage, beer, light	0.24	0	1.64	29	0	4	0	1.64
Alcoholic beverage, beer, light, BUD LIGHT	0.25	0	1.3	29	0	3	0	1.3
Alcoholic beverage, daiquiri, canned	0	0	15.7	125	0	40	0	15.7
Alcoholic beverage, daiquiri, prepared-from-recipe	0.06	0.06	6.94	186	0.1	5	0	6.84
Alcoholic beverage, beer, light, low carb	0.17	0	0.73	27	0	3	0	0.73
Alcoholic beverage, pina colada, canned	0.6	7.6	27.6	237	0.1	71	0	27.5
Beverages, almond milk, sweetened, vanilla flavor, ready-to-drink	0.42	1.04	6.59	38	0.4	63	0	6.19
Alcoholic beverage, pina colada, prepared-from-recipe	0.42	1.88	22.66	174	0.3	6	0	22.36
Alcoholic beverage, tequila sunrise, canned	0.3	0.1	11.3	110	0	57	0	11.3
Beverages, Energy drink, Citrus	0	0	11.27	45	0	10	0	11.27
Beverages, MONSTER energy drink, low carb	0	0	1.38	5	0	75	0	1.38
Beverages, Whiskey sour mix, powder	0.6	0.1	97.3	383	0	274	0	97.3
Alcoholic beverage, whiskey sour, prepared with water, whiskey and powder mix	0.1	0.02	15.85	164	0	47	0	15.85
Beverages, THE COCA-COLA COMPANY, NOS Zero, energy drink, sugar-free with guarana, fortified with vitamins B6 and B12	0	0	1.03	4	0	85	0	1.03
Alcoholic beverage, whiskey sour, canned	0	0	13.4	119	0.1	44	0	13.3
Beverages, Whiskey sour mix, bottled	0.1	0.1	21.4	87	0	102	0	21.4
Alcoholic beverage, whiskey sour, prepared from item 14028	0.06	0.06	12.82	153	0	61	0	12.82
Beverages, THE COCA-COLA COMPANY, NOS energy drink, Original, grape, loaded cherry, charged citrus, fortified with vitamins B6 and B12	0	0	11.25	44	0	85	0	11.25
Beverages, water, bottled, yumberry, pomegranate with anti-oxidants, zero calories	0	0	1.25	5	0	10	0	1.25
Beverages, ABBOTT, EAS whey protein powder	66.67	5.13	17.95	385	0	385	205	17.95
Alcoholic beverage, creme de menthe, 72 proof	0	0.3	41.6	371	0	5	0	41.6
Beverages, ABBOTT, EAS soy protein powder	47.62	3.57	43.94	405	0	452	0	43.94
Beverages, CYTOSPORT, Muscle Milk, ready-to-drink	5.87	2.01	2.06	49	0.2	95	2	1.86
Alcoholic beverage, distilled, all (gin, rum, vodka, whiskey) 80 proof	0	0	0	231	0	1	0	0
Beverages, OCEAN SPRAY, Cran-Energy, Cranberry Energy Juice Drink	0	0	3.75	15	0	21	0	3.75
Beverages, NESTLE, Boost plus, nutritional drink, ready-to-drink	5.38	5.38	17.29	138	1.2	77	4	16.09
Beverages, SLIMFAST, Meal replacement, High Protein Shake, Ready-To-Drink, 3-2-1 plan	6.59	2.88	0.85	58	0.4	72	4	0.45

Food Name ---> per 100 g	Protein (g)	Fat (g)	Carb (g)	Calories	Fiber (g)	Sodium (mg)	Cholesterol (mg)	Net Carb (g)
Beverages, UNILEVER, SLIMFAST, meal replacement, regular, ready-to-drink, 3-2-1 Plan	3.32	1.93	7.74	57	1.6	68	3	6.14
Beverages, UNILEVER, SLIMFAST Shake Mix, powder, 3-2-1 Plan	8.13	13.34	73.92	448	18.1	472	5	55.82
Beverages, FUZE, orange mango, fortified with vitamins A, C, E, B6	0.68	0.06	9.2	38	0.2	10	0	9
Alcoholic beverage, distilled, gin, 90 proof	0	0	0	263	0	2	0	0
Alcoholic beverage, distilled, rum, 80 proof	0	0	0	231	0	1	0	0
Alcoholic beverage, distilled, vodka, 80 proof	0	0	0	231	0	1	0	0
Alcoholic beverage, distilled, whiskey, 86 proof	0	0	0.1	250	0	0	0	0.1
Beverages, almond milk, chocolate, ready-to-drink	0.63	1.25	9.38	50	0.4	71	0	8.98
Beverages, UNILEVER, SLIMFAST Shake Mix, high protein, whey powder, 3-2-1 Plan,	27.87	11.62	50	368	18.2	495	6	31.8
Beverages, Acai berry drink, fortified	0.83	0.83	12.83	62	1.2	13	0	11.63
Alcoholic beverage, wine, dessert, sweet	0.2	0	13.69	160	0	9	0	13.69
Beverages, Whey protein powder isolate	58.14	1.16	29.07	359	0	372	12	29.07
Beverages, KELLOGG'S, SPECIAL K Protein Shake	3.2	1.6	9.2	64	1.7	73	4	7.5
Beverages, Energy Drink with carbonated water and high fructose corn syrup	0.42	0	15	62	0	48	0	15
Beverages, Energy Drink, sugar free	0.42	0	0.42	4	0	42	0	0.42
Beverages, ABBOTT, ENSURE, Nutritional Shake, Ready-to-Drink	3.8	2.53	16.88	105	0	84	2	16.88
Beverages, chocolate powder, no sugar added	9.09	9.09	63.64	373	9.1	636	0	54.54
Beverages, Orange juice, light, No pulp	0.21	0	5.42	21	0	4	0	5.42
Beverages, The COCA-COLA company, Hi-C Flashin' Fruit Punch	0	0	12.5	45	0	8	0	12.5
Beverages, Protein powder whey based	78.13	1.56	6.25	352	3.1	156	16	3.15
Beverages, Protein powder soy based	55.56	5.56	28.89	388	6.7	733	0	22.19
Beverages, KELLOGG'S SPECIAL K20 protein powder	35.2	0.6	58.4	380	37.5	280	4	20.9
Beverages, ZEVIA, cola	0	0	1.13	0	0	6	0	1.13
Beverages, ZEVIA, cola, caffeine free	0	0	1.13	0	0	6	0	1.13
Beverages, GEROLSTEINER BRUNNEN GmbH & Co. KG,Gerolsteiner naturally sparkling mineral water,	0	0	0	0	0	13	0	0
Beverages, ICELANDIC, Glacial Natural spring water	0	0	0	0	0	1	0	0
Beverages, yellow green colored citrus soft drink with caffeine	0	0	12.83	49	0	18	0	12.83
Beverages, rich chocolate, powder	0	0	92.96	372	0	636	0	92.96
Beverages, GEROLSTEINER BRUNNEN GmbH & Co. KG (Gerolsteiner), naturally sparkling, mineral bottled water	0	0	0	0	0	13	0	0
Beverages, chocolate malt, powder, prepared with fat free milk	3.25	0.17	8.64	49	0	77	2	8.64
Alcoholic beverage, wine, table, all	0.07	0	2.72	83	0	5	0	2.72
Beverages, V8 SPLASH Smoothies, Peach Mango	1.22	0	7.76	37	0	29	0	7.76
Beverages, V8 SPLASH Smoothies, Strawberry Banana	1.22	0	8.16	37	0	29	0	8.16
Beverages, V8 SPLASH Smoothies, Tropical Colada	1.22	0	8.54	41	0.4	20	0	8.14
Beverages, Coconut water, ready-to-drink, unsweetened	0.22	0	4.24	18	0	26	0	4.24
Beverages, almond milk, unsweetened, shelf stable	0.59	1.1	0.58	15	0	71	0	0.58

Food Name ---> per 100 g	Protein (g)	Fat (g)	Carb (g)	Calories	Fiber (g)	Sodium (mg)	Cholesterol (mg)	Net Carb (g)
Beverages, chocolate almond milk, unsweetened, shelf-stable, fortified with vitamin D2 and E	0.83	1.46	1.25	21	0.4	75	0	0.85
Beverages, The COCA-COLA company, Glaceau Vitamin Water, Revive Fruit Punch, fortified	0	0	0	0	0	0	0	0
Beverages, MINUTE MAID, Lemonada, Limeade	0	0	13.75	50	0	6	0	13.75
Alcoholic beverage, wine, table, red	0.07	0	2.61	85	0	4	0	2.61
Alcoholic Beverage, wine, table, red, Cabernet Sauvignon	0.07	0	2.6	83	0	0	0	2.6
Alcoholic Beverage, wine, table, red, Cabernet Franc	0.07	0	2.45	83	0	0	0	2.45
Alcoholic Beverage, wine, table, red, Pinot Noir	0.07	0	2.31	82	0	0	0	2.31
Alcoholic Beverage, wine, table, red, Syrah	0.07	0	2.58	83	0	0	0	2.58
Alcoholic Beverage, wine, table, red, Barbera	0.07	0	2.79	85	0	0	0	2.79
Alcoholic Beverage, wine, table, red, Zinfandel	0.07	0	2.86	88	0	0	0	2.86
Alcoholic Beverage, wine, table, red, Petite Sirah	0.07	0	2.68	85	0	0	0	2.68
Alcoholic Beverage, wine, table, red, Claret	0.07	0	3.01	83	0	0	0	3.01
Alcoholic beverage, wine, table, white	0.07	0	2.6	82	0	5	0	2.6
Alcoholic Beverage, wine, table, red, Lemberger	0.07	0	2.46	80	0	0	0	2.46
Alcoholic Beverage, wine, table, red, Sangiovese	0.07	0	2.62	86	0	0	0	2.62
Alcoholic Beverage, wine, table, red, Carignane	0.07	0	2.4	74	0	0	0	2.4
Alcoholic beverage, wine, table, white, Pinot Gris (Grigio)	0.07	0	2.06	83	0	0	0	2.06
Alcoholic beverage, wine, table, white, Chenin Blanc	0.07	0	3.31	80	0	0	0	3.31
Alcoholic beverage, wine, table, white, Fume Blanc	0.07	0	2.27	82	0	0	0	2.27
Beverages, Mixed vegetable and fruit juice drink, with added nutrients	0.04	0.01	7.47	29	0	21	0	7.47
Alcoholic beverage, wine, table, white, Muller Thurgau	0.07	0	3.48	76	0	0	0	3.48
Beverages, carbonated, club soda	0	0	0	0	0	21	0	0
Alcoholic beverage, wine, table, white, Gewurztraminer	0.07	0	2.6	81	0	0	0	2.6
Alcoholic beverage, wine, table, white, late harvest, Gewurztraminer	0.07	0	11.39	108	0	0	0	11.39
Alcoholic beverage, wine, table, white, Semillon	0.07	0	3.12	82	0	0	0	3.12
Carbonated beverage, cream soda	0	0	13.3	51	0	12	0	13.3
Alcoholic beverage, wine, table, white, Riesling	0.07	0	3.74	80	0	0	0	3.74
Alcoholic beverage, wine, table, white, Sauvignon Blanc	0.07	0	2.05	81	0	0	0	2.05
Alcoholic beverage, wine, table, white, late harvest	0.07	0	13.39	112	0	0	0	13.39
Beverages, carbonated, ginger ale	0	0	8.76	34	0	7	0	8.76
Beverages, NESTEA, tea, black, ready-to-drink, lemon	0	0	9.09	36	0	21	0	9.09
Alcoholic beverage, wine, table, white, Pinot Blanc	0.07	0	1.94	81	0	0	0	1.94
Alcoholic beverage, wine, table, white, Muscat	0.07	0	5.23	82	0	0	0	5.23
Beverages, carbonated, grape soda	0	0	11.2	43	0	15	0	11.2
Beverages, carbonated, low calorie, other than cola or pepper, without caffeine	0.1	0	0	0	0	6	0	0
Beverages, carbonated, lemon-lime soda, no caffeine	0.09	0	10.42	41	0	10	0	10.42
Beverages, carbonated, SPRITE, lemon-lime, without caffeine	0.05	0.02	10.14	40	0	9	0	10.14
Beverages, carbonated, low calorie, cola or pepper-type, with aspartame, without caffeine	0.12	0	0.12	1	0	4	0	0.12

Food Name ---> per 100 g	Protein (g)	Fat (g)	Carb (g)	Calories	Fiber (g)	Sodium (mg)	Cholesterol (mg)	Net Carb (g)
Beverages, carbonated, cola, without caffeine	0	0	10.58	41	0	4	0	10.58
Beverages, carbonated, cola, regular	0	0.25	10.36	42	0	3	0	10.36
Beverages, carbonated, reduced sugar, cola, contains caffeine and sweeteners	0	0	5.16	20	0	4	0	5.16
Beverages, carbonated, orange	0	0	12.3	48	0	12	0	12.3
Beverages, carbonated, low calorie, other than cola or pepper, with aspartame, contains caffeine	0.1	0	0	0	0	6	0	0
Alcoholic Beverage, wine, table, red, Burgundy	0.07	0	3.69	86	0	0	0	3.69
Beverages, carbonated, pepper-type, contains caffeine	0	0.1	10.4	41	0	10	0	10.4
Beverages, Energy drink, RED BULL	0.46	0	10.23	43	0	39	0	10.23
Beverages, carbonated, tonic water	0	0	8.8	34	0	12	0	8.8
Beverages, Energy drink, RED BULL, sugar free, with added caffeine, niacin, pantothenic acid, vitamins B6 and B12	0.25	0.08	0.7	5	0	83	0	0.7
Beverages, carbonated, root beer	0	0	10.6	41	0	13	0	10.6
Alcoholic Beverage, wine, table, red, Gamay	0.07	0	2.38	78	0	0	0	2.38
Alcoholic Beverage, wine, table, red, Mouvedre	0.07	0	2.64	88	0	0	0	2.64
Alcoholic beverage, wine, table, white, Chardonnay	0.07	0	2.16	84	0	5	0	2.16
Beverages, Kiwi Strawberry Juice Drink	0	0	12.26	47	0	11	0	12.26
Beverages, Apple juice drink, light, fortified with vitamin C	0	0.1	5.1	22	0	13	0	5.1
Beverages, chocolate drink, milk and soy based, ready to drink, fortified	4.22	1.69	17.3	101	1.3	63	4	16
Beverages, chocolate malt powder, prepared with 1% milk, fortified	3.32	0.97	8.81	57	0	60	5	8.81
Beverages, carbonated, limeade, high caffeine	0	0.11	4.16	18	0	40	0	4.16
Beverages, carbonated, low calorie, cola or pepper-types, with sodium saccharin, contains caffeine	0	0	0.1	0	0	16	0	0.1
Beverages, POWERADE, Zero, Mixed Berry	0	0	0.14	0	0	42	0	0.14
Beverages, Carob-flavor beverage mix, powder	1.8	0.2	93.3	372	8	103	0	85.3
Beverages, Carob-flavor beverage mix, powder, prepared with whole milk	3.16	3.11	8.68	75	0.4	46	10	8.28
Beverages, coconut milk, sweetened, fortified with calcium, vitamins A, B12, D2	0.21	2.08	2.92	31	0	19	0	2.92
Beverages, coffee, ready to drink, vanilla, light, milk based, sweetened	2.14	1.07	4.27	36	0	34	5	4.27
Beverages, Lemonade fruit juice drink light, fortified with vitamin E and C	0	0	5	21	0	5	0	5
Beverages, chocolate-flavor beverage mix, powder, prepared with whole milk	3.23	3.24	11.91	85	0.4	58	9	11.51
Beverages, coffee, ready to drink, milk based, sweetened	1.98	1.38	12.6	71	0	26	5	12.6
Beverages, coffee, brewed, breakfast blend	0.3	0	0.23	2	0	1	0	0.23
Beverages, chocolate syrup	2.1	1.13	65.1	279	2.6	72	0	62.5
Beverages, chocolate syrup, prepared with whole milk	3.07	2.96	12.78	90	0.3	47	9	12.48
Beverages, coffee, ready to drink, iced, mocha, milk based	1.48	0.98	11.42	60	0	31	0	11.42
Beverages, tea, Oolong, brewed	0	0	0.15	1	0	3	0	0.15
Beverages, Clam and tomato juice, canned	0.6	0.2	10.95	48	0.4	362	0	10.55
Beverages, tea, green, ready to drink, ginseng and honey, sweetened	0	0.18	7.16	30	0	2	0	7.16
Beverages, The COCA-COLA company, Minute Maid, Lemonade	0	0	12.08	46	0	6	0	12.08

Food Name ---> per 100 g	Protein (g)	Fat (g)	Carb (g)	Calories	Fiber (g)	Sodium (mg)	Cholesterol (mg)	Net Carb (g)
Beverages, tea, green, ready-to-drink, diet	0	0	0	0	0	6	0	0
Beverages, tea, green, ready-to-drink, citrus, diet, fortified with vitamin C	0	0	0.31	1	0	26	0	0.31
Beverages, Cocoa mix, powder	6.67	4	83.73	398	3.7	504	0	80.03
Beverages, Cocoa mix, powder, prepared with water	0.92	0.55	11.54	55	0.5	73	0	11.04
Beverages, Cocoa mix, NESTLE, Hot Cocoa Mix Rich Chocolate With Marshmallows	2.8	15	75	400	3.7	800	0	71.3
Beverages, Cocoa mix, no sugar added, powder	15.49	3	71.93	377	7.5	876	0	64.43
Cocoa mix, NESTLE, Rich Chocolate Hot Cocoa Mix	3	15	75	400	4	850	0	71
Beverages, tea, black, ready-to-drink, lemon, sweetened	0	0.22	10.8	45	0	3	0	10.8
Beverages, coffee, brewed, prepared with tap water, decaffeinated	0.1	0	0	0	0	2	0	0
Beverages, coffee, brewed, espresso, restaurant-prepared, decaffeinated	0.1	0.18	1.69	9	0	14	0	1.69
Beverages, coffee, instant, regular, half the caffeine	14.42	0.5	73.18	352	0	37	0	73.18
Beverages, coffee and cocoa, instant, decaffeinated, with whitener and low calorie sweetener	9	13.21	71.4	440	4.8	500	0	66.6
Beverages, tea, green, ready-to-drink, sweetened	0	0.22	6.2	27	0	21	0	6.2
Beverages, tea, ready-to-drink, lemon, diet	0	0	0.41	2	0	1	0	0.41
Beverages, coffee, brewed, prepared with tap water	0.12	0.02	0	1	0	2	0	0
Beverages, coffee, brewed, espresso, restaurant-prepared	0.12	0.18	1.67	9	0	14	0	1.67
Beverages, tea, black, ready-to-drink, lemon, diet	0	0	0.22	1	0	17	0	0.22
Beverages, coffee, instant, regular, powder	12.2	0.5	75.4	353	0	37	0	75.4
Beverages, coffee, instant, regular, prepared with water	0.1	0	0.34	2	0	4	0	0.34
Beverages, aloe vera juice drink, fortified with Vitamin C	0	0	3.75	15	0	8	0	3.75
Beverages, OCEAN SPRAY, Cran Grape	0.21	0	13.16	54	0.6	19	1	12.56
Beverages, coffee, instant, decaffeinated, powder	11.6	0.2	76	351	0	23	0	76
Beverages, coffee, instant, decaffeinated, prepared with water	0.12	0	0.43	2	0	4	0	0.43
Beverages, OCEAN SPRAY, Cranberry-Apple Juice Drink, bottled	0.29	0	13.68	56	0.6	19	0	13.08
Beverages, OCEAN SPRAY, Diet Cranberry Juice	0.07	0	0.8	4	0.6	7	0	0.2
Beverages, coffee, instant, with chicory	9.3	0.2	78.9	355	0.5	277	0	78.4
Beverages, coffee, instant, chicory	0.09	0	0.75	3	0	7	0	0.75
Beverages, coffee, instant, mocha, sweetened	5.29	15.87	74.04	460	1.9	317	0	72.14
Beverages, OCEAN SPRAY, Light Cranberry and Raspberry Flavored Juice	0.73	0	5.77	26	0.7	2	0	5.07
Beverages, OCEAN SPRAY, White Cranberry Strawberry Flavored Juice Drink	0.22	0.01	11.98	49	0.6	3	0	11.38
Beverages, KRAFT, coffee, instant, French Vanilla Cafe	2.5	19.2	74.6	481	1.4	399	0	73.2
Beverages, OCEAN SPRAY, Cran Raspberry Juice Drink	0.28	0	11.96	49	0.6	14	0	11.36
Beverages, OCEAN SPRAY, Cran Lemonade	0.07	0	11.12	45	0.6	52	0	10.52
Beverages, OCEAN SPRAY, Diet Cran Cherry	0.21	0	0.7	4	0.6	8	0	0.1
Beverages, coffee substitute, cereal grain beverage, powder	6.01	2.52	78.42	360	23.3	83	0	55.12
Beverages, coffee substitute, cereal grain beverage, prepared with water	0.1	0.04	1.3	6	0.4	5	0	0.9

Food Name ---> per 100 g	Protein (g)	Fat (g)	Carb (g)	Calories	Fiber (g)	Sodium (mg)	Cholesterol (mg)	Net Carb (g)
Beverages, cranberry-apple juice drink, bottled	0	0.11	15.85	63	0	2	0	15.85
Alcoholic beverage, malt beer, hard lemonade	0	0	10.07	68	0	5	0	10.07
Beverages, cranberry-apricot juice drink, bottled	0.2	0	16.2	64	0.1	2	0	16.1
Beverages, cranberry-grape juice drink, bottled	0.2	0.1	14	56	0.1	3	0	13.9
Cranberry juice cocktail, bottled	0	0.1	13.52	54	0	2	0	13.52
Cranberry juice cocktail, bottled, low calorie, with calcium, saccharin and corn sweetener	0.02	0.01	4.6	19	0	3	0	4.6
Beverages, Eggnog-flavor mix, powder, prepared with whole milk	2.93	3.02	14.2	95	0	55	11	14.2
Beverages, tea, green, instant, decaffeinated, lemon, unsweetened, fortified with vitamin C	0	0	94.45	378	0	0	0	94.45
Beverages, tea, black, ready to drink	0	0	0	0	0	2	0	0
Alcoholic beverage, beer, light, higher alcohol	0.25	0	0.77	46	0	4	0	0.77
Beverages, AMBER, hard cider	0	0	5.92	56	0	4	0	5.92
Alcoholic beverages, beer, higher alcohol	0.9	0	0.27	58	0	4	0	0.27
Beverages, Malt liquor beverage	0.35	0	0	40	0	3	0	0
Alcoholic beverages, wine, rose	0.36	0	3.8	83	0	5	0	3.8
Beverages, OCEAN SPRAY, Cran Pomegranate	0.07	0.01	12.56	47	0.6	12	0	11.96
Beverages, OCEAN SPRAY, Cran Cherry	0.19	0	12.76	46	0.6	7	0	12.16
Beverages, OCEAN SPRAY, Light Cranberry	0.22	0.01	4.72	19	0.7	15	0	4.02
Beverages, OCEAN SPRAY, White Cranberry Peach	0.13	0.01	11.88	45	0.6	11	0	11.28
Beverages, OCEAN SPRAY, Light Cranberry, Concord Grape	0.36	0.02	5.78	23	0.7	8	0	5.08
Beverages, tea, green, brewed, decaffeinated	0	0	0	0	0	0	0	0
Beverages, tea, green, ready to drink, unsweetened	0	0	0	0	0	7	0	0
Beverages, citrus fruit juice drink, frozen concentrate	1.2	0.1	40.2	162	0.2	3	0	40
Beverages, citrus fruit juice drink, frozen concentrate, prepared with water	0.34	0.03	11.42	46	0.1	4	0	11.32
Beverages, fruit punch drink, without added nutrients, canned	0	0	11.97	48	0	10	0	11.97
Beverages, Fruit punch drink, with added nutrients, canned	0	0	11.94	47	0.2	38	0	11.74
Beverages, Fruit punch drink, frozen concentrate	0.2	0	41.4	162	0.4	8	0	41
Beverages, Fruit punch drink, frozen concentrate, prepared with water	0.06	0	11.66	46	0.1	5	0	11.56
Beverages, coffee, instant, vanilla, sweetened, decaffeinated, with non dairy creamer	0	13.33	86.28	465	0	333	0	86.28
Beverages, Tropical Punch, ready-to-drink	0	0	2.5	10	0	13	0	2.5
Beverages, grape drink, canned	0	0	15.72	61	0	16	0	15.72
Beverages, tea, green, brewed, regular	0.22	0	0	1	0	1	0	0
Beverages, tea, black, ready-to-drink, peach, diet	0	0	0.25	1	0	5	0	0.25
Beverages, tea, black, ready to drink, decaffeinated, diet	0	0	0.83	0	0	4	0	0.83
Beverages, tea, black, ready to drink, decaffeinated	0	0	8.75	38	0	8	0	8.75
Beverages, grape juice drink, canned	0	0	14.55	57	0.1	9	0	14.45
Beverages, Cranberry juice cocktail	0	0.34	12.25	52	0	2	0	12.25
Beverages, OCEAN SPRAY, Ruby Red cranberry	0.07	0.01	11.58	45	0.6	11	0	10.98
Beverages, MOTTS, Apple juice light, fortified with vitamin C	0	0.1	5.1	22	0	13	0	5.1
Beverages, Lemonade, powder	0	1.05	97.57	376	0.4	51	0	97.17
Lemonade, powder, prepared with water	0	0.04	3.59	14	0	6	0	3.59
Beverages, SNAPPLE, tea, black and green, ready	0.1	0	0.1	2	0	3	0	0.1

39

Food Name ---> per 100 g	Protein (g)	Fat (g)	Carb (g)	Calories	Fiber (g)	Sodium (mg)	Cholesterol (mg)	Net Carb (g)
to drink, peach, diet								
Lemonade, frozen concentrate, white	0.22	0.7	49.89	196	0.3	7	0	49.59
Lemonade, frozen concentrate, white, prepared with water	0.07	0.04	10.42	40	0	4	0	10.42
Beverages, SNAPPLE, tea, black and green, ready to drink, lemon, diet	0.1	0	0.1	2	0	3	0	0.1
Beverages, lemonade-flavor drink, powder	0	1.01	97.9	380	0	130	0	97.9
Beverages, lemonade-flavor drink, powder, prepared with water	0	0.07	6.9	27	0	13	0	6.9
Limeade, frozen concentrate, prepared with water	0	0	13.79	52	0	3	0	13.79
Malt beverage, includes non-alcoholic beer	0.21	0.12	8.05	37	0	13	0	8.05
Beverages, OVALTINE, Classic Malt powder	0	0	93.33	372	0	636	0	93.33
Beverages, Malted drink mix, natural, with added nutrients, powder, prepared with whole milk	3.67	3.21	10.67	86	0	72	11	10.67
Beverages, Malted drink mix, natural, powder, dairy based.	14.29	9.52	71.21	428	0.1	405	24	71.11
Beverages, Malted drink mix, natural, powder, prepared with whole milk	3.86	3.62	10.23	88	0.1	79	12	10.13
Beverages, OVALTINE, chocolate malt powder	0	0	92.96	372	0	636	0	92.96
Beverages, Malted drink mix, chocolate, with added nutrients, powder, prepared with whole milk	3.29	3.26	11.19	87	0.4	87	10	10.79
Beverages, malted drink mix, chocolate, powder	5.1	4.76	86.94	411	4.8	190	1	82.14
Beverages, Malted drink mix, chocolate, powder, prepared with whole milk	3.37	3.29	11.2	85	0.5	60	10	10.7
Beverages, orange drink, canned, with added vitamin C	0	0.07	12.34	49	0	3	0	12.34
Beverages, orange and apricot juice drink, canned	0.3	0.1	12.7	51	0.1	2	0	12.6
Beverages, pineapple and grapefruit juice drink, canned	0.2	0.1	11.6	47	0.1	14	0	11.5
Beverages, pineapple and orange juice drink, canned	1.3	0	11.8	50	0.1	3	0	11.7
Shake, fast food, vanilla	3.37	6.52	19.59	148	0.9	81	23	18.69
Strawberry-flavor beverage mix, powder	0.1	0.2	99.1	389	0	38	0	99.1
Beverages, Strawberry-flavor beverage mix, powder, prepared with whole milk	3	3.1	12.3	88	0	48	12	12.3
Beverages, tea, black, brewed, prepared with tap water, decaffeinated	0	0	0.3	1	0	3	0	0.3
Beverages, tea, instant, decaffeinated, unsweetened	20.21	0	58.66	315	8.5	72	0	50.16
Beverages, tea, black, brewed, prepared with tap water	0	0	0.3	1	0	3	0	0.3
Beverages, tea, instant, decaffeinated, lemon, diet	3.3	0.6	85.4	338	0	412	0	85.4
Beverages, tea, instant, decaffeinated, lemon, sweetened	0.12	0.73	98.55	401	0	5	0	98.55
Beverages, tea, instant, unsweetened, powder	20.21	0	58.66	315	8.5	72	0	50.16
Beverages, tea, instant, unsweetened, prepared with water	0.06	0	0.17	1	0	4	0	0.17
Beverages, tea, instant, lemon, unsweetened	7.4	0.18	78.52	345	5	55	0	73.52
Beverages, tea, instant, lemon, sweetened, powder	0.12	0.73	98.55	401	0.7	5	0	97.85
Beverages, tea, instant, lemon, sweetened, prepared with water	0.01	0.06	8.61	35	0.1	2	0	8.51
Beverages, tea, instant, sweetened with sodium saccharin, lemon-flavored, powder	3.3	0.6	85.4	338	0	412	0	85.4
Beverages, tea, instant, lemon, diet	0.02	0	0.44	2	0	6	0	0.44
Beverages, tea, herb, other than chamomile, brewed	0	0	0.2	1	0	1	0	0.2
Beverages, water, bottled, PERRIER	0	0	0	0	0	1	0	0

Food Name ---> per 100 g	Protein (g)	Fat (g)	Carb (g)	Calories	Fiber (g)	Sodium (mg)	Cholesterol (mg)	Net Carb (g)
Beverages, water, bottled, POLAND SPRING	0	0	0	0	0	1	0	0
Beverages, cocoa mix, with aspartame, powder, prepared with water	1.21	0.23	5.61	29	0.6	72	0	5.01
Beverages, carbonated, cola, fast-food cola	0.07	0.02	9.56	37	0	4	0	9.56
Beverages, fruit punch juice drink, frozen concentrate	0.3	0.7	43.1	175	0.2	10	0	42.9
Beverages, fruit punch juice drink, frozen concentrate, prepared with water	0.07	0.17	11.4	42	0	5	0	11.4
Beverages, orange-flavor drink, breakfast type, powder	0	0	98.94	386	0.4	17	0	98.54
Beverages, orange-flavor drink, breakfast type, powder, prepared with water	0	0	12.65	49	0.1	5	0	12.55
Beverages, Orange-flavor drink, breakfast type, low calorie, powder	3.6	0	85.9	217	3.8	81	0	82.1
Beverages, water, tap, drinking	0	0	0	0	0	4	0	0
Beverages, water, tap, well	0	0	0	0	0	5	0	0
Alcoholic beverage, liqueur, coffee, 53 proof	0.1	0.3	46.8	336	0	8	0	46.8
Alcoholic beverage, liqueur, coffee with cream, 34 proof	2.8	15.7	20.9	327	0	92	58	20.9
Beverages, carbonated, low calorie, cola or pepper-type, with aspartame, contains caffeine	0.11	0.03	0.29	2	0	8	0	0.29
Beverages, coffee substitute, cereal grain beverage, powder, prepared with whole milk	3.3	3.3	5.6	65	0.1	49	13	5.5
Beverages, Dairy drink mix, chocolate, reduced calorie, with low-calorie sweeteners, powder	25	2.6	51.4	329	9.4	659	24	42
Beverages, dairy drink mix, chocolate, reduced calorie, with aspartame, powder, prepared with water and ice	2.19	0.23	4.51	29	0.8	61	2	3.71
Beverages, Orange-flavor drink, breakfast type, with pulp, frozen concentrate. Not manufactured anymore.	0.1	0.5	42.9	172	0.2	24	0	42.7
Beverages, Orange-flavor drink, breakfast type, with pulp, frozen concentrate, prepared with water	0.03	0.14	12.21	49	0	10	0	12.21
Beverages, Orange drink, breakfast type, with juice and pulp, frozen concentrate	0.4	0	39	153	0.1	26	0	38.9
Beverages, Orange drink, breakfast type, with juice and pulp, frozen concentrate, prepared with water	0.12	0	11.32	45	0	10	0	11.32
Beverages, shake, fast food, strawberry	3.4	2.8	18.9	113	0.4	83	11	18.5
Beverages, water, tap, municipal	0	0	0	0	0	3	0	0
Cranberry juice cocktail, frozen concentrate	0.05	0	51.45	201	0.2	4	0	51.25
Cranberry juice cocktail, frozen concentrate, prepared with water	0.01	0	11.81	47	0	4	0	11.81
Beverages, water, bottled, non-carbonated, DANNON	0	0	0	0	0	0	0	0
Beverages, water, bottled, non-carbonated, PEPSI, AQUAFINA	0	0	0	0	0	0	0	0
Beverages, The COCA-COLA company, DASANI, water, bottled, non-carbonated	0	0	0	0	0	0	0	0
Beverages, orange breakfast drink, ready-to-drink, with added nutrients	0	0	13.2	53	0.1	54	0	13.1
Beverages, water, bottled, non-carbonated, CALISTOGA	0	0	0	0	0	0	0	0
Beverages, water, bottled, non-carbonated, CRYSTAL GEYSER	0	0	0	0	0	1	0	0
Water, bottled, non-carbonated, NAYA	0	0	0	0	0	1	0	0
Beverages, water, bottled, non-carbonated,	0	0	0.03	0	0	1	0	0.03

Food Name ---> per 100 g	Protein (g)	Fat (g)	Carb (g)	Calories	Fiber (g)	Sodium (mg)	Cholesterol (mg)	Net Carb (g)
DANNON Fluoride To Go								
Beverages, drink mix, QUAKER OATS, GATORADE, orange flavor, powder	0	1.23	94.11	388	0	63	0	94.11
Beverages, PEPSICO QUAKER, Gatorade, G performance O 2, ready-to-drink.	0	0	6.43	26	0	39	0	6.43
Beverages, COCA-COLA, POWERADE, lemon-lime flavored, ready-to-drink	0	0.05	7.84	32	0	42	0	7.84
Beverages, Propel Zero, fruit-flavored, non-carbonated	0	0	1.14	5	0	33	0	1.14
Beverages, ARIZONA, tea, ready-to-drink, lemon	0	0	9.77	39	0	4	0	9.77
Beverages, LIPTON BRISK, tea, black, ready-to-drink, lemon	0	0	8.81	35	0	21	0	8.81
Whiskey sour mix, bottled, with added potassium and sodium	0.1	0.1	21.4	84	0	33	0	21.4
Alcoholic beverage, whiskey sour	0	0.03	13.17	149	0	20	0	13.17
Alcoholic beverage, distilled, all (gin, rum, vodka, whiskey) 94 proof	0	0	0	275	0	1	0	0
Alcoholic beverage, distilled, all (gin, rum, vodka, whiskey) 100 proof	0	0	0	295	0	1	0	0
Alcoholic beverage, liqueur, coffee, 63 proof	0.1	0.3	32.2	308	0	8	0	32.2
Alcoholic beverage, wine, dessert, dry	0.2	0	11.67	152	0	9	0	11.67
Carbonated beverage, low calorie, other than cola or pepper, with sodium saccharin, without caffeine	0	0	0.1	0	0	16	0	0.1
Beverages, Cocoa mix, low caloric, powder, with added calcium, phosphorus, aspartame, without added sodium or vitamin A	25.1	3	58	359	1.1	653	11	56.9
Beverages, fruit punch-flavor drink, powder, without added sodium, prepared with water	0	0.01	9.47	37	0	7	0	9.47
Lemonade, frozen concentrate, pink	0.22	0.69	48.86	192	0.3	4	0	48.56
Beverages, lemonade, frozen concentrate, pink, prepared with water	0.05	0.15	10.81	43	0.1	4	0	10.71
Beverages, tea, black, brewed, prepared with distilled water	0	0	0.3	1	0	0	0	0.3
Beverages, tea, herb, brewed, chamomile	0	0	0.2	1	0	1	0	0.2
Beverages, tea, instant, lemon, with added ascorbic acid	0.6	0.3	97.6	385	0	5	0	97.6
Alcoholic beverage, distilled, all (gin, rum, vodka, whiskey) 86 proof	0	0	0.1	250	0	1	0	0.1
Alcoholic beverage, distilled, all (gin, rum, vodka, whiskey) 90 proof	0	0	0	263	0	1	0	0
Carbonated beverage, chocolate-flavored soda	0	0	10.7	42	0	4	0	10.7
Beverages, Wine, non-alcoholic	0.5	0	1.1	6	0	7	0	1.1
Water, bottled, generic	0	0	0	0	0	2	0	0
Beverages, chocolate-flavor beverage mix for milk, powder, with added nutrients	4.55	2.27	90.28	400	4.5	136	0	85.78
Beverages, chocolate-flavor beverage mix for milk, powder, with added nutrients, prepared with whole milk	3.27	3.17	11.87	89	0.4	50	10	11.47
Beverages, water, bottled, non-carbonated, EVIAN	0	0	0	0	0	0	0	0
Beverages, Powerade Zero Ion4, calorie-free, assorted flavors	0	0	0	0	0	42	0	0
Beverages, WENDY'S, tea, ready-to-drink, unsweetened	0.22	0	0	1	0	3	0	0
Alcoholic Beverage, wine, table, red, Merlot	0.07	0	2.51	83	0	4	0	2.51
Water, non-carbonated, bottles, natural fruit flavors,	0	0	0.13	1	0	14	0	0.13

sweetened with low calorie sweetener

Food Name ---> per 100 g	Protein (g)	Fat (g)	Carb (g)	Calories	Fiber (g)	Sodium (mg)	Cholesterol (mg)	Net Carb (g)
Beverages, Water with added vitamins and minerals, bottles, sweetened, assorted fruit flavors	0	0	5.49	22	0	0	0	5.49
Beverages, V8 SPLASH Juice Drinks, Diet Berry Blend	0	0	1.23	4	0	14	0	1.23
Beverages, V8 SPLASH Juice Drinks, Diet Fruit Medley	0	0	1.26	4	0	13	0	1.26
Beverages, V8 SPLASH Juice Drinks, Diet Strawberry Kiwi	0	0	1.26	4	0	13	0	1.26
Beverages, V8 SPLASH Juice Drinks, Diet Tropical Blend	0	0	1.26	4	0	15	0	1.26
Beverages, V8 SPLASH Juice Drinks, Berry Blend	0	0	7.41	29	0	21	0	7.41
Beverages, V8 SPLASH Juice Drinks, Fruit Medley	0	0	7.82	33	0	21	0	7.82
Beverages, V8 SPLASH Juice Drinks, Guava Passion Fruit	0	0	7.82	33	0	14	0	7.82
Beverages, V8 SPLASH Juice Drinks, Mango Peach	0	0	8.23	33	0	16	0	8.23
Beverages, V8 SPLASH Juice Drinks, Orange Pineapple	0	0	7.41	29	0	21	0	7.41
Beverages, V8 SPLASH Juice Drinks, Orchard Blend	0	0	7.82	33	0	21	0	7.82
Beverages, V8 SPLASH Juice Drinks, Strawberry Banana	0	0	7.41	29	0	21	0	7.41
Beverages, V8 SPLASH Juice Drinks, Strawberry Kiwi	0	0	7.41	29	0	21	0	7.41
Beverages, V8 SPLASH Juice Drinks, Tropical Blend	0	0	7.41	29	0	21	0	7.41
Beverages, V8 V-FUSION Juices, Peach Mango	0.41	0	11.38	49	0	28	0	11.38
Beverages, V8 V-FUSION Juices, Strawberry Banana	0.41	0	11.79	49	0	28	0	11.79
Beverages, V8 V-FUSION Juices, Tropical	0.41	0	11.38	49	0	33	0	11.38
Beverages, V8 V- FUSION Juices, Acai Berry	0	0	10.98	45	0	28	0	10.98
Beverages, Energy drink, AMP	0.25	0.08	12.08	46	0	27	0	12.08
Beverages, Energy drink, FULL THROTTLE	0.25	0.08	12.08	46	0	35	0	12.08
Beverages, Energy Drink, Monster, fortified with vitamins C, B2, B3, B6, B12	0.47	0	11.28	47	0	77	0	11.28
Beverages, Energy drink, AMP, sugar free	0	0	1.03	2	0	31	0	1.03
Beverages, Energy drink, ROCKSTAR	0.34	0.22	12.7	58	0	16	0	12.7
Beverages, Energy drink, ROCKSTAR, sugar free	0.25	0.08	0.7	4	0	52	0	0.7
Beverages, Horchata, dry mix, unprepared, variety of brands, all with morro seeds	7.5	7.46	79.05	413	4	3	0	75.05
Beverages, Meal supplement drink, canned, peanut flavor	3.5	3.07	14.74	101	0	54	0	14.74
Beverages, Vegetable and fruit juice drink, reduced calorie, with low-calorie sweetener, added vitamin C	0	0	1.1	4	0	14	0	1.1
Beverages, milk beverage, reduced fat, flavored and sweetened, Ready-to-drink, added calcium, vitamin A and vitamin D	3.05	1.83	12.08	77	0.4	49	8	11.68
Beverages, vegetable and fruit juice blend, 100% juice, with added vitamins A, C, E	0.3	0.01	11.15	46	0	29	0	11.15
Beverages, fruit juice drink, reduced sugar, with vitamin E added	0	0.07	10	39	0	2	0	10
Water, with corn syrup and/or sugar and low calorie sweetener, fruit flavored	0	0	4.5	18	0	8	0	4.5

Food Name ---> per 100 g	Protein (g)	Fat (g)	Carb (g)	Calories	Fiber (g)	Sodium (mg)	Cholesterol (mg)	Net Carb (g)
Beverages, Horchata, as served in restaurant	0.48	0.71	11.52	54	0	14	0	11.52
Beverages, rice milk, unsweetened	0.28	0.97	9.17	47	0.3	39	0	8.87
Beverages, Energy drink, VAULT, citrus flavor	0	0	12.99	49	0	12	0	12.99
Beverages, Energy drink, VAULT Zero, sugar-free, citrus flavor	0.25	0.08	0.7	1	0	14	0	0.7
Beverages, PEPSICO QUAKER, Gatorade G2, low calorie	0.05	0.01	1.94	8	0	45	0	1.94
Beverages, Fruit flavored drink, less than 3% juice, not fortified with vitamin C	0	0	16.03	64	0	36	0	16.03
Beverages, Fruit flavored drink containing less than 3% fruit juice, with high vitamin C	0	0	6.67	27	0	36	0	6.67
Beverages, Fruit flavored drink, reduced sugar, greater than 3% fruit juice, high vitamin C, added calcium	0	0.37	6.67	29	0	25	0	6.67
Beverages, fruit juice drink, greater than 3% fruit juice, high vitamin C and added thiamin	0.13	0	13.16	54	0.1	61	0	13.06
Beverages, tea, hibiscus, brewed	0	0	0	0	0	4	0	0
Beverages, fruit juice drink, greater than 3% juice, high vitamin C	0.13	0.11	11.35	46	0.1	8	0	11.25
Beverages, nutritional shake mix, high protein, powder	53.57	10.71	20.38	392	0	1214	0	20.38
Beverages, fruit-flavored drink, dry powdered mix, low calorie, with aspartame	0.45	0.04	87.38	218	0.1	404	0	87.28
Beverages, Orange juice drink	0.2	0	13.41	54	0.2	2	0	13.21
Alcoholic beverage, wine, cooking	0.5	0	6.3	50	0	626	0	6.3
Alcoholic beverage, wine, light	0.07	0	1.17	49	0	7	0	1.17
Beverages, fruit-flavored drink, powder, with high vitamin C with other added vitamins, low calorie	0.25	0.16	91	227	2.2	14	0	88.8
Beverages, Chocolate-flavored drink, whey and milk based	0.64	0.4	10.68	49	0.6	91	0	10.08
Beverages, coffee, instant, with whitener, reduced calorie	1.96	29.1	59.94	509	0.5	0	0	59.44
Beverages, cranberry-apple juice drink, low calorie, with vitamin C added	0.1	0	4.7	19	0.1	5	0	4.6
Alcoholic beverage, rice (sake)	0.5	0	5	134	0	2	0	5
Beverages, ABBOTT, ENSURE PLUS, ready-to-drink	5.16	4.52	19.88	141	0	95	2	19.88
Beverages, Cocktail mix, non-alcoholic, concentrated, frozen	0.08	0.01	71.6	287	0	0	0	71.6

Baby Products

Food Name ---> per serving	Weigh (g)	Measure	Calories	Total Carb (g)	Net Carb (g)	Sodium (mg)
Babyfood, apple yogurt dessert, strained	15	1 tbsp	14	2.92	2.82	3
Babyfood, apple-banana juice	31.2	1 fl oz	16	3.84	3.74	1
Babyfood, apples with ham, strained	15	1 tbsp	9	1.64	1.34	1
Babyfood, apples, dices, toddler	28.35	1 oz	14	3.28	2.78	1
Babyfood, Baby MUM MUM Rice Biscuits	8	4.0 biscuit	31	6.66	6.66	25
Babyfood, baked product, finger snacks cereal fortified	1.7	1 cookie	7	1.3	1.3	0
Babyfood, banana apple dessert, strained	15	1 tbsp	10	2.44	2.34	1
Babyfood, banana juice with low fat yogurt	31.5	1 fl oz	27	5.53	5.43	12
Babyfood, banana no tapioca, strained	15	1 tbsp	14	3.2	3	0
Babyfood, banana with mixed berries, strained	99	1 packet	91	21.1	20.1	0
Babyfood, beverage, GERBER, GRADUATES, FRUIT SPLASHERS	113	4.0 oz	33	8.31	8.31	12
Babyfood, carrots and beef, strained	15	1 tbsp	9	0.85	0.45	10
Babyfood, carrots, toddler	28.35	1 oz	6	1.48	0.78	14
Babyfood, cereal, barley, dry fortified	2.4	1 tbsp	9	1.67	1.47	1
Babyfood, cereal, barley, prepared with whole milk	28.35	1 oz	24	2.82	2.62	12
Babyfood, cereal, brown rice, dry, instant	3.7	1 tbsp	15	3.18	2.98	0
Babyfood, cereal, egg yolks and bacon, junior	28.35	1 oz	22	1.76	1.46	14
Babyfood, cereal, high protein, prepared with whole milk	28.35	1 oz	31	3.29	3.29	14
Babyfood, cereal, high protein, with apple and orange, dry	2.4	1 tbsp	9	1.38	1.18	2
Babyfood, cereal, high protein, with apple and orange, prepared with whole milk	28.35	1 oz	32	3.8	3.8	16
Babyfood, cereal, mixed, dry fortified	2.5	1 tbsp	10	1.96	1.76	1
Babyfood, cereal, mixed, prepared with whole milk	28.35	1 oz	27	3.49	3.29	12
Babyfood, cereal, mixed, with applesauce and bananas, junior, fortified	28.35	1 oz	24	5.33	5.03	1
Babyfood, cereal, mixed, with applesauce and bananas, strained	28.35	1 oz	23	5.21	4.91	1
Babyfood, cereal, mixed, with bananas, dry	2.5	1 tbsp	10	1.93	1.73	0
Babyfood, cereal, mixed, with bananas, prepared with whole milk	28.35	1 oz	24	2.83	2.73	14
Babyfood, cereal, mixed, with honey, prepared with whole milk	28.35	1 oz	33	4.51	4.51	14
Babyfood, cereal, oatmeal, dry fortified	3.2	1 tbsp	13	2.35	2.15	1
Babyfood, cereal, oatmeal, prepared with whole milk	28.35	1 oz	33	4.34	4.04	13
Babyfood, cereal, oatmeal, with applesauce and bananas, junior, fortified	28.35	1 oz	22	4.54	4.24	1
Babyfood, cereal, oatmeal, with applesauce and bananas, strained	28.35	1 oz	21	4.43	4.13	1

Food Name ---> per serving	Weight (g)	Measure	Calories	Total Carb (g)	Net Carb (g)	Sodium (mg)
Babyfood, cereal, oatmeal, with bananas, dry	15	1 serv	60	11.71	10.91	5
Babyfood, cereal, oatmeal, with bananas, prepared with whole milk	28.35	1 oz	24	2.83	2.73	14
Babyfood, cereal, oatmeal, with honey, dry	2.4	1 tbsp	9	1.66	1.66	1
Babyfood, cereal, oatmeal, with honey, prepared with whole milk	28.35	1 oz	33	4.34	4.34	14
Babyfood, cereal, rice with pears and apple, dry, instant fortified	15	1 serv	58	13.28	12.88	0
Babyfood, cereal, rice, dry fortified	2.5	1 tbsp	10	2.08	2.08	1
Babyfood, cereal, rice, prepared with whole milk	28.35	1 oz	24	2.92	2.92	12
Babyfood, cereal, rice, with applesauce and bananas, strained	16	1 tbsp	13	2.74	2.54	1
Babyfood, cereal, rice, with bananas, dry	2.5	1 tbsp	10	2	2	0
Babyfood, cereal, rice, with bananas, prepared with whole milk	28.35	1 oz	24	2.97	2.97	13
Babyfood, cereal, rice, with honey, prepared with whole milk	28.35	1 oz	33	4.85	4.85	14
Babyfood, cereal, whole wheat, with apples, dry fortified	15	0.5 oz	60	12.48	11.48	10
Babyfood, cereal, with egg yolks, junior	28.35	1 oz	15	2.01	1.71	9
Babyfood, cereal, with egg yolks, strained	28.35	1 oz	14	1.98	1.68	9
Babyfood, cereal, with eggs, strained	28.35	1 oz	16	2.27	2.27	11
Babyfood, cherry cobbler, junior	28.35	1 oz	22	5.44	5.34	0
Babyfood, cookie, baby, fruit	8	1 cookie	35	5.9	5.6	1
Babyfood, cookies	28.35	1 oz	123	19.02	18.92	85
Babyfood, cookies, arrowroot	28.35	1 oz	120	21.38	21.28	90
Babyfood, corn and sweet potatoes, strained	28.35	1 oz	19	4.32	3.82	4
Babyfood, crackers, vegetable	0.7	1 cracker	3	0.47	0.47	4
Babyfood, dessert, banana pudding, strained	15	1 tbsp	10	2.12	2.02	8
Babyfood, dessert, banana yogurt, strained	15	1 tbsp	12	2.6	2.5	2
Babyfood, dessert, blueberry yogurt, strained	15	1 tbsp	12	2.56	2.46	2
Babyfood, dessert, cherry vanilla pudding, junior	28.35	1 oz	20	5.22	5.12	0
Babyfood, dessert, cherry vanilla pudding, strained	28.35	1 oz	19	5.05	4.95	0
Babyfood, dessert, custard pudding, vanilla, junior	229	1 cup	197	40.26	39.76	60
Babyfood, dessert, custard pudding, vanilla, strained	229	1 cup	195	36.64	36.64	0
Babyfood, dessert, dutch apple, junior	28.35	1 oz	22	5.44	5.04	1
Babyfood, dessert, dutch apple, strained	28.35	1 oz	21	5.6	5.2	0
Babyfood, dessert, fruit dessert, without ascorbic acid, junior	15	1 tbsp	9	2.58	2.48	0
Babyfood, dessert, fruit dessert, without ascorbic acid, strained	15	1 tbsp	9	2.4	2.3	0
Babyfood, dessert, fruit pudding, orange, strained	28.35	1 oz	23	5.02	4.82	6

Food Name ---> per serving	Weight (g)	Measure	Calories	Total Carb (g)	Net Carb (g)	Sodium (mg)
Babyfood, dessert, fruit pudding, pineapple, strained	15	1 tbsp	12	34	2.94	0
Babyfood, dessert, peach cobbler, junior	15	1 tbsp	10	2.75	2.65	0
Babyfood, dessert, peach cobbler, strained	15	1 tbsp	10	2.67	2.57	1
Babyfood, dessert, peach melba, junior	28.35	1 oz	17	4.65	4.65	3
Babyfood, dessert, peach melba, strained	28.35	1 oz	17	4.68	4.68	3
Babyfood, dessert, peach yogurt	15	1 tbsp	12	2.64	2.54	2
Babyfood, dessert, tropical fruit, junior	28.35	1 oz	17	4.65	4.65	2
Babyfood, dinner, apples and chicken, strained	28.35	1 oz	18	38	2.58	3
Babyfood, dinner, beef and rice, toddler	28.35	1 oz	23	2.49	2.49	9
Babyfood, dinner, beef lasagna, toddler	28.35	1 oz	22	2.83	2.83	12
Babyfood, dinner, beef noodle, junior	16	1 tbsp	9	1.17	0.97	4
Babyfood, dinner, beef noodle, strained	16	1 tbsp	10	1.31	1.11	2
Babyfood, dinner, beef with vegetables	113	4 oz	108	7.19	5.19	43
Babyfood, dinner, broccoli and chicken, junior	29	1 tbsp	18	1.84	1.44	5
Babyfood, dinner, chicken and rice	16	1 tbsp	8	1.47	1.27	4
Babyfood, dinner, chicken noodle, junior	16	1 tbsp	12	1.25	0.95	4
Babyfood, dinner, chicken noodle, strained	16	1 tbsp	12	1.25	0.95	4
Babyfood, dinner, chicken soup, strained	113	1 jar	56	8.14	6.94	18
Babyfood, dinner, chicken stew, toddler	16	1 tbsp	12	12	0.92	4
Babyfood, dinner, macaroni and cheese, junior	28.35	1 oz	17	2.32	2.22	52
Babyfood, dinner, macaroni and cheese, strained	28.35	1 oz	19	2.54	2.34	25
Babyfood, dinner, macaroni and tomato and beef, junior	16	1 tbsp	9	1.5	1.3	6
Babyfood, dinner, macaroni and tomato and beef, strained	16	1 tbsp	10	1.51	1.31	6
Babyfood, dinner, macaroni, beef and tomato sauce, toddler	16	1 tbsp	13	1.84	1.64	6
Babyfood, dinner, mixed vegetable, junior	99	1 serv	34	7.8	6.8	40
Babyfood, dinner, mixed vegetable, strained	28.35	1 oz	12	2.69	2.69	11
Babyfood, dinner, pasta with vegetables	113	1 jar, (4 oz)	68	9.49	7.79	12
Babyfood, dinner, spaghetti and tomato and meat, junior	16	1 tbsp	11	1.83	1.63	5
Babyfood, dinner, spaghetti and tomato and meat, toddler	28.35	1 oz	21	36	36	68
Babyfood, dinner, sweet potatoes and chicken, strained	16	1 tbsp	12	1.77	1.57	4
Babyfood, dinner, turkey and rice, junior	16	1 tbsp	9	1.53	1.33	4
Babyfood, dinner, turkey and rice, strained	16	1 tbsp	8	1.27	1.17	3
Babyfood, dinner, turkey, rice, and vegetables, toddler	28.35	1 oz	17	2.13	1.93	50
Babyfood, dinner, vegetables and beef, junior	256	1 cup	197	22.63	19.33	79
Babyfood, dinner, vegetables and beef, strained	256	1 cup	197	22.63	19.33	79

Food Name ---> per serving	Weight (g)	Measure	Calories	Total Carb (g)	Net Carb (g)	Sodium (mg)
Babyfood, dinner, vegetables and chicken, junior	256	1 cup	136	22.17	19.37	87
Babyfood, dinner, vegetables and dumplings and beef, junior	28.35	1 oz	14	2.27	2.27	15
Babyfood, dinner, vegetables and dumplings and beef, strained	28.35	1 oz	14	2.18	2.18	14
Babyfood, dinner, vegetables and lamb, junior	28.35	1 oz	14	2.01	1.71	4
Babyfood, dinner, vegetables and noodles and turkey, junior	28.35	1 oz	15	2.15	1.85	5
Babyfood, dinner, vegetables and noodles and turkey, strained	28.35	1 oz	12	1.93	1.63	6
Babyfood, dinner, vegetables and turkey, junior	256	1 cup	136	19.33	17.03	115
Babyfood, dinner, vegetables and turkey, strained	256	1 cup	123	19.51	15.71	51
Babyfood, dinner, vegetables chicken, strained	256	1 cup	151	21.56	16.16	61
Babyfood, dinner, vegetables, noodles and chicken, junior	28.35	1 oz	18	2.58	2.28	7
Babyfood, dinner, vegetables, noodles and chicken, strained	28.35	1 oz	18	2.24	1.94	6
Babyfood, fortified cereal bar, fruit filling	19	1 bar	65	134	12.74	30
Babyfood, fruit and vegetable, apple and sweet potato	113	1 jar, (4 oz)	72	17.29	15.69	3
Babyfood, fruit dessert, mango with tapioca	15	1 tbsp	10	2.85	2.65	1
Babyfood, fruit supreme dessert	15	1 tbsp	11	2.58	2.28	0
Babyfood, fruit, apple and blueberry, junior	28.35	1 oz	18	4.71	4.21	0
Babyfood, fruit, apple and blueberry, strained	28.35	1 oz	17	4.62	4.12	0
Babyfood, fruit, apple and raspberry, junior	28.35	1 oz	16	4.37	3.77	0
Babyfood, fruit, apple and raspberry, strained	28.35	1 oz	16	4.42	3.82	0
Babyfood, fruit, applesauce and apricots, junior	16	1 tbsp	8	1.98	1.68	0
Babyfood, fruit, applesauce and apricots, strained	16	1 tbsp	7	1.86	1.56	0
Babyfood, fruit, applesauce and cherries, junior	28.35	1 oz	14	4	3.7	0
Babyfood, fruit, applesauce and cherries, strained	28.35	1 oz	14	4	3.7	0
Babyfood, fruit, applesauce and pineapple, junior	28.35	1 oz	11	2.98	2.58	1
Babyfood, fruit, applesauce and pineapple, strained	28.35	1 oz	10	2.86	2.46	1
Babyfood, fruit, applesauce with banana, junior	16	1 tbsp	11	2.59	2.29	0
Babyfood, fruit, applesauce, junior	16	1 tbsp	6	1.65	1.35	0
Babyfood, fruit, applesauce, strained	16	1 tbsp	7	1.73	1.43	0
Babyfood, fruit, apricot with tapioca, junior	15	1 tbsp	9	2.6	2.4	0
Babyfood, fruit, apricot with tapioca, strained	15	1 tbsp	9	2.44	2.24	0

Food Name ---> per serving	Weight (g)	Measure	Calories	Total Carb (g)	Net Carb (g)	Sodium (mg)
Babyfood, fruit, banana and strawberry, junior	140	1 bottle	153	36.09	34.09	1
Babyfood, fruit, bananas and pineapple with tapioca, junior	15	1 tbsp	10	2.76	2.56	0
Babyfood, fruit, bananas and pineapple with tapioca, strained	15	1 tbsp	10	2.67	2.47	0
Babyfood, fruit, bananas with apples and pears, strained	15	1 tbsp	12	2.9	2.7	0
Babyfood, fruit, bananas with tapioca, junior	15	1 tbsp	10	2.67	2.47	0
Babyfood, fruit, bananas with tapioca, strained	15	1 tbsp	8	2.29	2.09	0
Babyfood, fruit, guava and papaya with tapioca, strained	28.35	1 oz	18	4.82	4.82	1
Babyfood, fruit, papaya and applesauce with tapioca, strained	28.35	1 oz	20	5.36	4.96	1
Babyfood, fruit, peaches, junior	17	1 tbsp	11	2.46	2.26	1
Babyfood, fruit, peaches, strained	17	1 tbsp	11	2.46	2.26	1
Babyfood, fruit, pears and pineapple, junior	16	1 tbsp	7	1.82	1.42	0
Babyfood, fruit, pears and pineapple, strained	16	1 tbsp	7	1.74	1.34	0
Babyfood, fruit, pears, junior	16	1 tbsp	7	1.86	1.46	0
Babyfood, fruit, pears, strained	16	1 tbsp	7	1.73	1.33	0
Babyfood, fruit, plums with tapioca, without ascorbic acid, junior	15	1 tbsp	11	38	2.88	0
Babyfood, fruit, plums with tapioca, without ascorbic acid, strained	15	1 tbsp	11	2.96	2.76	0
Babyfood, fruit, prunes with tapioca, without ascorbic acid, junior	28.35	1 oz	20	5.3	4.5	1
Babyfood, fruit, prunes with tapioca, without ascorbic acid, strained	15	1 tbsp	10	2.77	2.37	1
Babyfood, fruit, tutti frutti, junior	15	1 tbsp	10	2.4	2.3	3
Babyfood, fruit, tutti frutti, strained	15	1 tbsp	10	2.32	2.22	4
Babyfood, GERBER, 2nd Foods, apple, carrot and squash, organic	99	1 serv	63	14.67	13.47	20
Babyfood, GERBER, 3rd Foods, apple, mango and kiwi	170	1 serv	82	21.9	18.5	3
Babyfood, GERBER, Banana with orange medley	113	1 jar	78	236	20.66	11
Babyfood, GERBER, GRADUATES Lil Biscuits Vanilla Wheat	28.35	1 oz	115	20.55	18.85	73
Babyfood, grape juice, no sugar, canned	118	4.0 fl oz	73	18.15	18.15	12
Babyfood, green beans and turkey, strained	14	1 tbsp	7	0.75	0.55	2
Babyfood, green beans, dices, toddler	28.35	1 oz	8	1.62	1.22	10
Babyfood, juice treats, fruit medley, toddler	28	1 packet	97	24.27	24.27	25
Babyfood, juice, apple	31.7	1 fl oz	15	3.71	3.71	3
Babyfood, juice, apple - cherry	31.2	1 fl oz	15	3.49	3.39	1
Babyfood, juice, apple and grape	31.2	1 fl oz	14	3.54	3.54	0
Babyfood, juice, apple and peach	31.2	1 fl oz	13	3.28	3.28	0
Babyfood, juice, apple and prune	31.2	1 fl oz	22	5.65	5.65	2
Babyfood, juice, apple-sweet potato	30.8	1 fl oz	87	3.51	3.31	6
Babyfood, juice, apple, with calcium	189	1 serv	14	20.98	20.18	2

Food Name ---> per serving	Weight (g)	Measure	Calories	Total Carb (g)	Net Carb (g)	Sodium (mg)
Babyfood, juice, fruit punch, with calcium	31.2	1 fl oz	16	3.96	3.86	1
Babyfood, juice, mixed fruit	31.2	1 fl oz	15	3.65	3.65	2
Babyfood, juice, orange	31.2	1 fl oz	14	3.18	3.18	0
Babyfood, juice, orange and apple	31.2	1 fl oz	13	3.15	3.15	1
Babyfood, juice, orange and apple and banana	31.2	1 fl oz	15	3.59	3.59	0
Babyfood, juice, orange and apricot	31.2	1 fl oz	14	3.4	3.4	2
Babyfood, juice, orange and banana	31.2	1 fl oz	16	3.71	3.71	1
Babyfood, juice, orange and pineapple	31.2	1 fl oz	15	3.65	3.65	1
Babyfood, juice, orange-carrot	30.8	1 fl oz	13	35	2.95	3
Babyfood, juice, pear	31.2	1 fl oz	13	3.7	3.7	2
Babyfood, juice, prune and orange	31.2	1 fl oz	22	5.24	5.24	1
Babyfood, macaroni and cheese, toddler	113	1 cont.	93	12.66	12.06	298
Babyfood, mashed cheddar potatoes and broccoli, toddlers	170	1 cont.	82	12.7	10.7	299
Babyfood, meat, beef with vegetables, toddler	179	1 jar	124	15.61	12.41	47
Babyfood, meat, beef, junior	28.35	1 oz	23	0.69	0.69	12
Babyfood, meat, beef, strained	14.7	1 tbsp	12	0.36	0.36	6
Babyfood, meat, chicken sticks, junior	10	1 stick	19	0.15	0.15	27
Babyfood, meat, chicken, junior	15	1 tbsp	22	0	0	7
Babyfood, meat, chicken, strained	15	1 tbsp	20	0.01	0.01	7
Babyfood, meat, ham, junior	28.35	1 oz	27	15	15	12
Babyfood, meat, ham, strained	15	1 tbsp	15	0.56	0.56	7
Babyfood, meat, lamb, junior	28.35	1 oz	32	0	0	12
Babyfood, meat, lamb, strained	22	1 tbsp	21	0.19	0.19	9
Babyfood, meat, meat sticks, junior	10	1 stick	18	0.11	0.11	27
Babyfood, meat, pork, strained	28.35	1 oz	35	0	0	12
Babyfood, meat, turkey sticks, junior	10	1 stick	19	0.14	0.14	30
Babyfood, meat, turkey, junior	19	1 tbsp	21	0.27	0.27	9
Babyfood, meat, turkey, strained	15	1 tbsp	17	0.21	0.21	7
Babyfood, meat, veal, strained	16	1 tbsp	13	0.24	0.24	6
Babyfood, mixed fruit juice with low fat yogurt	31.5	1 fl oz	23	4.62	4.52	11
Babyfood, mixed fruit yogurt, strained	15	1 tbsp	11	2.43	2.33	2
Babyfood, Multigrain whole grain cereal, dry fortified	16	3 tbsp	65	12.81	11.71	5
Babyfood, oatmeal cereal with fruit, dry, instant, toddler fortified	5.3	1 tbsp	21	3.93	3.53	0
Babyfood, peaches, dices, toddler	28.35	1 oz	14	3.35	3.15	3
Babyfood, pears, dices, toddler	28.35	1 oz	16	3.86	3.56	2
Babyfood, peas and brown rice	230	1 cup	147	26.43	20.63	14
Babyfood, peas, dices, toddler	28.35	1 oz	18	2.92	1.82	14
Babyfood, plums, bananas and rice, strained	28.35	1 oz	16	3.6	3.2	0
Babyfood, potatoes, toddler	163	1 cup	85	19.12	17.62	93
Babyfood, pretzels	28.35	1 oz	113	23.3	22.6	76
Babyfood, prunes, without vitamin c, strained	15	1 tbsp	15	3.53	3.13	0
Babyfood, ravioli, cheese filled, with tomato sauce	16	1 tbsp	16	2.61	2.61	45
Babyfood, rice and apples, dry	2.5	1 tbsp	10	2.17	2.07	0

Food Name ---> per serving	Weight (g)	Measure	Calories	Total Carb (g)	Net Carb (g)	Sodium (mg)
Babyfood, rice cereal, dry, EARTHS BEST ORGANIC WHOLE GRAIN, fortified only with iron	18	4.0 tbsp	69	14.05	13.95	1
Babyfood, snack, GERBER GRADUATE FRUIT STRIPS, Real Fruit Bars	9.9	1 bar	33	7.58	7.38	1
Babyfood, Snack, GERBER, GRADUATES, LIL CRUNCHIES, baked whole grain corn snack	7	18.0 piece	35	4.31	4.31	35
Babyfood, snack, GERBER, GRADUATES, YOGURT MELTS	7	1 serv	27	5.03	4.83	20
Babyfood, tropical fruit medley	88	1 serv	40	10.75	9.65	0
Babyfood, vegetable and brown rice, strained	230	1 cup	159	27.83	25.33	32
Babyfood, vegetable, butternut squash and corn	113	4 oz	56	10.46	8.16	6
Babyfood, vegetable, green beans and potatoes	113	4 oz	70	10.17	8.57	20
Babyfood, vegetables, beets, strained	224	1 cup	76	17.25	12.95	186
Babyfood, vegetables, carrots, junior	224	1 cup	72	16.13	12.33	110
Babyfood, vegetables, carrots, strained	224	1 cup	58	13.44	9.64	155
Babyfood, vegetables, corn, creamed, junior	240	1 cup	156	39	34	125
Babyfood, vegetables, corn, creamed, strained	113	1 jar	64	15.93	13.53	49
Babyfood, vegetables, garden vegetable, strained	28.35	1 oz	9	1.93	1.53	9
Babyfood, vegetables, green beans, junior	240	1 cup	58	13.92	9.32	12
Babyfood, vegetables, green beans, strained	240	1 cup	65	15.1	9.8	17
Babyfood, vegetables, mix vegetables junior	99	3.5 oz serv	36	8.12	6.62	--
Babyfood, vegetables, mix vegetables strained	28.35	1 oz	10	2.34	1.94	0
Babyfood, vegetables, peas, strained	16	1 tbsp	8	1.34	14	1
Babyfood, vegetables, spinach, creamed, strained	240	1 cup	89	13.68	9.38	118
Babyfood, vegetables, squash, junior	16	1 tbsp	4	0.92	0.82	1
Babyfood, vegetables, squash, strained	16	1 tbsp	4	0.92	0.82	1
Babyfood, vegetables, sweet potatoes strained	224	1 cup	128	29.57	26.17	49
Babyfood, vegetables, sweet potatoes, junior	224	1 cup	134	31.36	27.96	40
Babyfood, water, bottled, GERBER, without added fluoride	113	1 serv	0	0	0	--
Babyfood, yogurt, whole milk, with fruit, multigrain cereal and added DHA fortified	31	1 oz	30	4.1	4	13
Babyfood, yogurt, whole milk, with fruit, multigrain cereal and added iron fortified	16	1 tbsp	15	2.08	1.98	6
Child formula, ABBOTT NUTRITION, PEDIASURE, ready-to-feed	31	1 fl oz	31	3.46	3.46	11
Child formula, ABBOTT NUTRITION, PEDIASURE, ready-to-feed, with iron and fiber	31	1 fl oz	31	3.5	3.3	11

Food Name ---> per serving	Weight (g)	Measure	Calories	Total Carb (g)	Net Carb (g)	Sodium (mg)
Clif Z bar	36	1 bar	150	26.9	23.9	135
Fluid replacement, electrolyte solution (include PEDIALYTE)	31.2	1 fl oz	3	0.76	0.76	32
Infant formula, ABBOTT NUTRITION, ALIMENTUM ADVANCE, with iron, powder, not reconstituted, with DHA and ARA	8.7	1 scoop	45	4.52	4.52	19
Infant formula, ABBOTT NUTRITION, SIMILAC NEOSURE, ready-to-feed, with ARA and DHA	30.5	1 fl oz	21	2.12	2.12	7
Infant formula, ABBOTT NUTRITION, SIMILAC, ADVANCE, with iron, liquid concentrate, not reconstituted	31.4	1 fl oz	40	4.25	4.25	10
Infant formula, ABBOTT NUTRITION, SIMILAC, ADVANCE, with iron, powder, not reconstituted	8.5	1 scoop	44	4.65	4.65	11
Infant formula, ABBOTT NUTRITION, SIMILAC, ADVANCE, with iron, ready-to-feed	30.4	1 fl oz	20	2.06	2.06	5
Infant formula, ABBOTT NUTRITION, SIMILAC, ALIMENTUM, ADVANCE, ready-to-feed, with ARA and DHA	30.5	1 fl oz	20	2.06	2.06	9
Infant formula, ABBOTT NUTRITION, SIMILAC, ALIMENTUM, with iron, ready-to-feed	30.5	1 fl oz	20	2.06	2.06	9
Infant formula, ABBOTT NUTRITION, SIMILAC, Expert Care, Diarrhea, ready-to- feed with ARA and DHA	30.4	1 fl oz	20	2.03	1.83	9
Infant formula, ABBOTT NUTRITION, SIMILAC, For Spit Up, powder, with ARA and DHA	9.5	1 scoop	49	5.22	5.22	15
Infant formula, ABBOTT NUTRITION, SIMILAC, For Spit Up, ready-to-feed, with ARA and DHA	30.4	1 fl oz	20	2.19	2.19	6
Infant formula, ABBOTT NUTRITION, SIMILAC, GO AND GROW, powder, with ARA and DHA	9.6	1 scoop	49	5.01	5.01	15
Infant formula, ABBOTT NUTRITION, SIMILAC, GO AND GROW, ready-to-feed, with ARA and DHA	153	5.0 fl oz	101	10.24	10.24	31
Infant formula, ABBOTT NUTRITION, SIMILAC, ISOMIL, ADVANCE with iron, liquid concentrate	31.4	1 fl oz	40	4.15	4.15	18
Infant formula, ABBOTT NUTRITION, SIMILAC, ISOMIL, ADVANCE with iron, powder, not reconstituted	8.7	1 scoop	45	4.66	4.66	20
Infant formula, ABBOTT NUTRITION, SIMILAC, ISOMIL, ADVANCE with iron, ready-to-feed	30.5	1 fl oz	20	2.04	2.04	9
Infant formula, ABBOTT NUTRITION, SIMILAC, ISOMIL, with iron, liquid concentrate	31.4	1 fl oz	40	4.15	4.15	18
Infant formula, ABBOTT NUTRITION, SIMILAC, ISOMIL, with iron, powder, not reconstituted	8.7	1 scoop	45	4.66	4.66	20

Food Name ---> per serving	Weight (g)	Measure	Calories	Total Carb (g)	Net Carb (g)	Sodium (mg)
Infant formula, ABBOTT NUTRITION, SIMILAC, ISOMIL, with iron, ready-to-feed	30.5	1 fl oz	20	2.04	2.04	9
Infant formula, ABBOTT NUTRITION, SIMILAC, NEOSURE, powder, with ARA and DHA	30.5	1 fl oz	159	15.78	15.78	52
Infant formula, ABBOTT NUTRITION, SIMILAC, PM 60/40, powder not reconstituted	8.7	1 scoop	46	4.78	4.78	11
Infant formula, ABBOTT NUTRITION, SIMILAC, SENSITIVE (LACTOSE FREE) ready-to-feed, with ARA and DHA	30.5	1 fl oz	21	2.26	2.26	6
Infant formula, ABBOTT NUTRITION, SIMILAC, SENSITIVE, (LACTOSE FREE), liquid concentrate, with ARA and DHA	30.5	1 fl oz	39	4.16	4.16	12
Infant formula, ABBOTT NUTRITION, SIMILAC, SENSITIVE, (LACTOSE FREE), powder, with ARA and DHA	30.5	1 fl oz	159	16.98	16.98	48
Infant formula, ABBOTT NUTRITION, SIMILAC, with iron, liquid concentrate, not reconstituted	31.4	1 fl oz	40	4.32	4.32	10
Infant formula, ABBOTT NUTRITION, SIMILAC, with iron, powder, not reconstituted	8.5	1 scoop	44	4.65	4.65	11
Infant Formula, GERBER GOOD START 2, GENTLE PLUS, powder	9.4	1 scoop	46	5.37	5.37	13
Infant Formula, GERBER GOOD START 2, GENTLE PLUS, ready-to-feed	30.4	1 fl oz	20	2.31	2.31	5
Infant formula, GERBER, GOOD START 2 SOY, with iron, powder	9.4	1 scoop	47	5.23	5.23	19
Infant formula, GERBER, GOOD START 2 Soy, with iron, ready-to-feed	30.4	1 fl oz	20	2.17	2.17	8
Infant formula, GERBER, GOOD START 2, PROTECT PLUS, powder	9.4	1 scoop	47	5.29	5.29	13
Infant formula, GERBER, GOOD START 2, PROTECT PLUS, ready-to-feed	30.4	1 fl oz	20	2.25	2.25	5
Infant formula, GERBER, GOOD START, PROTECT PLUS, powder	9.4	1 scoop	48	5.36	5.36	13
Infant formula, GERBER, GOOD START, PROTECT PLUS, ready-to-feed	30.4	1 fl oz	20	2.18	2.18	5
Infant formula, MEAD JOHNSON, Enfamil 24, ready to feed, with ARA and DHA	30.5	1 fl oz	22	2.11	2.11	6
Infant formula, MEAD JOHNSON, Enfamil Enspire Powder, with ARA and DHA, not reconstituted	8.8	1 scoop	45	5.03	5.03	12
Infant formula, MEAD JOHNSON, Enfamil for Supplementing, powder, with ARA and DHA, not reconstituted	8.7	1 serv	45	4.85	4.85	16
Infant formula, MEAD JOHNSON, Enfamil for Supplementing, ready to feed, with ARA and DHA	103	100.0 ml	70	7.83	7.83	25

Food Name ---> per serving	Weight (g)	Measure	Calories	Total Carb (g)	Net Carb (g)	Sodium (mg)
Infant Formula, MEAD JOHNSON, ENFAMIL GENTLEASE, with iron, prepared from powder	30.5	1 fl oz	21	2.32	2.32	7
Infant formula, MEAD JOHNSON, ENFAMIL LIPIL, with iron, ready-to-feed, with ARA and DHA	106	100 ml	68	7.53	7.53	19
Infant formula, MEAD JOHNSON, Enfamil Premature 30 Calories, ready to feed, with ARA and DHA	30.5	1 fl oz	31	3.39	3.39	21
Infant formula, MEAD JOHNSON, Enfamil Premature High Protein 24 Calories, ready to feed, with ARA and DHA	30.4	1 fl oz	25	2.63	2.63	17
Infant formula, MEAD JOHNSON, Enfamil Reguline Powder, with ARA and DHA, not reconstituted	8.7	1 scoop	45	4.86	4.86	16
Infant formula, MEAD JOHNSON, Enfamil Reguline, ready to feed, with ARA and DHA	30.5	1 fl oz	21	2.32	2.32	7
Infant formula, MEAD JOHNSON, ENFAMIL, AR, powder, with ARA and DHA	9	1 scoop	45	5.17	5.17	18
Infant formula, MEAD JOHNSON, ENFAMIL, AR, ready-to-feed, with ARA and DHA	106	100 ml	75	9.25	8.85	28
Infant Formula, MEAD JOHNSON, ENFAMIL, ENFACARE, ready-to-feed, with ARA and DHA	30.8	1 fl oz	22	2.38	2.38	8
Infant formula, MEAD JOHNSON, ENFAMIL, ENFACARE, with iron, powder, with ARA and DHA	9.9	1 scoop	50	5.33	5.33	18
Infant formula, MEAD JOHNSON, ENFAMIL, ENFAGROW, GENTLEASE, Toddler transitions, with ARA and DHA, powder	9	1 scoop	45	4.82	4.82	18
Infant formula, MEAD JOHNSON, ENFAMIL, Enfagrow, Soy, Toddler ready-to-feed	30.4	1 fl oz	20	2.32	2.32	7
Infant formula, MEAD JOHNSON, ENFAMIL, ENFAGROW, Soy, Toddler transitions, with ARA and DHA, powder	9.4	1 scoop	45	5.26	5.26	16
Infant Formula, MEAD JOHNSON, ENFAMIL, GENTLEASE, with ARA and DHA powder not reconstituted	8.7	1 scoop	45	4.92	4.92	16
Infant formula, MEAD JOHNSON, ENFAMIL, Infant, ready-to-feed, with ARA and DHA	106	100 ml	72	8.33	8.33	19
Infant formula, MEAD JOHNSON, ENFAMIL, Infant, with iron, liquid concentrate, with ARA and DHA, reconstituted	31.3	1 fl oz	21	2.46	2.46	6
Infant formula, MEAD JOHNSON, ENFAMIL, Infant, with iron, powder, with ARA and DHA	8.8	1 scope	45	4.95	4.95	12

Food Name ---> per serving	Weight (g)	Measure	Calories	Total Carb (g)	Net Carb (g)	Sodium (mg)
Infant formula, MEAD JOHNSON, ENFAMIL, LIPIL, low iron, liquid concentrate, with ARA and DHA	31.3	1 fl oz	41	4.46	4.46	12
Infant formula, MEAD JOHNSON, ENFAMIL, LIPIL, low iron, ready to feed, with ARA and DHA	106	100 ml	68	7.61	7.61	19
Infant Formula, MEAD JOHNSON, ENFAMIL, Newborn, with ARA and DHA, powder	8.7	1 scoop	45	5.01	5.01	12
Infant Formula, MEAD JOHNSON, ENFAMIL, Newborn, with DHA and ARA, ready-to-feed	30.5	1 fl oz	21	2.38	2.38	5
Infant formula, MEAD JOHNSON, ENFAMIL, NUTRAMIGEN AA, ready-to-feed	30.4	1 fl oz	20	2.06	2.06	9
Infant formula, MEAD JOHNSON, ENFAMIL, NUTRAMIGEN WITH LGG, with iron, powder, not reconstituted, with ARA and DHA	9	1 scoop	46	4.82	4.82	22
Infant formula, MEAD JOHNSON, ENFAMIL, NUTRAMIGEN, PurAmino, powder, not reconstituted	9.4	1 scoop	48	5.23	5.23	22
Infant Formula, MEAD JOHNSON, ENFAMIL, NUTRAMIGEN, with iron, liquid concentrate not reconstituted, with ARA and DHA	31.6	1 fl oz	21	2.28	2.28	10
Infant formula, MEAD JOHNSON, ENFAMIL, NUTRAMIGEN, with iron, ready-to-feed, with ARA and DHA	107	100 ml	73	7.71	7.71	33
Infant formula, MEAD JOHNSON, ENFAMIL, Premature, 20 calories ready-to-feed Low iron	30.4	1 fl oz	20	2.19	2.19	12
Infant formula, MEAD JOHNSON, ENFAMIL, Premature, 24 calories ready-to-feed Low iron	30	5.0 fl oz	20	2.16	2.16	11
Infant formula, MEAD JOHNSON, ENFAMIL, Premature, with iron, 20 calories, ready-to-feed	30.4	1 fl oz	19	1.88	1.88	14
Infant formula, MEAD JOHNSON, ENFAMIL, Premature, with iron, 24 calories, ready-to-feed	30.4	1 fl oz	25	2.7	2.7	17
Infant Formula, MEAD JOHNSON, ENFAMIL, Premium LIPIL, Infant, Liquid concentrate, not reconstituted	31.4	1 fl oz	41	4.53	4.53	11
Infant Formula, MEAD JOHNSON, ENFAMIL, Premium LIPIL, Infant, powder	8.7	1 scoop	44	4.96	4.96	12
Infant Formula, MEAD JOHNSON, ENFAMIL, Premium, Infant, Liquid concentrate, not reconstituted	31.4	1 fl oz	41	4.5	4.5	11
Infant Formula, MEAD JOHNSON, ENFAMIL, Premium, Infant, powder	8.7	1 scoop	44	4.96	4.96	12
Infant Formula, MEAD JOHNSON, ENFAMIL, Premium, Infant, ready-to-feed	30.5	1 fl oz	20	2.25	2.25	5

Food Name ---> per serving	Weight (g)	Measure	Calories	Total Carb (g)	Net Carb (g)	Sodium (mg)
Infant formula, MEAD JOHNSON, ENFAMIL, PROSOBEE, liquid concentrate, reconstituted, with ARA and DHA	31.3	1 fl oz	21	2.37	2.37	7
Infant formula, MEAD JOHNSON, ENFAMIL, PROSOBEE, with iron, powder, not reconstituted, with ARA and DHA	8.8	1 scoop	45	4.8	4.8	16
Infant formula, MEAD JOHNSON, ENFAMIL, with iron, powder	8.3	1 scoop	43	4.66	4.66	12
Infant formula, MEAD JOHNSON, Gentlease, ready to feed, with ARA and DHA	30	1 fl oz	20	2.28	2.28	--
Infant formula, MEAD JOHNSON, NEXT STEP PROSOBEE, powder, not reconstituted	9.3	1 scoop	45	5.31	5.31	16
Infant formula, MEAD JOHNSON, NEXT STEP, PROSOBEE LIPIL, powder, with ARA and DHA	28	3 scoop	134	15.99	15.99	48
Infant formula, MEAD JOHNSON, NEXT STEP, PROSOBEE, LIPIL, ready to feed, with ARA and DHA	103	100 ml	69	8.33	8.33	24
Infant formula, MEAD JOHNSON, Pregestimil 20 Calories, ready to feed, with ARA and DHA	1	100.0 ml	1	0.07	0.07	0
Infant formula, MEAD JOHNSON, Pregestimil 24 Calories, ready to feed, with ARA and DHA	104	100.0 ml	75	6.19	6.19	38
Infant formula, MEAD JOHNSON, PREGESTIMIL, with iron, powder, with ARA and DHA, not reconstituted	8.8	1 scoop	45	4.59	4.59	21
Infant formula, MEAD JOHNSON, PREGESTIMIL, with iron, with ARA and DHA, prepared from powder	104	1 serv 100 ml	70	6.8	6.8	32
Infant formula, MEAD JOHNSON, PROSOBEE, with iron, ready to feed, with ARA and DHA	106	1 serv 100 ml	68	6.86	6.86	25
Infant formula, MEAD JOHNSON, PROSOBEE, with iron, ready-to-feed	106	1 Serv 100 ml	67	6.48	6.48	24
Infant formula, MEAD JOHNSON,NEXT STEP PROSOBEE, prepared from powder	30.5	1 fl oz	20	2.46	2.46	7
Infant formula, NESTLE, GOOD START ESSENTIALS SOY, with iron, powder	8.5	1 scoop	43	4.73	4.73	15
Infant formula, NESTLE, GOOD START SOY, with ARA and DHA, powder	9.4	1 scoop	47	5.23	5.23	19
Infant formula, NESTLE, GOOD START SOY, with DHA and ARA, liquid concentrate	29.2	1 fl oz	39	4.3	4.3	15
Infant formula, NESTLE, GOOD START SOY, with DHA and ARA, ready-to-feed	29	1 oz	19	2.07	2.07	8

Food Name ---> per serving	Weight (g)	Measure	Calories	Total Carb (g)	Net Carb (g)	Sodium (mg)
Infant formula, NESTLE, GOOD START SUPREME, with iron, DHA and ARA, prepared from liquid concentrate	31.4	1 fl oz	21	2.32	2.32	6
Infant formula, NESTLE, GOOD START SUPREME, with iron, DHA and ARA, ready-to-feed	30.5	1 fl oz	20	2.25	2.25	5
Infant formula, NESTLE, GOOD START SUPREME, with iron, liquid concentrate, not reconstituted	31.4	1 fl oz	40	4.46	4.46	11
Infant formula, NESTLE, GOOD START SUPREME, with iron, powder	8.7	1 scoop	44	4.99	4.99	12
Infant formula, PBM PRODUCTS, store brand, liquid concentrate, not reconstituted	31.4	1 fl oz	41	4.36	4.36	9
Infant formula, PBM PRODUCTS, store brand, powder	8.4	1 scoop	44	4.7	4.7	10
Infant formula, PBM PRODUCTS, store brand, ready-to-feed	30.4	1 fl oz	19	1.94	1.94	4
Infant formula, PBM PRODUCTS, store brand, soy, liquid concentrate, not reconstituted	31.4	1 fl oz	40	3.82	3.82	11
Infant formula, PBM PRODUCTS, store brand, soy, powder	8.7	1 scoop	44	4.54	4.54	13
Infant formula, PBM PRODUCTS, store brand, soy, ready-to-feed	30.4	1 fl oz	19	1.85	1.85	5
Toddler drink, MEAD JOHNSON, PurAmino Toddler Powder, with ARA and DHA, not reconstituted	7.2	1 scoop	37	4.01	4.01	17
Toddler formula, MEAD JOHNSON, ENFAGROW PREMIUM (formerly ENFAMIL, LIPIL, NEXT STEP), ready-to-feed	29.2	1 fl oz	19	2.1	2.1	7
Toddler formula, MEAD JOHNSON, ENFAGROW, Toddler Transitions, with ARA and DHA, powder	9	1 scoop	45	4.75	4.75	16
Toddler formula, MEAD JOHNSON, Nutramigen Toddler with LGG Powder, with ARA and DHA, not reconstituted	9.3	1 scoop	45	5.76	5.76	17
Zwieback	28.35	1 oz	121	214	20.34	64

Beef and Beef Products

Food Name ---> per 100 g	Protein (g)	Fat (g)	Carb (g)	Calories	Fiber (g)	Sodium (mg)	Cholesterol (mg)	Net Carb (g)
Beef, grass-fed, strip steaks, lean only, raw	23.07	2.69	0	117	0	55	55	0
Beef, carcass, separable lean and fat, choice, raw	17.32	24.05	0	291	0	59	74	0
Beef, carcass, separable lean and fat, select, raw	17.48	22.55	0	278	0	59	74	0
Beef, retail cuts, separable fat, raw	8.21	70.89	0	674	0	26	99	0
Beef, retail cuts, separable fat, cooked	10.65	70.33	0	680	0	23	95	0
Beef, brisket, whole, separable lean only, all grades, raw	20.72	7.37	0	155	0	79	62	0
Beef, grass-fed, ground, raw	19.42	12.73	0	198	0	68	62	0
Beef, brisket, flat half, separable lean and fat, trimmed to 1/8" fat, select, cooked, braised	28.97	17.37	0	280	0	49	107	0
Beef, flank, steak, separable lean and fat, trimmed to 0" fat, choice, raw	21.22	8.29	0	165	0	54	68	0
Beef, flank, steak, separable lean and fat, trimmed to 0" fat, choice, cooked, braised	26.98	16.44	0	263	0	70	72	0
Beef, flank, steak, separable lean and fat, trimmed to 0" fat, choice, cooked, broiled	27.55	9.31	0	202	0	53	81	0
Beef, flank, steak, separable lean only, trimmed to 0" fat, choice, raw	21.72	6.29	0	149	0	57	69	0
Beef, flank, steak, separable lean only, trimmed to 0" fat, choice, cooked, braised	28.02	13	0	237	0	72	71	0
Beef, flank, steak, separable lean only, trimmed to 0" fat, choice, cooked, broiled	27.82	8.32	0	194	0	56	80	0
Beef, rib, eye, small end (ribs 10-12), separable lean and fat, trimmed to 0" fat, choice, raw	17.51	22.07	0	274	0	56	68	0
Beef, rib, eye, small end (ribs 10-12), separable lean and fat, trimmed to 0" fat, choice, cooked, broiled	26.58	16.76	0	265	0	53	88	0
Beef, rib, eye, small end (ribs 10-12), separable lean only, trimmed to 0" fat, choice, raw	20.13	8.3	0	161	0	63	59	0
Beef, rib, eye, small end (ribs 10-12), separable lean only, trimmed to 0" fat, choice, cooked, broiled	28.88	9.01	0	205	0	60	90	0
Beef, rib, shortribs, separable lean and fat, choice, raw	14.4	36.23	0	388	0	49	76	0
Beef, rib, shortribs, separable lean and fat, choice, cooked, braised	21.57	41.98	0	471	0	50	94	0
Beef, rib, shortribs, separable lean only, choice, raw	19.05	10.19	0	173	0	65	59	0
Beef, rib, shortribs, separable lean only, choice, cooked, braised	30.76	18.13	0	295	0	58	93	0
Beef, round, full cut, separable lean only, trimmed to 1/4" fat, choice, cooked, broiled	29.21	7.31	0	191	0	64	78	0
Beef, round, full cut, separable lean only, trimmed to 1/4" fat, select, cooked, broiled	29.25	5.22	0	172	0	64	78	0
Beef, brisket, flat half, separable lean and fat, trimmed to 0" fat, choice, cooked, braised	32.21	9.24	0	221	0	52	92	0
USDA Commodity, beef, canned	20.52	17.57	0	246	0	187	77	0
Beef, shank crosscuts, separable lean only, trimmed to 1/4" fat, choice, raw	21.75	3.85	0	128	0	63	39	0
Beef, shank crosscuts, separable lean only,	33.68	6.36	0	201	0	64	78	0

trimmed to 1/4" fat, choice, cooked, simmered

Food Name ---> per 100 g	Protein (g)	Fat (g)	Carb (g)	Calories	Fiber (g)	Sodium (mg)	Cholesterol (mg)	Net Carb (g)
Beef, short loin, porterhouse steak, separable lean only, trimmed to 1/8" fat, choice, raw	22.13	7.39	0	161	0	56	59	0
Beef, short loin, porterhouse steak, separable lean only, trimmed to 1/8" fat, choice, cooked, grilled	27.65	11.36	0	221	0	67	85	0
Beef, short loin, t-bone steak, bone-in, separable lean only, trimmed to 1/8" fat, choice, raw	22.1	7.27	0	160	0	35	59	0
Beef, short loin, t-bone steak, bone-in, separable lean only, trimmed to 1/8" fat, choice, cooked, grilled	27.48	11.05	0	217	0	68	81	0
Beef, rib eye, small end (ribs 10-12), separable lean only, trimmed to 0" fat, select, raw	21.17	6.57	0	149	0	52	60	0
Beef, chuck, under blade pot roast, boneless, separable lean only, trimmed to 0" fat, all grades, cooked, braised	30.54	10.46	0	216	0	65	104	0
Beef, chuck, under blade pot roast or steak, boneless, separable lean only, trimmed to 0" fat, all grades, raw	21.13	6.07	0.31	140	0	81	66	0.31
Beef, chuck, under blade pot roast or steak, boneless, separable lean only, trimmed to 0" fat, choice, raw	21.19	6.51	0.39	145	0	80	65	0.39
Beef, ground, patties, frozen, cooked, broiled	23.05	21.83	0	295	0	77	84	0
Beef, variety meats and by-products, brain, raw	10.86	10.3	1.05	143	0	126	3010	1.05
Beef, variety meats and by-products, brain, cooked, pan-fried	12.57	15.83	0	196	0	158	1995	0
Beef, variety meats and by-products, brain, cooked, simmered	11.67	10.53	1.48	151	0	108	3100	1.48
Beef, variety meats and by-products, heart, raw	17.72	3.94	0.14	112	0	98	124	0.14
Beef, variety meats and by-products, heart, cooked, simmered	28.48	4.73	0.15	165	0	59	212	0.15
Beef, variety meats and by-products, kidneys, raw	17.4	3.09	0.29	99	0	182	411	0.29
Beef, variety meats and by-products, kidneys, cooked, simmered	27.27	4.65	0	158	0	94	716	0
Beef, variety meats and by-products, liver, raw	20.36	3.63	3.89	135	0	69	275	3.89
Beef, variety meats and by-products, liver, cooked, braised	29.08	5.26	5.13	191	0	79	396	5.13
Beef, variety meats and by-products, liver, cooked, pan-fried	26.52	4.68	5.16	175	0	77	381	5.16
Beef, variety meats and by-products, lungs, raw	16.2	2.5	0	92	0	198	242	0
Beef, variety meats and by-products, lungs, cooked, braised	20.4	3.7	0	120	0	101	277	0
Beef, variety meats and by-products, mechanically separated beef, raw	14.97	23.52	0	276	0	57	209	0
Beef, variety meats and by-products, pancreas, raw	15.7	18.6	0	235	0	67	205	0
Beef, variety meats and by-products, pancreas, cooked, braised	27.1	17.2	0	271	0	60	262	0
Beef, variety meats and by-products, spleen, raw	18.3	3	0	105	0	85	263	0
Beef, variety meats and by-products, spleen, cooked, braised	25.1	4.2	0	145	0	57	347	0
Beef, variety meats and by-products, suet, raw	1.5	94	0	854	0	7	68	0
Beef, variety meats and by-products, thymus, raw	12.18	20.35	0	236	0	96	223	0
Beef, variety meats and by-products, thymus, cooked, braised	21.85	24.98	0	319	0	116	294	0
Beef, variety meats and by-products, tongue, raw	14.9	16.09	3.68	224	0	69	87	3.68

Food Name ---> per 100 g	Protein (g)	Fat (g)	Carb (g)	Calories	Fiber (g)	Sodium (mg)	Cholesterol (mg)	Net Carb (g)
Beef, variety meats and by-products, tongue, cooked, simmered	19.29	22.3	0	284	0	65	132	0
Beef, variety meats and by-products, tripe, raw	12.07	3.69	0	85	0	97	122	0
Beef, sandwich steaks, flaked, chopped, formed and thinly sliced, raw	16.5	27	0	309	0	68	71	0
Beef, brisket, flat half, separable lean only, trimmed to 0" fat, choice, cooked, braised	32.62	8.07	0	212	0	52	99	0
Beef, cured, breakfast strips, raw or unheated	12.5	38.8	0.7	406	0	955	82	0.7
Beef, cured, breakfast strips, cooked	31.3	34.4	1.4	449	0	2253	119	1.4
Beef, cured, corned beef, brisket, raw	14.68	14.9	0.14	198	0	1217	54	0.14
Beef, cured, corned beef, brisket, cooked	18.17	18.98	0.47	251	0	973	98	0.47
Beef, chuck, under blade pot roast or steak, boneless, separable lean only, trimmed to 0" fat, select, raw	21.03	5.41	0.19	134	0	81	66	0.19
Beef, chuck, under blade center steak, boneless, Denver Cut, separable lean only, trimmed to 0" fat, all grades, cooked, grilled	26.5	12.64	0.14	220	0	73	93	0.14
Beef, chuck, under blade center steak, boneless, Denver Cut, separable lean only, trimmed to 0" fat, choice, cooked, grilled	26.49	13.42	0.28	228	0	73	89	0.28
Beef, chuck, under blade center steak, boneless, Denver Cut, separable lean only, trimmed to 0" fat, select, cooked, grilled	26.53	11.46	0	209	0	74	98	0
Beef, chuck, under blade center steak, boneless, Denver Cut, separable lean only, trimmed to 0" fat, all grades, raw	19.42	9.99	0.49	170	0	77	69	0.49
Beef, chuck, under blade center steak, boneless, Denver Cut, separable lean only, trimmed to 0" fat, choice, raw	19.23	10.96	0.67	178	0	76	70	0.67
Beef, composite of trimmed retail cuts, separable lean and fat, trimmed to 0" fat, all grades, cooked	28.4	12.42	0	230	0	62	89	0
Beef, composite of trimmed retail cuts, separable lean and fat, trimmed to 0" fat, choice, cooked	28.17	12.53	0	233	0	62	86	0
Beef, composite of trimmed retail cuts, separable lean and fat, trimmed to 0" fat, select, cooked	28.61	9.18	0	203	0	62	85	0
Beef, composite of trimmed retail cuts, separable lean only, trimmed to 0" fat, all grades, cooked	29.9	8.37	0	203	0	64	90	0
Beef, composite of trimmed retail cuts, separable lean only, trimmed to 0" fat, choice, cooked	29.51	8.87	0	206	0	63	89	0
Beef, composite of trimmed retail cuts, separable lean only, trimmed to 0" fat, select, cooked	29.88	7.12	0	188	0	64	89	0
Beef, brisket, whole, separable lean and fat, trimmed to 0" fat, all grades, cooked, braised	26.79	19.52	0	291	0	65	93	0
Beef, brisket, whole, separable lean only, trimmed to 0" fat, all grades, cooked, braised	29.75	10.08	0	218	0	70	93	0
Beef, brisket, flat half, separable lean and fat, trimmed to 0" fat, all grades, cooked, braised	32.9	8.01	0	213	0	54	92	0
Beef, brisket, flat half, separable lean only, trimmed to 0" fat, all grades, cooked, braised	33.26	6.99	0	205	0	54	100	0
Beef, brisket, point half, separable lean and fat, trimmed to 0" fat, all grades, cooked, braised	23.53	28.5	0	358	0	68	92	0
Beef, brisket, point half, separable lean only, trimmed to 0" fat, all grades, cooked, braised	28.05	13.8	0	244	0	77	91	0
Beef, chuck, arm pot roast, separable lean and fat, trimmed to 0" fat, all grades, cooked, braised	28.94	19.17	0	297	0	47	116	0
Beef, chuck, arm pot roast, separable lean and fat,	29.23	17.56	0	283	0	48	115	0

trimmed to 0" fat, select, cooked, braised

Food Name ---> per 100 g	Protein (g)	Fat (g)	Carb (g)	Calories	Fiber (g)	Sodium (mg)	Cholesterol (mg)	Net Carb (g)
Beef, chuck, arm pot roast, separable lean only, trimmed to 0" fat, choice, cooked, braised	33.36	7.67	0	212	0	54	100	0
Beef, chuck, arm pot roast, separable lean only, trimmed to 0" fat, select, cooked, braised	33.37	5.8	0	195	0	55	98	0
Beef, chuck, blade roast, separable lean and fat, trimmed to 0" fat, all grades, cooked, braised	27.18	24.14	0	334	0	65	104	0
Beef, chuck, under blade pot roast, boneless, separable lean and fat, trimmed to 0" fat, choice, cooked, braised	26.39	21.48	0	306	0	61	100	0
Beef, chuck, under blade pot roast, boneless, separable lean and fat, trimmed to 0" fat, select, cooked, braised	27.17	19.02	0	288	0	64	98	0
Beef, chuck, blade roast, separable lean only, trimmed to 0" fat, all grades, cooked, braised	31.06	13.3	0	253	0	71	106	0
Beef, chuck, under blade pot roast, boneless, separable lean only, trimmed to 0" fat, choice, cooked, braised	30.45	11.14	0	231	0	63	105	0
Beef, chuck, under blade pot roast, boneless, separable lean only, trimmed to 0" fat, select, cooked, braised	30.68	9.44	0	216	0	67	102	0
Beef, rib, large end (ribs 6-9), separable lean and fat, trimmed to 0" fat, choice, cooked, roasted	22.8	30.49	0	372	0	64	85	0
Beef, rib, large end (ribs 6-9), separable lean and fat, trimmed to 0" fat, select, cooked, roasted	23.48	25.54	0	331	0	65	84	0
Beef, rib, large end (ribs 6-9), separable lean only, trimmed to 0" fat, all grades, cooked, roasted	27.53	13.4	0	238	0	73	81	0
Beef, rib, large end (ribs 6-9), separable lean only, trimmed to 0" fat, choice, cooked, roasted	27.53	15	0	253	0	73	81	0
Beef, rib, large end (ribs 6-9), separable lean only, trimmed to 0" fat, select, cooked, roasted	27.53	11.4	0	220	0	73	81	0
Beef, rib, small end (ribs 10-12), separable lean and fat, trimmed to 0" fat, all grades, cooked, broiled	27.27	14.74	0	249	0	56	89	0
Beef, rib, small end (ribs 10-12), separable lean and fat, trimmed to 0" fat, choice, cooked, broiled	24.73	22.84	0	312	0	64	83	0
Beef, rib, small end (ribs 10-12), separable lean and fat, trimmed to 0" fat, select, cooked, broiled	24.91	19.79	0	285	0	64	83	0
Beef, rib, small end (ribs 10-12), separable lean only, trimmed to 0" fat, all grades, cooked, broiled	29.41	7.53	0	193	0	61	91	0
Beef, rib, small end (ribs 10-12), separable lean only, trimmed to 0" fat, choice, cooked, broiled	28.04	11.7	0	225	0	69	80	0
Beef, rib, small end (ribs 10-12), separable lean only, trimmed to 0" fat, select, cooked, broiled	28.04	8.7	0	198	0	69	80	0
Beef, round, bottom round, steak, separable lean and fat, trimmed to 0" fat, all grades, cooked, braised	33.56	8.86	0	223	0	44	95	0
Beef, round, bottom round, roast, separable lean and fat, trimmed to 0" fat, all grades, cooked, roasted	27.42	7.72	0	187	0	36	79	0
Beef, round, bottom round, steak, separable lean and fat, trimmed to 0" fat, choice, cooked, braised	32.73	10	0	230	0	42	96	0
Beef, round, bottom round, roast, separable lean and fat, trimmed to 0" fat, choice, cooked, roasted	26.76	9.37	0	199	0	35	81	0
Beef, round, bottom round, steak, separable lean and fat, trimmed to 0" fat, select, cooked, braised	34.39	7.72	0	217	0	45	93	0

Food Name ---> per 100 g	Protein (g)	Fat (g)	Carb (g)	Calories	Fiber (g)	Sodium (mg)	Cholesterol (mg)	Net Carb (g)
Beef, round, bottom round, roast, separable lean and fat, trimmed to 0" fat, select, cooked, roasted	28.08	6.06	0	175	0	37	77	0
Beef, round, bottom round, steak, separable lean only, trimmed to 0" fat, all grades, cooked, braised	34	7.67	0	214	0	44	93	0
Beef, round, bottom round, roast, separable lean only, trimmed to 0" fat, all grades, cooked, roasted	27.76	6.48	0	177	0	36	77	0
Beef, round, bottom round, steak, separable lean only, trimmed to 0" fat, choice, cooked, braised	33.08	9.03	0	223	0	43	95	0
Beef, round, bottom round, roast, separable lean only, trimmed to 0" fat, choice, cooked, roasted	27.23	7.63	0	185	0	36	78	0
Beef, round, bottom round, steak, separable lean only, trimmed to 0" fat, select, cooked, braised	34.93	6.3	0	206	0	46	91	0
Beef, round, bottom round roast, separable lean only, trimmed to 0" fat, select, cooked, roasted	28.29	5.33	0	169	0	38	76	0
Beef, round, eye of round roast, boneless, separable lean and fat, trimmed to 0" fat, all grades, cooked, roasted	29.66	4.46	0	167	0	67	76	0
Beef, round, eye of round roast, boneless, separable lean and fat, trimmed to 0" fat, choice, cooked, roasted	29.79	4.83	0	171	0	66	74	0
Beef, round, eye of round roast, boneless, separable lean and fat, trimmed to 0" fat, select, cooked, roasted	29.45	3.97	0	162	0	63	79	0
Beef, round, eye of round roast, boneless, separable lean only, trimmed to 0" fat, all grades, cooked, roasted	29.85	3.9	0	163	0	67	76	0
Beef, round, eye of round roast, boneless, separable lean only, trimmed to 0" fat, choice, cooked, roasted	29.94	4.26	0	166	0	66	74	0
Beef, round, eye of round roast, boneless, separable lean only, trimmed to 0" fat, select, cooked, roasted	29.52	3.43	0	157	0	63	79	0
Beef, round, tip round, roast, separable lean and fat, trimmed to 0" fat, all grades, cooked, roasted	26.79	8.21	0	188	0	35	78	0
Beef, round, tip round, roast, separable lean and fat, trimmed to 0" fat, choice, cooked, roasted	27.01	8.9	0	196	0	35	80	0
Beef, round, tip round, roast, separable lean and fat, trimmed to 0" fat, select, cooked, roasted	26.57	7.53	0	181	0	35	76	0
Beef, round, tip round, roast, separable lean only, trimmed to 0" fat, all grades, cooked, roasted	27.53	6.2	0	174	0	36	74	0
Beef, round, tip round, roast, separable lean only, trimmed to 0" fat, choice, cooked, roasted	27.68	6.42	0	176	0	36	76	0
Beef, round, tip round, roast, separable lean only, trimmed to 0" fat, select, cooked, roasted	27.37	4.38	0	149	0	36	71	0
Beef, round, top round, separable lean and fat, trimmed to 0" fat, all grades, cooked, braised	35.62	6.31	0	209	0	45	90	0
Beef, round, top round, separable lean and fat, trimmed to 0" fat, choice, cooked, braised	35.62	7.09	0	216	0	45	90	0
Beef, round, top round, separable lean and fat, trimmed to 0" fat, select, cooked, braised	35.62	5.33	0	200	0	45	90	0
Beef, round, top round, separable lean only, trimmed to 0" fat, choice, cooked, braised	36.12	5.8	0	207	0	45	90	0
Beef, round, top round, separable lean only, trimmed to 0" fat, select, cooked, braised	36.12	4	0	190	0	45	90	0
Beef, loin, tenderloin steak, boneless, separable lean and fat, trimmed to 0" fat, all grades, cooked, grilled	30.5	8.91	0	211	0	57	93	0

Food Name ---> per 100 g	Protein (g)	Fat (g)	Carb (g)	Calories	Fiber (g)	Sodium (mg)	Cholesterol (mg)	Net Carb (g)
Beef, loin, tenderloin steak, boneless, separable lean and fat, trimmed to 0" fat, choice, cooked, grilled	30.21	9.71	0	217	0	58	93	0
Beef, loin, tenderloin steak, boneless, separable lean and fat, trimmed to 0" fat, select, cooked, grilled	30.93	7.7	0	202	0	54	93	0
Beef, loin, tenderloin steak, boneless, separable lean only, trimmed to 0" fat, all grades, cooked, grilled	30.7	8.32	0	198	0	59	93	0
Beef, loin, tenderloin steak, boneless, separable lean only, trimmed to 0" fat, choice, cooked, grilled	30.45	9.03	0	211	0	71	93	0
Beef, loin, tenderloin steak, boneless, separable lean only, trimmed to 0" fat, select, cooked, grilled	31.09	7.25	0	198	0	55	93	0
Beef, loin, top loin steak, boneless, lip off, separable lean and fat, trimmed to 0" fat, all grades, cooked, grilled	28.57	11.15	0	223	0	59	81	0
Beef, loin, top loin steak, boneless, lip off, separable lean and fat, trimmed to 0" fat, choice, cooked, grilled	28.19	12.51	0	233	0	59	88	0
Beef, loin, top loin steak, boneless, lip off, separable lean and fat, trimmed to 0" fat, select, cooked, grilled	29.16	9.12	0	207	0	57	85	0
Beef, loin, top loin steak, boneless, lip off, separable lean only, trimmed to 0" fat, all grades, cooked, grilled	29.53	8.41	0	202	0	61	91	0
Beef, loin, top loin steak, boneless, lip off, separable lean only, trimmed to 0" fat, choice, cooked, grilled	29.22	9.52	0	211	0	59	87	0
Beef, loin, top loin steak, boneless, lip off, separable lean only, trimmed to 0" fat, select, cooked, grilled	29.99	6.74	0	189	0	58	86	0
Beef, top sirloin, steak, separable lean and fat, trimmed to 0" fat, all grades, cooked, broiled	29.33	9.67	0	212	0	61	88	0
Beef, top sirloin, steak, separable lean and fat, trimmed to 0" fat, choice, cooked, broiled	29.02	10.54	0	219	0	58	89	0
Beef, top sirloin, steak, separable lean and fat, trimmed to 0" fat, select, cooked, broiled	29.65	8.8	0	206	0	63	87	0
Beef, top sirloin, steak, separable lean only, trimmed to 0" fat, all grades, cooked, broiled	30.55	5.79	0	183	0	64	82	0
Beef, top sirloin, steak, separable lean only, trimmed to 0" fat, choice, cooked, broiled	30.29	6.55	0	188	0	63	83	0
Beef, top sirloin, steak, separable lean only, trimmed to 0" fat, select, cooked, broiled	30.8	5.03	0	177	0	66	81	0
Beef, short loin, porterhouse steak, separable lean and fat, trimmed to 0" fat, all grades, cooked, broiled	23.96	19.27	0	276	0	65	67	0
Beef, short loin, porterhouse steak, separable lean and fat, trimmed to 0" fat, USDA choice, cooked, broiled	23.61	20.15	0	283	0	65	69	0
Beef, short loin, porterhouse steak, separable lean and fat, trimmed to 0" fat, USDA select, cooked, broiled	24.47	17.98	0	267	0	65	64	0
Beef, short loin, porterhouse steak, separable lean only, trimmed to 1/8" fat, all grades, raw	22.32	6.6	0	155	0	51	58	0
Beef, short loin, porterhouse steak, separable lean only, trimmed to 1/8" fat, all grades, cooked,	28.16	10.32	0	213	0	68	82	0

grilled

Food Name ---> per 100 g	Protein (g)	Fat (g)	Carb (g)	Calories	Fiber (g)	Sodium (mg)	Cholesterol (mg)	Net Carb (g)
Beef, short loin, porterhouse steak, separable lean only, trimmed to 0" fat, all grades, cooked, broiled	26.07	11.18	0	212	0	69	62	0
Beef, short loin, porterhouse steak, separable lean only, trimmed to 0" fat, choice, cooked, broiled	25.51	12.8	0	224	0	69	91	0
Beef, short loin, porterhouse steak, separable lean only, trimmed to 1/8" fat, select, raw	22.61	5.41	0	145	0	43	57	0
Beef, short loin, porterhouse steak, separable lean only, trimmed to 1/8" fat, select, cooked, grilled	28.92	8.76	0	203	0	67	78	0
Beef, short loin, porterhouse steak, separable lean only, trimmed to 0" fat, select, cooked, broiled	26.89	8.81	0	194	0	69	84	0
Beef, short loin, t-bone steak, separable lean and fat, trimmed to 0" fat, all grades, cooked, broiled	24.18	15.93	0	247	0	67	60	0
Beef, short loin, t-bone steak, separable lean and fat, trimmed to 0" fat, USDA choice, cooked, broiled	24.05	17.26	0	258	0	67	61	0
Beef, short loin, t-bone steak, separable lean and fat, trimmed to 0" fat, USDA select, cooked, broiled	24.38	14	0	230	0	68	59	0
Beef, short loin, t-bone steak, bone-in, separable lean only, trimmed to 1/8" fat, all grades, raw	22.22	6.5	0	153	0	42	59	0
Beef, short loin, t-bone steak, bone-in, separable lean only, trimmed to 1/8" fat, all grades, cooked, grilled	27.86	10.37	0	212	0	67	82	0
Beef, short loin, t-bone steak, separable lean only, trimmed to 0" fat, choice, cooked, broiled	25.98	9.61	0	198	0	71	83	0
Beef, short loin, t-bone steak, bone-in, separable lean only, trimmed to 1/8" fat, select, raw	22.41	5.34	0	144	0	57	59	0
Beef, short loin, t-bone steak, bone-in, separable lean only, trimmed to 1/8" fat, select, cooked, grilled	28.45	9.35	0	206	0	66	83	0
Beef, short loin, t-bone steak, separable lean only, trimmed to 0" fat, select, cooked, broiled	26	7.36	0	177	0	71	80	0
Beef, brisket, flat half, separable lean only, trimmed to 0" fat, select, cooked, braised	33.9	5.92	0	198	0	56	102	0
Beef, round, tip round, roast, separable lean and fat, trimmed to 0" fat, all grades, raw	20.48	7.01	0	151	0	55	62	0
Beef, round, tip round, roast, separable lean and fat, trimmed to 0" fat, choice, raw	20.16	7.73	0	156	0	51	63	0
Beef, round, tip round, roast, separable lean and fat, trimmed to 0" fat, select, raw	20.8	6.28	0	145	0	58	61	0
Beef, rib, eye, small end (ribs 10- 12) separable lean only, trimmed to 0" fat, select, cooked, broiled	29.93	6.05	0	182	0	63	95	0
Beef, round, top round steak, boneless, separable lean only, trimmed to 0" fat, all grades, cooked, grilled	30.09	3.77	0	162	0	75	86	0
Beef, round, top round steak, boneless, separable lean only, trimmed to 0" fat, choice, cooked, grilled	30.24	4.11	0	166	0	78	85	0
Beef, round, top round steak, boneless, separable lean only, trimmed to 0" fat, select, cooked, grilled	29.81	3.37	0	158	0	76	88	0
Beef, ground, 70% lean meat / 30% fat, crumbles, cooked, pan-browned	25.56	17.86	0	270	0	96	89	0
Beef, ground, 70% lean meat / 30% fat, loaf, cooked, baked	23.87	15.37	0	241	0	73	88	0

Food Name ---> per 100 g	Protein (g)	Fat (g)	Carb (g)	Calories	Fiber (g)	Sodium (mg)	Cholesterol (mg)	Net Carb (g)
Beef, ground, 70% lean meat / 30% fat, patty cooked, pan-broiled	22.86	15.54	0	238	0	92	84	0
Beef, ground, 70% lean meat / 30% fat, patty, cooked, broiled	25.38	18.66	0	277	0	81	88	0
Beef, ground, 70% lean meat / 30% fat, raw	14.35	30	0	332	0	66	78	0
Beef, chuck, under blade center steak, boneless, Denver Cut, separable lean only, trimmed to 0" fat, select, raw	19.71	8.54	0.21	157	0	77	68	0.21
Beef, shoulder top blade steak, boneless, separable lean only, trimmed to 0" fat, all grades, cooked, grilled	28.15	9.23	0	196	0	87	95	0
Beef, shoulder top blade steak, boneless, separable lean only, trimmed to 0" fat, choice, cooked, grilled	28.28	9.83	0	202	0	85	93	0
Beef, shoulder top blade steak, boneless, separable lean only, trimmed to 0" fat, select, cooked, grilled	27.96	8.34	0	187	0	89	98	0
Beef, shoulder top blade steak, boneless, separable lean only, trimmed to 0" fat, all grades, raw	20.36	6.42	0	139	0	83	69	0
Beef, shoulder top blade steak, boneless, separable lean only, trimmed to 0" fat, choice, raw	20.35	6.88	0	143	0	82	68	0
Beef, shoulder top blade steak, boneless, separable lean only, trimmed to 0" fat, select, raw	20.39	5.73	0	133	0	87	71	0
Beef, brisket, flat half, boneless separable lean only, trimmed to 0" fat, all grades, raw	21.47	5.11	0	132	0	83	67	0
Beef, brisket, flat half, boneless, separable lean only, trimmed to 0" fat, choice, raw	21.28	5.75	0	137	0	82	67	0
Beef, brisket, flat half, boneless, separable lean only, trimmed to 0" fat, select, raw	21.74	4.14	0	124	0	85	69	0
Beef, shoulder top blade steak, boneless, separable lean and fat, trimmed to 0" fat, all grades, cooked, grilled	27.59	11.07	0	210	0	85	95	0
Beef, shoulder pot roast or steak, boneless, separable lean only, trimmed to 0" fat, all grades, raw	21.64	4.09	0	123	0	73	65	0
Beef, shoulder pot roast or steak, boneless, separable lean only, trimmed to 0" fat, choice, raw	21.45	4.35	0.11	125	0	74	64	0.11
Beef, shoulder pot roast or steak, boneless, separable lean only, trimmed to 0" fat, select, raw	21.93	3.7	0	121	0	71	68	0
Beef, shoulder top blade steak, boneless, separable lean and fat, trimmed to 0" fat, choice, cooked, grilled	27.51	12.26	0	220	0	84	92	0
Beef, chuck eye roast, boneless, America's Beef Roast, separable lean and fat, trimmed to 0" fat, all grades, raw	19.18	11.48	0	180	0	81	69	0
Beef, chuck eye roast, boneless, America's Beef Roast, separable lean and fat, trimmed to 0" fat, choice, raw	19.14	12.02	0	185	0	80	67	0
Beef, chuck eye roast, boneless, America's Beef Roast, separable lean and fat, trimmed to 0" fat, select, raw	19.25	10.67	0	173	0	82	73	0
Beef, composite of trimmed retail cuts, separable lean and fat, trimmed to 1/8" fat, all grades, raw	20.01	14.42	0	214	0	52	72	0
Beef, composite of trimmed retail cuts, separable lean and fat, trimmed to 1/8" fat, all grades, cooked	26.11	16.59	0	259	0	50	87	0
Beef, composite of trimmed retail cuts, separable lean and fat, trimmed to 1/8" fat, choice, raw	19.79	15.42	0	222	0	50	72	0

Food Name ---> per 100 g	Protein (g)	Fat (g)	Carb (g)	Calories	Fiber (g)	Sodium (mg)	Cholesterol (mg)	Net Carb (g)
Beef, composite of trimmed retail cuts, separable lean and fat, trimmed to 1/8" fat, choice, cooked	25.85	17.68	0	268	0	49	89	0
Beef, composite of trimmed retail cuts, separable lean and fat, trimmed to 1/8" fat, select, raw	19.06	12.4	0	192	0	51	68	0
Beef, composite of trimmed retail cuts, separable lean and fat, trimmed to 1/8" fat, select, cooked	26.06	15.09	0	245	0	51	85	0
Beef, brisket, whole, separable lean and fat, trimmed to 1/8" fat, all grades, raw	18.42	19.06	0	251	0	69	68	0
Beef, brisket, whole, separable lean and fat, trimmed to 1/8" fat, all grades, cooked, braised	25.85	24.5	0	331	0	64	93	0
Beef, brisket, flat half, separable lean and fat, trimmed to 1/8" fat, all grades, raw	17.94	22.18	0	277	0	59	92	0
Beef, brisket, flat half, separable lean and fat, trimmed to 1/8" fat, all grades, cooked, braised	28.82	18.42	0	289	0	48	106	0
Beef, brisket, point half, separable lean and fat, trimmed to 1/8" fat, all grades, raw	17.65	20.98	0	265	0	72	71	0
Beef, brisket, point half, separable lean and fat, trimmed to 1/8" fat, all grades, cooked, braised	24.4	27.17	0	349	0	69	92	0
Beef, chuck, arm pot roast, separable lean and fat, trimmed to 1/8" fat, all grades, raw	19.23	17.98	0	244	0	62	91	0
Beef, chuck, arm pot roast, separable lean and fat, trimmed to 1/8" fat, all grades, cooked, braised	30.12	19.22	0	302	0	50	120	0
Beef, chuck, arm pot roast, separable lean and fat, trimmed to 1/8" fat, choice, raw	19.14	18.57	0	249	0	63	89	0
Beef, chuck, arm pot roast, separable lean and fat, trimmed to 1/8" fat, choice, cooked, braised	30.2	19.93	0	309	0	49	121	0
Beef, chuck, arm pot roast, separable lean and fat, trimmed to 1/8" fat, select, raw	19.33	17.39	0	239	0	62	93	0
Beef, chuck, arm pot roast, separable lean and fat, trimmed to 1/8" fat, select, cooked, braised	30.05	18.5	0	295	0	50	119	0
Beef, chuck, blade roast, separable lean and fat, trimmed to 1/8" fat, all grades, raw	17.16	19.41	0	248	0	68	71	0
Beef, chuck, blade roast, separable lean and fat, trimmed to 1/8" fat, all grades, cooked, braised	26.78	25.12	0	341	0	65	104	0
Beef, chuck, blade roast, separable lean and fat, trimmed to 1/8" fat, choice, raw	16.98	21.31	0	265	0	67	72	0
Beef, chuck, blade roast, separable lean and fat, trimmed to 1/8" fat, choice, cooked, braised	26.37	27.26	0	359	0	64	103	0
Beef, chuck, blade roast, separable lean and fat, trimmed to 1/8" fat, select, raw	17.37	17.33	0	230	0	69	71	0
Beef, chuck, blade roast, separable lean and fat, trimmed to 1/8" fat, select, cooked, braised	27.33	22.35	0	318	0	66	104	0
Beef, chuck eye roast, boneless, America's Beef Roast, separable lean only, trimmed to 0" fat, all grades, cooked, roasted	26.65	8.46	0	183	0	80	83	0
Beef, chuck eye roast, boneless, America's Beef Roast, separable lean only, trimmed to 0" fat, choice, cooked, roasted	26.41	9.36	0	190	0	79	84	0
Beef, chuck eye roast, boneless, America's Beef Roast, separable lean only, trimmed to 0" fat, select, cooked, roasted	27.02	7.12	0	172	0	81	81	0
Beef, rib, whole (ribs 6-12), separable lean and fat, trimmed to 1/8" fat, all grades, raw	16.53	26.1	0	306	0	55	70	0
Beef, rib, whole (ribs 6-12), separable lean and fat, trimmed to 1/8" fat, all grades, cooked, broiled	22.42	26.75	0	337	0	63	82	0
Beef, rib, whole (ribs 6-12), separable lean and fat, trimmed to 1/8" fat, all grades, cooked, roasted	22.77	28.11	0	351	0	64	84	0

Food Name ---> per 100 g	Protein (g)	Fat (g)	Carb (g)	Calories	Fiber (g)	Sodium (mg)	Cholesterol (mg)	Net Carb (g)
Beef, rib, whole (ribs 6-12), separable lean and fat, trimmed to 1/8" fat, choice, raw	16.34	27.93	0	322	0	54	71	0
Beef, rib, whole (ribs 6-12), separable lean and fat, trimmed to 1/8" fat, choice, cooked, broiled	22.26	28.5	0	352	0	63	82	0
Beef, rib, whole (ribs 6-12), separable lean and fat, trimmed to 1/8" fat, choice, cooked, roasted	22.6	29.79	0	365	0	64	84	0
Beef, rib, whole (ribs 6-12), separable lean and fat, trimmed to 1/8" fat, select, raw	16.75	23.95	0	288	0	55	70	0
Beef, rib, whole (ribs 6-12), separable lean and fat, trimmed to 1/8" fat, select, cooked, broiled	22.73	24.2	0	315	0	64	81	0
Beef, rib, whole (ribs 6-12), separable lean and fat, trimmed to 1/8" fat, select, cooked, roasted	23.1	25.63	0	330	0	65	84	0
Beef, rib, whole (ribs 6-12), separable lean and fat, trimmed to 1/8" fat, prime, raw	16.15	31.66	0	355	0	53	72	0
Beef, rib, whole (ribs 6-12), separable lean and fat, trimmed to 1/8" fat, prime, cooked, broiled	21.95	32.38	0	386	0	62	85	0
Beef, rib, whole (ribs 6-12), separable lean and fat, trimmed to 1/8" fat, prime, cooked, roasted	22.57	33.7	0	400	0	65	85	0
Beef, rib, large end (ribs 6-9), separable lean and fat, trimmed to 1/8" fat, all grades, raw	16.26	27.29	0	316	0	55	71	0
Beef, rib, large end (ribs 6-9), separable lean and fat, trimmed to 1/8" fat, all grades, cooked, broiled	21.55	27.22	0	338	0	64	80	0
Beef, rib, large end (ribs 6-9), separable lean and fat, trimmed to 1/8" fat, all grades, cooked, roasted	23.01	28.51	0	355	0	64	85	0
Beef, rib, large end (ribs 6-9), separable lean and fat, trimmed to 1/8" fat, choice, raw	16.03	29.34	0	333	0	54	72	0
Beef, rib, large end (ribs 6-9), separable lean and fat, trimmed to 1/8" fat, choice, cooked, broiled	20.86	31.18	0	370	0	63	81	0
Beef, rib, large end (ribs 6-9), separable lean and fat, trimmed to 1/8" fat, choice, cooked, roasted	22.5	31.28	0	378	0	63	85	0
Beef, rib, large end (ribs 6-9), separable lean and fat, trimmed to 1/8" fat, select, raw	16.52	24.85	0	295	0	56	70	0
Beef, rib, large end (ribs 6-9), separable lean and fat, trimmed to 1/8" fat, select, cooked, broiled	21.55	25.71	0	324	0	64	80	0
Beef, rib, large end (ribs 6-9), separable lean and fat, trimmed to 1/8" fat, select, cooked, roasted	23.4	25.84	0	333	0	65	84	0
Beef, rib, large end (ribs 6-9), separable lean and fat, trimmed to 1/8" fat, prime, raw	15.77	33.26	0	367	0	53	73	0
Beef, rib, large end (ribs 6-9), separable lean and fat, trimmed to 1/8" fat, prime, cooked, broiled	20.65	34.97	0	404	0	62	86	0
Beef, rib, large end (ribs 6-9), separable lean and fat, trimmed to 1/8" fat, prime, cooked, roasted	22.86	32.74	0	393	0	64	85	0
Beef, rib, small end (ribs 10-12), separable lean and fat, trimmed to 1/8" fat, all grades, raw	19.33	19.06	0	254	0	49	81	0
Beef, rib, small end (ribs 10-12), separable lean and fat, trimmed to 1/8" fat, all grades, cooked, broiled	25.85	20.04	0	291	0	53	97	0
Beef, rib, small end (ribs 10-12), separable lean and fat, trimmed to 1/8" fat, all grades, cooked, roasted	22.54	27.14	0	341	0	63	83	0
Beef, rib, small end (ribs 10-12), separable lean and fat, trimmed to 1/8" fat, choice, raw	19.09	20.13	0	263	0	48	80	0
Beef, rib, small end (ribs 10-12), separable lean and fat, trimmed to 1/8" fat, choice, cooked, broiled	24.53	22.09	0	304	0	49	94	0
Beef, rib, small end (ribs 10-12), separable lean and fat, trimmed to 1/8" fat, choice, cooked,	22.28	29.21	0	359	0	63	83	0

roasted

Food Name ---> per 100 g	Protein (g)	Fat (g)	Carb (g)	Calories	Fiber (g)	Sodium (mg)	Cholesterol (mg)	Net Carb (g)
Beef, rib, small end (ribs 10-12), separable lean and fat, trimmed to 1/8" fat, select, raw	19.56	18	0	246	0	49	85	0
Beef, rib, small end (ribs 10-12), separable lean and fat, trimmed to 1/8" fat, select, cooked, broiled	27.17	18	0	278	0	58	103	0
Beef, rib, small end (ribs 10-12), separable lean and fat, trimmed to 1/8" fat, select, cooked, roasted	22.76	25.02	0	323	0	64	83	0
Beef, rib, small end (ribs 10-12), separable lean and fat, trimmed to 1/8" fat, prime, raw	16.74	29.18	0	335	0	53	70	0
Beef, rib, small end (ribs 10-12), separable lean and fat, trimmed to 1/8" fat, prime, cooked, broiled	24.13	27.86	0	354	0	63	83	0
Beef, rib, small end (ribs 10-12), separable lean and fat, trimmed to 1/8" fat, prime, cooked, roasted	22.15	35.12	0	411	0	65	84	0
Beef, shoulder top blade steak, boneless, separable lean and fat, trimmed to 0" fat, select, cooked, grilled	27.7	9.29	0	194	0	88	98	0
Beef, shoulder top blade steak, boneless, separable lean and fat, trimmed to 0" fat, all grades, raw	20.16	7.25	0	146	0	82	69	0
Beef, round, full cut, separable lean and fat, trimmed to 1/8" fat, choice, raw	20.56	11.92	0	195	0	54	62	0
Beef, round, full cut, separable lean and fat, trimmed to 1/8" fat, choice, cooked, broiled	27.54	12.98	0	235	0	62	79	0
Beef, round, full cut, separable lean and fat, trimmed to 1/8" fat, select, raw	20.56	10.68	0	184	0	54	62	0
Beef, round, full cut, separable lean and fat, trimmed to 1/8" fat, select, cooked, broiled	27.58	11.08	0	218	0	62	79	0
Beef, round, bottom round, steak, separable lean and fat, trimmed to 1/8" fat, all grades, raw	20.7	11.54	0	192	0	56	73	0
Beef, round, bottom round, steak, separable lean and fat, trimmed to 1/8" fat, all grades, cooked, braised	32.76	11.87	0	247	0	43	100	0
Beef, round, bottom round, roast, separable lean and fat, trimmed to 1/8" fat, all grades, cooked, roasted	26.41	11.64	0	218	0	35	85	0
Beef, round, bottom round, steak, separable lean and fat, trimmed to 1/8" fat, choice, raw	20.71	12.15	0	198	0	53	75	0
Beef, round, bottom round, steak, separable lean and fat, trimmed to 1/8" fat, choice, cooked, braised	32.85	12.56	0	254	0	42	101	0
Beef, round, bottom round, roast, separable lean and fat, trimmed to 1/8" fat, choice, cooked, roasted	26.05	12.44	0	223	0	34	86	0
Beef, round, bottom round, steak, separable lean and fat, trimmed to 1/8" fat, select, raw	20.68	10.93	0	187	0	60	72	0
Beef, round, bottom round, steak, separable lean and fat, trimmed to 1/8" fat, select, cooked, braised	32.67	11.19	0	240	0	43	98	0
Beef, round, bottom round, roast, separable lean and fat, trimmed to 1/8" fat, select, cooked, roasted	26.77	10.85	0	212	0	35	84	0
Beef, round, eye of round, roast, separable lean and fat, trimmed to 1/8" fat, all grades, raw	21.49	8.24	0	166	0	58	68	0
Beef, round, eye of round, roast, separable lean	28.31	9.65	0	208	0	37	84	0

Food Name ---> per 100 g	Protein (g)	Fat (g)	Carb (g)	Calories	Fiber (g)	Sodium (mg)	Cholesterol (mg)	Net Carb (g)
and fat, trimmed to 1/8" fat, all grades, cooked, roasted								
Beef, round, eye of round, roast, separable lean and fat, trimmed to 1/8" fat, choice, raw	21.68	8.91	0	173	0	55	70	0
Beef, round, eye of round, roast, separable lean and fat, trimmed to 1/8" fat, choice, cooked, roasted	28.48	10.05	0	212	0	37	86	0
Beef, round, eye of round, roast, separable lean and fat, trimmed to 1/8" fat, select, raw	21.3	7.57	0	159	0	62	66	0
Beef, round, eye of round, roast, separable lean and fat, trimmed to 1/8" fat, select, cooked, roasted	28.13	9.26	0	204	0	37	83	0
Beef, round, tip round, separable lean and fat, trimmed to 1/8" fat, all grades, raw	19.6	11.67	0	189	0	58	65	0
Beef, round, tip round, roast, separable lean and fat, trimmed to 1/8" fat, all grades, cooked, roasted	27.45	11.34	0	219	0	63	82	0
Beef, round, tip round, separable lean and fat, trimmed to 1/8" fat, choice, raw	19.48	12.83	0	199	0	58	65	0
Beef, round, tip round, roast, separable lean and fat, trimmed to 1/8" fat, choice, cooked, roasted	27.27	12.34	0	228	0	63	82	0
Beef, round, tip round, separable lean and fat, trimmed to 1/8" fat, select, raw	19.74	10.39	0	178	0	58	64	0
Beef, round, tip round, roast, separable lean and fat, trimmed to 1/8" fat, select, cooked, roasted	27.63	10.24	0	210	0	64	82	0
Beef, shoulder top blade steak, boneless, separable lean and fat, trimmed to 0" fat, choice, raw	20.07	7.94	0	152	0	81	68	0
Beef, round, top round, separable lean only, trimmed to 1/8" fat, choice, cooked, pan-fried	33.93	8.33	2.03	228	0	65	102	2.03
Beef, round, top round, steak, separable lean and fat, trimmed to 1/8" fat, all grades, raw	22.06	7.93	0	166	0	60	69	0
Beef, round, top round, separable lean and fat, trimmed to 1/8" fat, all grades, cooked, braised	34.34	10.13	0	238	0	45	90	0
Beef, round, top round steak, separable lean and fat, trimmed to 1/8" fat, all grades, cooked, broiled	30.67	9	0	204	0	41	90	0
Beef, round, top round, steak, separable lean and fat, trimmed to 1/8" fat, choice, raw	21.94	8.19	0	168	0	57	69	0
Beef, round, top round, separable lean and fat, trimmed to 1/8" fat, choice, cooked, braised	34.09	11.61	0	250	0	45	90	0
Beef, round, top round, steak, separable lean and fat, trimmed to 1/8" fat, choice, cooked, broiled	30.7	10.27	0	224	0	40	92	0
Beef, round, top round, separable lean and fat, trimmed to 1/8" fat, choice, cooked, pan-fried	32.99	13.83	0	266	0	68	97	0
Beef, round, top round, steak, separable lean and fat, trimmed to 1/8" fat, select, raw	22.18	7.68	0	164	0	63	68	0
Beef, round, top round, separable lean and fat, trimmed to 1/8" fat, select, cooked, braised	34.6	8.54	0	225	0	45	90	0
Beef, round, top round, steak, separable lean and fat, trimmed to 1/8" fat, select, cooked, broiled	30.63	7.73	0	201	0	41	87	0
Beef, round, top round, separable lean and fat, trimmed to 1/8" fat, prime, raw	22.24	8.67	0	173	0	51	59	0
Beef, round, top round, steak, separable lean and fat, trimmed to 1/8" fat, prime, cooked, broiled	31.27	10.1	0	225	0	61	84	0
Beef, shoulder top blade steak, boneless, separable lean and fat, trimmed to 0" fat, select, raw	20.28	6.21	0	137	0	86	71	0
Beef, brisket, flat half, boneless, separable lean and fat, trimmed to 0" fat, all grades, raw	20.32	9.29	0	165	0	80	67	0

Food Name ---> per 100 g	Protein (g)	Fat (g)	Carb (g)	Calories	Fiber (g)	Sodium (mg)	Cholesterol (mg)	Net Carb (g)
Beef, short loin, porterhouse steak, separable lean and fat, trimmed to 1/8" fat, choice, raw	20.36	14.58	0	218	0	52	61	0
Beef, short loin, porterhouse steak, separable lean and fat, trimmed to 1/8" fat, choice, cooked, grilled	24.85	19.78	0	284	0	63	85	0
Beef, short loin, t-bone steak, separable lean and fat, trimmed to 1/8" fat, choice, raw	20	15.83	0	228	0	35	62	0
Beef, short loin, t-bone steak, separable lean and fat, trimmed to 1/8" fat, choice, cooked, grilled	24.21	21.13	0	294	0	63	82	0
Beef, short loin, top loin, steak, separable lean and fat, trimmed to 1/8" fat, all grades, raw	20.61	15.49	0	228	0	52	81	0
Beef, loin, top loin, separable lean and fat, trimmed to 1/8" fat, all grades, cooked, grilled	26.44	16.78	0	264	0	54	88	0
Beef, loin, top loin, separable lean and fat, trimmed to 1/8" fat, choice, raw	19.32	17.1	0	237	0	54	82	0
Beef, short loin, top loin, steak, separable lean and fat, trimmed to 1/8" fat, choice, cooked, grilled	26.16	18.45	0	278	0	52	97	0
Beef, loin, top loin, separable lean and fat, trimmed to 1/8" fat, select, raw	20.59	15.04	0	224	0	52	80	0
Beef, loin, top loin, separable lean and fat, trimmed to 1/8" fat, select, cooked, grilled	26.72	15.11	0	250	0	57	79	0
Beef, short loin, top loin, steak, separable lean and fat, trimmed to 1/8" fat, prime, raw	19	22.17	0	281	0	53	67	0
Beef, short loin, top loin, separable lean and fat, trimmed to 1/8" fat, prime, cooked, broiled	25.92	22.12	0	310	0	64	79	0
Beef, tenderloin, steak, separable lean and fat, trimmed to 1/8" fat, all grades, raw	19.61	18.16	0	247	0	50	85	0
Beef, tenderloin, steak, separable lean and fat, trimmed to 1/8" fat, all grades, cooked, broiled	26.46	17.12	0	267	0	54	97	0
Beef, tenderloin, roast, separable lean and fat, trimmed to 1/8" fat, all grades, cooked, roasted	23.9	24.6	0	324	0	57	85	0
Beef, tenderloin, steak, separable lean and fat, trimmed to 1/8" fat, choice, raw	19.82	17.88	0	246	0	50	85	0
Beef, tenderloin, steak, separable lean and fat, trimmed to 1/8" fat, choice, cooked, broiled	26.43	17.78	0	273	0	52	99	0
Beef, tenderloin, roast, separable lean and fat, trimmed to 1/8" fat, choice, cooked, roasted	23.9	25.39	0	331	0	65	85	0
Beef, tenderloin, steak, separable lean and fat, trimmed to 1/8" fat, select, raw	19.37	18.46	0	249	0	50	86	0
Beef, tenderloin, steak, separable lean and fat, trimmed to 1/8" fat, select, cooked, broiled	26.48	16.53	0	262	0	57	96	0
Beef, tenderloin, roast, separable lean and fat, trimmed to 1/8" fat, select, cooked, roasted	23.9	23.7	0	316	0	57	85	0
Beef, tenderloin, separable lean and fat, trimmed to 1/8" fat, prime, raw	18.15	21.83	0	274	0	49	70	0
Beef, tenderloin, steak, separable lean and fat, trimmed to 1/8" fat, prime, cooked, broiled	25.26	22.21	0	308	0	59	86	0
Beef, tenderloin, roast, separable lean and fat, trimmed to 1/8" fat, prime, cooked, roasted	24.04	26.67	0	343	0	55	88	0
Beef, top sirloin, steak, separable lean and fat, trimmed to 1/8" fat, all grades, raw	20.3	12.71	0	201	0	52	75	0
Beef, top sirloin, steak, separable lean and fat, trimmed to 1/8" fat, all grades, cooked, broiled	26.96	14.23	0	243	0	56	92	0
Beef, top sirloin, steak, separable lean and fat, trimmed to 1/8" fat, choice, raw	19.92	14.28	0	214	0	51	78	0
Beef, top sirloin, steak, separable lean and fat,	26.8	15.75	0	257	0	54	96	0

Food Name ---> per 100 g	Protein (g)	Fat (g)	Carb (g)	Calories	Fiber (g)	Sodium (mg)	Cholesterol (mg)	Net Carb (g)
trimmed to 1/8" fat, choice, cooked, broiled								
Beef, top sirloin, steak, separable lean and fat, trimmed to 1/8" fat, choice, cooked, pan-fried	28.77	21.06	0	313	0	71	98	0
Beef, top sirloin, steak, separable lean and fat, trimmed to 1/8" fat, select, raw	20.68	11.13	0	189	0	53	72	0
Beef, top sirloin, steak, separable lean and fat, trimmed to 1/8" fat, select, cooked, broiled	27.12	12.71	0	230	0	57	89	0
Beef, chuck, clod roast, separable lean only, trimmed to 0" fat, choice, cooked, roasted	25.95	6.69	0	171	0	74	87	0
Beef, chuck, clod roast, separable lean only, trimmed to 0" fat, select, cooked, roasted	28.09	5.82	0	172	0	74	90	0
Beef, shoulder steak, boneless, separable lean only, trimmed to 0" fat, choice, cooked, grilled	28.54	6.25	0	178	0	68	81	0
Beef, shoulder steak, boneless, separable lean only, trimmed to 0" fat, select, cooked, grilled	28.71	5.17	0	169	0	68	83	0
Beef, flank, steak, separable lean and fat, trimmed to 0" fat, all grades, cooked, broiled	27.66	8.23	0	192	0	56	79	0
Beef, flank, steak, separable lean and fat, trimmed to 0" fat, select, cooked, broiled	27.78	7.15	0	183	0	58	78	0
Beef, brisket, flat half, separable lean and fat, trimmed to 0" fat, select, cooked, braised	33.59	6.77	0	205	0	57	93	0
Beef, rib eye, small end (ribs 10-12), separable lean and fat, trimmed to 0" fat, select, cooked, broiled	27.95	12.71	0	234	0	59	92	0
Beef, rib eye, small end (ribs 10-12), separable lean and fat, trimmed to 0" fat, all grades, cooked, broiled	27.27	14.74	0	249	0	56	89	0
Beef, bottom sirloin, tri-tip roast, separable lean and fat, trimmed to 0" fat, all grades, cooked, roasted	26.05	11.07	0	211	0	53	83	0
Beef, bottom sirloin, tri-tip roast, separable lean and fat, trimmed to 0" fat, all grades, raw	20.64	8.55	0	165	0	52	66	0
Beef, bottom sirloin, tri-tip roast, separable lean and fat, trimmed to 0" fat, choice, cooked, roasted	25.66	12.36	0	221	0	50	85	0
Beef, bottom sirloin, tri-tip roast, separable lean and fat, trimmed to 0" fat, choice, raw	20.64	9.51	0	174	0	51	68	0
Beef, bottom sirloin, tri-tip roast, separable lean and fat, trimmed to 0" fat, select, cooked, roasted	26.44	9.78	0	201	0	56	81	0
Beef, bottom sirloin, tri-tip roast, separable lean and fat, trimmed to 0" fat, select, raw	20.64	7.68	0	157	0	53	65	0
Beef, round, top round steak, boneless, separable lean and fat, trimmed to 0" fat, all grades, cooked, grilled	29.96	4.28	0	167	0	75	86	0
Beef, chuck, mock tender steak, separable lean only, trimmed to 0" fat, choice, cooked, broiled	25.74	5.69	0	161	0	73	94	0
Beef, chuck, mock tender steak, separable lean only, trimmed to 0" fat, select, cooked, broiled	26.13	5.02	0	157	0	68	99	0
Beef, chuck, top blade, separable lean only, trimmed to 0" fat, choice, cooked, broiled	26.11	11.65	0	217	0	68	93	0
Beef, chuck, top blade, separable lean only, trimmed to 0" fat, select, cooked, broiled	26.16	8	0	184	0	68	94	0
Beef, round, top round steak, boneless, separable lean and fat, trimmed to 0" fat, choice, cooked, grilled	30.12	4.62	0	170	0	78	86	0
Beef, round, top round steak, boneless, separable lean and fat, trimmed to 0" fat, select, cooked, grilled	29.7	3.85	0	162	0	76	88	0

Food Name ---> per 100 g	Protein (g)	Fat (g)	Carb (g)	Calories	Fiber (g)	Sodium (mg)	Cholesterol (mg)	Net Carb (g)
Beef, flank, steak, separable lean and fat, trimmed to 0" fat, all grades, raw	21.22	7.17	0	155	0	54	65	0
Beef, flank, steak, separable lean and fat, trimmed to 0" fat, select, raw	21.22	6.06	0	145	0	54	62	0
Beef, chuck eye roast, boneless, America's Beef Roast, separable lean only, trimmed to 0" fat, all grades, raw	20.61	6.01	0	137	0	85	69	0
Beef, chuck eye roast, boneless, America's Beef Roast, separable lean only, trimmed to 0" fat, choice, raw	20.67	6.21	0	139	0	85	67	0
Beef, chuck eye roast, boneless, America's Beef Roast, separable lean only, trimmed to 0" fat, select, raw	20.52	5.71	0	133	0	86	74	0
Beef, brisket, flat half, boneless, separable lean and fat, trimmed to 0" fat, choice, raw	20.15	9.86	0	169	0	79	67	0
Beef, plate, inside skirt steak, separable lean only, trimmed to 0" fat, all grades, cooked, broiled	26.66	10.06	0	205	0	76	85	0
Beef, plate, outside skirt steak, separable lean only, trimmed to 0" fat, all grades, cooked, broiled	24.18	14.37	0	233	0	94	91	0
Beef, chuck, short ribs, boneless, separable lean only, trimmed to 0" fat, choice, cooked, braised	28.84	14.95	0	250	0	75	102	0
Beef, chuck, short ribs, boneless, separable lean only, trimmed to 0" fat, select, cooked, braised	28.79	12.08	0	224	0	75	108	0
Beef, chuck, short ribs, boneless, separable lean only, trimmed to 0" fat, all grades, cooked, braised	28.82	13.8	0	240	0	75	105	0
Beef, brisket, flat half, boneless, separable lean and fat, trimmed to 0" fat, select, raw	20.57	8.45	0	158	0	82	69	0
Beef, loin, bottom sirloin butt, tri-tip roast, separable lean only, trimmed to 0" fat, all grades, cooked, roasted	26.75	8.34	0	182	0	55	78	0
Beef, shoulder pot roast or steak, boneless, separable lean and fat, trimmed to 0" fat, all grades, raw	21.39	4.97	0	130	0	72	66	0
Beef, short loin, porterhouse steak, separable lean and fat, trimmed to 1/8" fat, all grades, raw	20.49	14.06	0	214	0	48	61	0
Beef, short loin, porterhouse steak, separable lean and fat, trimmed to 1/8" fat, all grades, cooked, grilled	25.4	18.57	0	276	0	64	83	0
Beef, short loin, porterhouse steak, separable lean and fat, trimmed to 1/8" fat, select, raw	20.69	13.27	0	208	0	42	60	0
Beef, short loin, porterhouse steak, separable lean and fat, trimmed to 1/8" fat, select, cooked, grilled	26.21	16.75	0	263	0	63	79	0
Beef, short loin, t-bone steak, separable lean and fat, trimmed to 1/8" fat, all grades, raw	20.11	15.18	0	223	0	40	62	0
Beef, short loin, t-bone steak, separable lean and fat, trimmed to 1/8" fat, all grades, cooked, grilled	24.6	20.36	0	289	0	62	83	0
Beef, short loin, t-bone steak, separable lean and fat, trimmed to 1/8" fat, select, raw	20.28	14.19	0	215	0	52	62	0
Beef, short loin, t-bone steak, separable lean and fat, trimmed to 1/8" fat, select, cooked, grilled	25.18	19.22	0	281	0	62	84	0
Beef, round, knuckle, tip side, steak, separable lean and fat, trimmed to 0" fat, choice, raw	21.41	4.66	0	133	0	62	61	0
Beef, round, knuckle, tip side, steak, separable lean and fat, trimmed to 0" fat, choice, cooked, grilled	28.79	5.71	0	174	0	55	82	0
Beef, round, knuckle, tip side, steak, separable lean and fat , trimmed to 0" fat, select, raw	21.96	3.24	0	124	0	57	61	0

Food Name ---> per 100 g	Protein (g)	Fat (g)	Carb (g)	Calories	Fiber (g)	Sodium (mg)	Cholesterol (mg)	Net Carb (g)
Beef, round, knuckle, tip side, steak, separable lean and fat, trimmed to 0" fat, select, cooked, grilled	29.24	3.91	0	160	0	52	78	0
Beef, chuck, shoulder clod, shoulder tender, medallion, separable lean and fat, trimmed to 0" fat, choice, raw	20.51	6.36	0	145	0	59	56	0
Beef, chuck, shoulder clod, shoulder tender, medallion, separable lean and fat, trimmed to 0" fat, choice, cooked, grilled	26.07	7.68	0	181	0	60	76	0
Beef, chuck, shoulder clod, shoulder tender, medallion, separable lean and fat, trimmed to 0" fat, select, raw	20.93	5.79	0	142	0	60	58	0
Beef, chuck, shoulder clod, shoulder top and center steaks, separable lean and fat, trimmed to 0" fat, choice, raw	20.39	6.12	0	143	0	61	57	0
Beef, chuck, shoulder clod, shoulder top and center steaks, separable lean and fat, trimmed to 0" fat, choice, cooked, grilled	26.07	8.11	0	184	0	59	74	0
Beef, chuck, shoulder clod, shoulder top and center steaks, separable lean and fat, trimmed to 0" fat, select, raw	21.13	5.51	0	140	0	58	58	0
Beef, chuck, shoulder clod, shoulder top and center steaks, separable lean and fat, trimmed to 0" fat, select, cooked, grilled	26.66	6.94	0	176	0	62	77	0
Beef, chuck, shoulder clod, top blade, steak, separable lean and fat, trimmed to 0" fat, choice, raw	18.75	11.33	0	182	0	74	65	0
Beef, chuck, shoulder clod, top blade, steak, separable lean and fat, trimmed to 0" fat, choice, cooked, grilled	24.7	13.59	0	228	0	78	83	0
Beef, chuck, shoulder clod, top blade, steak, separable lean and fat, trimmed to 0" fat, select, raw	19.38	9.22	0	166	0	75	66	0
Beef, chuck, shoulder clod, top blade, steak, separable lean and fat, trimmed to 0" fat, select, cooked, grilled	25.29	11.52	0	212	0	76	83	0
Beef, round, knuckle, tip center, steak, separable lean and fat, trimmed to 0" fat, choice, raw	20.74	6.85	0	150	0	54	58	0
Beef, round, knuckle, tip center, steak, separable lean and fat, trimmed to 0" fat, choice, cooked, grilled	26.88	8.13	0	188	0	51	75	0
Beef, round, knuckle, tip center, steak, separable lean and fat, trimmed to 0" fat, select, raw	20.98	5.21	0	137	0	53	59	0
Beef, round, knuckle, tip center, steak, separable lean and fat, trimmed to 0" fat, select, cooked, grilled	26.61	5.32	0	162	0	53	74	0
Beef, round, outside round, bottom round, steak, separable lean and fat, trimmed to 0" fat, choice, raw	21.24	6.59	0	150	0	63	61	0
Beef, round, outside round, bottom round, steak, separable lean and fat, trimmed to 0" fat, choice, cooked, grilled	27.22	8.3	0	191	0	57	78	0
Beef, round, outside round, bottom round, steak, separable lean and fat, trimmed to 0" fat, select, raw	22.15	3.83	0	129	0	62	61	0
Beef, round, outside round, bottom round, steak, separable lean and fat, trimmed to 0" fat, select,	28.01	5.17	0	166	0	60	75	0

cooked, grilled

Food Name ---> per 100 g	Protein (g)	Fat (g)	Carb (g)	Calories	Fiber (g)	Sodium (mg)	Cholesterol (mg)	Net Carb (g)
Beef, chuck, shoulder clod, shoulder tender, medallion, separable lean and fat, trimmed to 0" fat, all grades, raw	20.54	6.22	0	144	0	58	57	0
Beef, chuck, shoulder clod, shoulder tender, medallion, separable lean and fat, trimmed to 0" fat, all grades, cooked, grilled	26.22	7.2	0	177	0	59	78	0
Beef, round, knuckle, tip side, steak, separable lean and fat, trimmed to 0" fat, all grades, raw	21.69	4	0	129	0	61	61	0
Beef, round, knuckle, tip side, steak, separable lean and fat, trimmed to 0" fat, all grades, cooked, grilled	29.08	4.84	0	168	0	54	80	0
Beef, chuck, shoulder clod, shoulder top and center steaks, separable lean and fat, trimmed to 0" fat, all grades, raw	20.67	5.88	0	141	0	60	57	0
Beef, chuck, shoulder clod, shoulder top and center steaks, separable lean and fat, trimmed to 0" fat, all grades, cooked, grilled	26.3	7.66	0	182	0	60	76	0
Beef, chuck, shoulder clod, top blade, steak, separable lean and fat, trimmed to 0" fat, all grades, raw	18.99	10.52	0	176	0	74	66	0
Beef, chuck, shoulder clod, top blade, steak, separable lean and fat, trimmed to 0" fat, all grades, cooked, grilled	24.93	12.79	0	222	0	77	83	0
Beef, round, knuckle, tip center, steak, separable lean and fat, trimmed to 0" fat, all grades, raw	20.93	5.89	0	143	0	54	59	0
Beef, round, knuckle, tip center, steak, separable lean and fat, trimmed to 0" fat, all grades, cooked, grilled	27.12	6.78	0	177	0	52	77	0
Beef, round, outside round, bottom round, steak, separable lean and fat, trimmed to 0" fat, all grades, raw	21.59	5.53	0	142	0	62	61	0
Beef, round, outside round, bottom round, steak, separable lean and fat, trimmed to 0" fat, all grades, cooked, grilled	27.52	7.1	0	182	0	58	77	0
Beef, chuck, shoulder clod, shoulder tender, medallion, separable lean and fat, trimmed to 0" fat, select, cooked, grilled	26.45	6.43	0	172	0	58	80	0
Beef, chuck, short ribs, boneless, separable lean only, trimmed to 0" fat, choice, raw	19.38	10.7	0.29	175	0	81	73	0.29
Beef, chuck, short ribs, boneless, separable lean only, trimmed to 0" fat, select, raw	20.14	8.99	0	161	0	93	80	0
Beef, chuck, short ribs, boneless, separable lean only, trimmed to 0" fat, all grades, raw	19.68	10.02	0.05	169	0	85	76	0.05
Beef, chuck eye Country-Style ribs, boneless, separable lean only, trimmed to 0" fat, choice, cooked, braised	30.95	12.22	0	234	0	69	100	0
Beef, chuck eye Country-Style ribs, boneless, separable lean only, trimmed to 0" fat, select, cooked, braised	32.1	10.24	0	221	0	70	99	0
Beef, chuck eye Country-Style ribs, boneless, separable lean only, trimmed to 0" fat, all grades, cooked, braised	31.41	11.43	0	228	0	69	99	0
Beef, chuck eye Country-Style ribs, boneless, separable lean only, trimmed to 0" fat, choice, raw	20.87	7.67	0	152	0	81	70	0
Beef, chuck eye Country-Style ribs, boneless, separable lean only, trimmed to 0" fat, select, raw	21.1	5.89	0	137	0	82	71	0

Food Name ---> per 100 g	Protein (g)	Fat (g)	Carb (g)	Calories	Fiber (g)	Sodium (mg)	Cholesterol (mg)	Net Carb (g)
Beef, chuck eye Country-Style ribs, boneless, separable lean only, trimmed to 0" fat, all grades, raw	20.96	6.95	0	146	0	82	70	0
Beef, chuck eye steak, boneless, separable lean only, trimmed to 0" fat, choice, cooked, grilled	27.97	11.47	0	215	0	75	86	0
Beef, chuck eye steak, boneless, separable lean only, trimmed to 0" fat, select, cooked, grilled	27.88	9.77	0	199	0	74	91	0
Beef, chuck eye steak, boneless, separable lean only, trimmed to 0" fat, all grades, cooked, grilled	27.94	10.79	0	209	0	75	88	0
Beef, chuck eye steak, boneless, separable lean only, trimmed to 0" fat, choice, raw	21.31	8.29	0	160	0	70	66	0
Beef, chuck eye steak, boneless, separable lean only, trimmed to 0" fat, select, raw	21.28	6.47	0	143	0	73	69	0
Beef, chuck eye steak, boneless, separable lean only, trimmed to 0" fat, all grades, raw	21.29	7.56	0	153	0	70	67	0
Beef, shoulder pot roast, boneless, separable lean only, trimmed to 0" fat, choice, cooked, braised	31.32	8.3	0	200	0	60	97	0
Beef, shoulder pot roast, boneless, separable lean only, trimmed to 0" fat, select, cooked, braised	31.71	7.02	0	190	0	63	99	0
Beef, shoulder pot roast, boneless, separable lean only, trimmed to 0" fat, all grades, cooked, braised	31.48	7.78	0	196	0	61	98	0
Beef, chuck, mock tender steak, boneless, separable lean only, trimmed to 0" fat, choice, cooked, braised	33.55	6.94	0	197	0	67	113	0
Beef, chuck, mock tender steak, boneless, separable lean only, trimmed to 0" fat, select, cooked, braised	32.96	5.44	0	181	0	70	117	0
Beef, chuck, mock tender steak, boneless, separable lean only, trimmed to 0" fat, all grades, cooked, braised	33.31	6.34	0	190	0	68	115	0
Beef, chuck, mock tender steak, boneless, separable lean only, trimmed to 0" fat, choice, raw	21.36	4.6	0	127	0	83	67	0
Beef, chuck, mock tender steak, boneless, separable lean only, trimmed to 0" fat, select, raw	21.22	3.53	0	117	0	76	68	0
Beef, chuck, mock tender steak, boneless, separable lean only, trimmed to 0" fat, all grades, raw	21.3	4.17	0	123	0	81	67	0
Beef, chuck for stew, separable lean and fat, all grades, cooked, braised	32.41	6.82	0	191	0	67	99	0
Beef, chuck for stew, separable lean and fat, select, cooked, braised	32.29	6.34	0	186	0	68	102	0
Beef, chuck for stew, separable lean and fat, choice, cooked, braised	32.49	7.14	0	194	0	65	96	0
Beef, chuck for stew, separable lean and fat, all grades, raw	21.75	4.48	0.16	128	0	80	64	0.16
Beef, chuck for stew, separable lean and fat, select, raw	21.9	3.99	0.21	124	0	81	66	0.21
Beef, chuck for stew, separable lean and fat, choice, raw	21.64	4.81	0.12	130	0	79	63	0.12
Beef, chuck, under blade steak, boneless, separable lean only, trimmed to 0" fat, choice, cooked, braised	30.91	10.91	0	222	0	65	106	0
Beef, chuck, under blade steak, boneless, separable lean only, trimmed to 0" fat, select, cooked, braised	32.01	9.66	0	215	0	66	108	0
Beef, chuck, under blade steak, boneless, separable lean only, trimmed to 0" fat, all grades,	31.35	10.41	0	219	0	65	107	0

Food Name ---> per 100 g	Protein (g)	Fat (g)	Carb (g)	Calories	Fiber (g)	Sodium (mg)	Cholesterol (mg)	Net Carb (g)
cooked, braised								
Beef, chuck, under blade pot roast, boneless, separable lean and fat, trimmed to 0" fat, all grades, cooked, braised	26.7	20.49	0	291	0	62	99	0
Beef, rib eye steak, boneless, lip-on, separable lean only, trimmed to 1/8" fat, all grades, cooked, grilled	27.97	10.57	0	207	0	59	79	0
Beef, rib eye roast, bone-in, lip-on, separable lean only, trimmed to 1/8" fat, choice, cooked, roasted	27.18	14.55	0	240	0	68	83	0
Beef, chuck, under blade pot roast or steak, boneless, separable lean and fat, trimmed to 0" fat, all grades, raw	19.17	13.26	0	196	0	76	66	0
Beef, chuck, under blade pot roast or steak, boneless, separable lean and fat, trimmed to 0" fat, choice, raw	19.15	13.93	0	202	0	76	66	0
Beef, chuck, under blade pot roast or steak, boneless, separable lean and fat, trimmed to 0" fat, select, raw	19.2	12.27	0	187	0	77	67	0
Beef, chuck, under blade center steak, boneless, Denver Cut, separable lean and fat, trimmed to 0" fat, all grades, cooked, grilled	26.18	13.54	0.21	227	0	73	93	0.21
Beef, chuck, under blade center steak, boneless, Denver Cut, separable lean and fat, trimmed to 0" fat, choice, cooked, grilled	26.1	14.41	0.4	236	0	73	89	0.4
Beef, chuck, under blade center steak, boneless, Denver Cut, separable lean and fat, trimmed to 0" fat, select, cooked, grilled	26.3	12.25	0	215	0	73	98	0
Beef, chuck, under blade center steak, boneless, Denver Cut, separable lean and fat, trimmed to 0" fat, all grades, raw	18.99	11.64	0.36	182	0	76	69	0.36
Beef, chuck, under blade center steak, boneless, Denver Cut, separable lean and fat, trimmed to 0" fat, choice, raw	18.85	12.4	0.53	189	0	75	70	0.53
Beef, chuck, under blade center steak, boneless, Denver Cut, separable lean and fat, trimmed to 0" fat, select, raw	19.2	10.5	0.09	172	0	76	68	0.09
Beef, shoulder pot roast or steak, boneless, separable lean and fat, trimmed to 0" fat, choice, raw	21.17	5.33	0.07	133	0	74	64	0.07
Beef, shoulder pot roast or steak, boneless, separable lean and fat, trimmed to 0" fat, select, raw	21.72	4.44	0	127	0	70	68	0
Beef, chuck eye roast, boneless, America's Beef Roast, separable lean and fat, trimmed to 0" fat, all grades, cooked, roasted	24.63	15.29	0	236	0	76	83	0
Beef, chuck eye roast, boneless, America's Beef Roast, separable lean and fat, trimmed to 0" fat, choice, cooked, roasted	24.47	15.87	0	241	0	75	84	0
Beef, chuck eye roast, boneless, America's Beef Roast, separable lean and fat, trimmed to 0" fat, select, cooked, roasted	24.86	14.41	0	229	0	76	81	0
Beef, chuck, under blade steak, boneless, separable lean and fat, trimmed to 0" fat, all grades, cooked, braised	28.23	18	0	275	0	65	96	0
Beef, chuck, under blade steak, boneless, separable lean and fat, trimmed to 0" fat, choice, cooked, braised	27.6	19.3	0	284	0	64	98	0

Food Name ---> per 100 g	Protein (g)	Fat (g)	Carb (g)	Calories	Fiber (g)	Sodium (mg)	Cholesterol (mg)	Net Carb (g)
Beef, chuck, under blade steak, boneless, separable lean and fat, trimmed to 0" fat, select, cooked, braised	29.18	16.05	0	261	0	66	94	0
Beef, chuck, mock tender steak, boneless, separable lean and fat, trimmed to 0" fat, all grades, cooked, braised	32.07	10.18	0	220	0	67	113	0
Beef, chuck, mock tender steak, boneless, separable lean and fat, trimmed to 0" fat, choice, cooked, braised	32.21	10.74	0	225	0	66	112	0
Beef, chuck, mock tender steak, boneless, separable lean and fat, trimmed to 0" fat, select, cooked, braised	31.86	9.34	0	211	0	69	115	0
Beef, chuck, mock tender steak, boneless, separable lean and fat, trimmed to 0" fat, all grades, raw	21.13	4.79	0	128	0	80	67	0
Beef, chuck, mock tender steak, boneless, separable lean and fat, trimmed to 0" fat, choice, raw	21.19	5.18	0	131	0	82	67	0
Beef, chuck, mock tender steak, boneless, separable lean and fat, trimmed to 0" fat, select, raw	21.05	4.2	0	122	0	76	68	0
Beef, chuck, short ribs, boneless, separable lean and fat, trimmed to 0" fat, all grades, cooked, braised	25.48	22.58	0	305	0	70	100	0
Beef, chuck, short ribs, boneless, separable lean and fat, trimmed to 0" fat, choice, cooked, braised	25.26	24.05	0	317	0	70	98	0
Beef, chuck, short ribs, boneless, separable lean and fat, trimmed to 0" fat, select, cooked, braised	25.81	20.38	0	287	0	71	104	0
Beef, chuck, short ribs, boneless, separable lean and fat, trimmed to 0" fat, all grades, raw	17.48	18.33	0	235	0	78	75	0
Beef, chuck, short ribs, boneless, separable lean and fat, trimmed to 0" fat, choice, raw	17.22	19.03	0	240	0	75	73	0
Beef, chuck, short ribs, boneless, separable lean and fat, trimmed to 0" fat, select, raw	17.87	17.28	0	227	0	85	78	0
Beef, shoulder pot roast, boneless, separable lean and fat, trimmed to 0" fat, all grades, cooked, braised	31.03	8.92	0	204	0	61	98	0
Beef, shoulder pot roast, boneless, separable lean and fat, trimmed to 0" fat, choice, cooked, braised	30.93	9.25	0	207	0	60	98	0
Beef, shoulder pot roast, boneless, separable lean and fat, trimmed to 0" fat, select, cooked, braised	31.18	8.41	0	200	0	62	98	0
Beef, chuck eye Country-Style ribs, boneless, separable lean and fat, trimmed to 0" fat, all grades, cooked, braised	27.69	20.55	0	296	0	65	96	0
Beef, chuck eye Country-Style ribs, boneless, separable lean and fat, trimmed to 0" fat, choice, cooked, braised	27.16	21.56	0	303	0	65	96	0
Beef, chuck eye Country-Style ribs, boneless, separable lean and fat, trimmed to 0" fat, select, cooked, braised	28.47	19.03	0	285	0	66	95	0
Beef, chuck eye Country-Style ribs, boneless, separable lean and fat, trimmed to 0" fat, all grades, raw	18.97	14.32	0	205	0	77	70	0
Beef, chuck eye Country-Style ribs, boneless, separable lean and fat, trimmed to 0" fat, choice, raw	18.87	14.99	0	210	0	76	70	0
Beef, chuck eye Country-Style ribs, boneless,	19.1	13.33	0	196	0	77	71	0

Food Name ---> per 100 g	Protein (g)	Fat (g)	Carb (g)	Calories	Fiber (g)	Sodium (mg)	Cholesterol (mg)	Net Carb (g)
separable lean and fat, trimmed to 0" fat, select, raw								
Beef, chuck eye steak, boneless, separable lean and fat, trimmed to 0" fat, all grades, cooked, grilled	24.98	19.64	0	277	0	71	87	0
Beef, chuck eye steak, boneless, separable lean and fat, trimmed to 0" fat, choice, cooked, grilled	24.95	20.35	0	283	0	71	86	0
Beef, chuck eye steak, boneless, separable lean and fat, trimmed to 0" fat, select, cooked, grilled	25.03	18.57	0	267	0	70	89	0
Beef, chuck eye steak, boneless, separable lean and fat, trimmed to 0" fat, all grades, raw	18.86	16.35	0	223	0	66	68	0
Beef, chuck eye steak, boneless, separable lean and fat, trimmed to 0" fat, choice, raw	18.86	16.85	0	227	0	66	68	0
Beef, chuck eye steak, boneless, separable lean and fat, trimmed to 0" fat, select, raw	18.86	15.6	0	216	0	68	68	0
Beef, rib eye roast, bone-in, lip-on, separable lean only, trimmed to 1/8" fat, all grades, cooked, roasted	27.12	13.64	0	231	0	69	80	0
Beef, rib eye roast, bone-in, lip-on, separable lean only, trimmed to 1/8" fat, select, cooked, roasted	27.03	12.29	0	219	0	70	77	0
Beef, rib eye steak, boneless, lip-on, separable lean only, trimmed to 1/8" fat, choice, cooked, grilled	27.3	11.97	0	217	0	60	80	0
Beef, rib eye steak, boneless, lip-on, separable lean only, trimmed to 1/8" fat, select, cooked, grilled	28.98	8.48	0	192	0	59	77	0
Beef, rib eye steak/roast, bone-in, lip-on, separable lean only, trimmed to 1/8" fat, all grades, raw	21.22	9.04	0	166	0	64	64	0
Beef, rib eye steak/roast, bone-in, lip-on, separable lean only, trimmed to 1/8" fat, choice, raw	20.93	9.97	0	173	0	65	65	0
Beef, rib eye steak/roast, bone-in, lip-on, separable lean only, trimmed to 1/8" fat, select, raw	21.65	7.64	0	155	0	63	62	0
Beef, rib eye steak/roast, boneless, lip-on, separable lean only, trimmed to 1/8" fat, all grades, raw	21.99	7.54	0	156	0	56	66	0
Beef, rib eye steak/roast, boneless, lip-on, separable lean only, trimmed to 1/8" fat, choice, raw	21.62	8.29	0	161	0	56	63	0
Beef, rib eye steak/roast, boneless, lip-on, separable lean only, trimmed to 1/8" fat, select, raw	22.55	6.41	0	148	0	55	70	0
Beef, rib eye steak, bone-in, lip-on, separable lean only, trimmed to 1/8" fat, all grades, cooked, grilled	27.4	12.43	0	221	0	67	80	0
Beef, rib eye steak, bone-in, lip-on, separable lean only, trimmed to 1/8" fat, choice, cooked, grilled	27.03	13.44	0	229	0	67	82	0
Beef, rib eye steak, bone-in, lip-on, separable lean only, trimmed to 1/8" fat, select, cooked, grilled	27.96	10.91	0	210	0	67	78	0
Beef, rib eye roast, boneless, lip-on, separable lean only, trimmed to 1/8" fat, all grades, cooked, roasted	28.21	11.68	0	218	0	56	80	0
Beef, rib eye roast, boneless, lip-on, separable lean only, trimmed to 1/8" fat, choice, cooked, roasted	27.87	13.01	0	229	0	54	81	0
Beef, rib eye roast, boneless, lip-on, separable lean	28.72	9.68	0	202	0	59	79	0

only, trimmed to 1/8" fat, select, cooked, roasted

Food Name ---> per 100 g	Protein (g)	Fat (g)	Carb (g)	Calories	Fiber (g)	Sodium (mg)	Cholesterol (mg)	Net Carb (g)
Beef, plate steak, boneless, inside skirt, separable lean only, trimmed to 0" fat, all grades, cooked, grilled	29.99	12.69	0	234	0	63	92	0
Beef, plate steak, boneless, inside skirt, separable lean only, trimmed to 0" fat, all grades, raw	21.17	8.82	0	164	0	66	64	0
Beef, plate steak, boneless, inside skirt, separable lean only, trimmed to 0" fat, choice, cooked, grilled	29.56	13.72	0	242	0	64	93	0
Beef, plate steak, boneless, inside skirt, separable lean only, trimmed to 0" fat, choice, raw	20.89	9.76	0	171	0	67	64	0
Beef, plate steak, boneless, inside skirt, separable lean only, trimmed to 0" fat, select, cooked, grilled	30.64	11.16	0	223	0	62	91	0
Beef, plate steak, boneless, inside skirt, separable lean only, trimmed to 0" fat, select, raw	21.61	7.41	0	153	0	66	63	0
Beef, plate steak, boneless, outside skirt, separable lean only, trimmed to 0" fat, all grades, cooked, grilled	27.68	19.01	0	282	0	71	102	0
Beef, plate steak, boneless, outside skirt, separable lean only, trimmed to 0" fat, all grades, raw	18.74	14.53	0.19	206	0	67	69	0.19
Beef, plate steak, boneless, outside skirt, separable lean only, trimmed to 0" fat, choice, cooked, grilled	27.03	20.28	0	291	0	71	105	0
Beef, plate steak, boneless, outside skirt, separable lean only, trimmed to 0" fat, choice, raw	18.47	15.26	0.17	212	0	68	70	0.17
Beef, plate steak, boneless, outside skirt, separable lean only, trimmed to 0" fat, select, cooked, grilled	28.65	17.1	0	268	0	70	99	0
Beef, plate steak, boneless, outside skirt, separable lean only, trimmed to 0" fat, select, raw	19.14	13.44	0.23	198	0	65	69	0.23
Beef, rib eye steak, boneless, lip off, separable lean only, trimmed to 0" fat, all grades, cooked, grilled	28.11	10.37	0	206	0	59	79	0
Beef, rib eye steak, boneless, lip off, separable lean only, trimmed to 0" fat, all grades, raw	21.85	7.41	0	154	0	56	66	0
Beef, rib eye steak, boneless, lip off, separable lean only, trimmed to 0" fat, choice, cooked, grilled	27.39	11.75	0	215	0	60	80	0
Beef, rib eye steak, boneless, lip off, separable lean only, trimmed to 0" fat, choice, raw	21.44	8.5	0	162	0	56	63	0
Beef, rib eye steak, boneless, lip off, separable lean only, trimmed to 0" fat, select, cooked, grilled	29.18	8.31	0	191	0	59	77	0
Beef, rib eye steak, boneless, lip off, separable lean only, trimmed to 0" fat, select, raw	22.46	5.78	0	142	0	55	70	0
Beef, rib, back ribs, bone-in, separable lean only, trimmed to 0" fat, all grades, cooked, braised	28.36	20.57	0	299	0	68	90	0
Beef, rib, back ribs, bone-in, separable lean only, trimmed to 0" fat, all grades, raw	19.11	17.91	0.46	239	0	60	70	0.46
Beef, rib, back ribs, bone-in, separable lean only, trimmed to 0" fat, choice, cooked, braised	27.75	21.72	0	306	0	68	91	0
Beef, rib, back ribs, bone-in, separable lean only, trimmed to 0" fat, choice, raw	18.72	19.36	0.64	252	0	61	72	0.64
Beef, rib, back ribs, bone-in, separable lean only, trimmed to 0" fat, select, cooked, braised	29.28	18.84	0	287	0	68	89	0
Beef, rib, back ribs, bone-in, separable lean only, trimmed to 0" fat, select, raw	19.71	15.73	0.2	221	0	59	67	0.2
Beef, rib eye steak, bone-in, lip-on, separable lean and fat, trimmed to 1/8" fat, choice, cooked,	22.71	24.7	0	313	0	60	83	0

grilled

Food Name ---> per 100 g	Protein (g)	Fat (g)	Carb (g)	Calories	Fiber (g)	Sodium (mg)	Cholesterol (mg)	Net Carb (g)
Beef, rib eye steak, bone-in, lip-on, separable lean and fat, trimmed to 1/8" fat, select, cooked, grilled	23.19	23.47	0	304	0	59	80	0
Beef, rib eye steak, bone-in, lip-on, separable lean and fat, trimmed to 1/8" fat, all grades, cooked, grilled	22.9	24.2	0	309	0	60	82	0
Beef, rib eye roast, bone-in, lip-on, separable lean and fat, trimmed to 1/8" fat, choice, cooked, roasted	23.53	23.61	0	307	0	62	83	0
Beef, rib eye roast, bone-in, lip-on, separable lean and fat, trimmed to 1/8" fat, select, cooked, roasted	23.36	21.85	0	290	0	64	79	0
Beef, rib eye roast, bone-in, lip-on, separable lean and fat, trimmed to 1/8" fat, all grades, cooked, roasted	23.47	22.91	0	300	0	63	82	0
Beef, rib eye steak/roast, bone-in, lip-on, separable lean and fat, trimmed to 1/8" fat, all grades, raw	18.13	20.31	0	255	0	56	69	0
Beef, rib eye steak/roast, bone-in, lip-on, separable lean and fat, trimmed to 1/8" fat, choice, raw	17.92	20.96	0	260	0	57	70	0
Beef, rib eye steak/roast, bone-in, lip-on, separable lean and fat, trimmed to 1/8" fat, select, raw	18.44	19.34	0	248	0	55	68	0
Beef, rib eye steak, boneless, lip-on, separable lean and fat, trimmed to 1/8" fat, choice, cooked, grilled	22.92	23.52	0	303	0	54	81	0
Beef, rib eye steak, boneless, lip-on, separable lean and fat, trimmed to 1/8" fat, select, cooked, grilled	24.83	19.25	0	273	0	54	79	0
Beef, rib eye steak, boneless, lip-on, separable lean and fat, trimmed to 1/8" fat, all grades, cooked, grilled	23.69	21.81	0	291	0	54	80	0
Beef, rib eye roast, boneless, lip-on, separable lean and fat, trimmed to 1/8" fat, all grades, cooked, roasted	24.3	21.66	0	292	0	52	81	0
Beef, rib eye roast, boneless, lip-on, separable lean and fat, trimmed to 1/8" fat, choice, cooked, roasted	23.92	22.98	0	303	0	51	82	0
Beef, rib eye roast, boneless, lip-on, separable lean and fat, trimmed to 1/8" fat, select, cooked, roasted	24.85	19.68	0	277	0	54	80	0
Beef, rib eye steak/roast, boneless, lip-on, separable lean and fat, trimmed to 1/8" fat, all grades, raw	18.85	18.73	0	244	0	50	70	0
Beef, rib eye steak/roast, boneless, lip-on, separable lean and fat, trimmed to 1/8" fat, choice, raw	18.39	19.95	0	253	0	50	68	0
Beef, rib eye steak/roast, boneless, lip-on, separable lean and fat, trimmed to 1/8" fat, select, raw	19.55	16.9	0	230	0	50	74	0
Beef, plate steak, boneless, inside skirt, separable lean and fat, trimmed to 0" fat, all grades, cooked, grilled	29.36	14.2	0	245	0	63	92	0
Beef, plate steak, boneless, inside skirt, separable lean and fat, trimmed to 0" fat, choice, cooked, grilled	28.9	15.3	0	253	0	63	93	0

Food Name ---> per 100 g	Protein (g)	Fat (g)	Carb (g)	Calories	Fiber (g)	Sodium (mg)	Cholesterol (mg)	Net Carb (g)
Beef, plate steak, boneless, inside skirt, separable lean and fat, trimmed to 0" fat, select, cooked, grilled	30.06	12.54	0	233	0	61	91	0
Beef, plate steak, boneless, inside skirt, separable lean and fat, trimmed to 0" fat, all grades, raw	20.38	11.71	0	187	0	64	65	0
Beef, plate steak, boneless, inside skirt, separable lean and fat, trimmed to 0" fat, choice, raw	20.06	12.78	0	195	0	65	65	0
Beef, plate steak, boneless, inside skirt, separable lean and fat, trimmed to 0" fat, select, raw	20.87	10.11	0	174	0	65	65	0
Beef, ground, unspecified fat content, cooked	25.07	14.53	0.62	240	0	85	84	0.62
Beef, plate steak, boneless, outside skirt, separable lean and fat, trimmed to 0" fat, all grades, cooked, grilled	27.06	20.47	0	292	0	70	102	0
Beef, plate steak, boneless, outside skirt, separable lean and fat, trimmed to 0" fat, choice, cooked, grilled	26.46	21.62	0	300	0	70	104	0
Beef, plate steak, boneless, outside skirt, separable lean and fat, trimmed to 0" fat, select, cooked, grilled	27.95	18.75	0	281	0	69	98	0
Beef, plate steak, boneless, outside skirt, separable lean and fat, trimmed to 0" fat, all grades, raw	17.98	17.59	0.35	232	0	65	71	0.35
Beef, plate steak, boneless, outside skirt, separable lean and fat, trimmed to 0" fat, choice, raw	17.69	18.44	0.35	238	0	65	71	0.35
Beef, plate steak, boneless, outside skirt, separable lean and fat, trimmed to 0" fat, select, raw	18.43	16.31	0.36	222	0	63	70	0.36
Beef, rib eye steak, boneless, lip off, separable lean and fat, trimmed to 0" fat, all grades, cooked, grilled	24.85	19.02	0	271	0	58	78	0
Beef, rib eye steak, boneless, lip off, separable lean and fat, trimmed to 0" fat, choice, cooked, grilled	23.89	21.1	0	285	0	58	80	0
Beef, rib eye steak, boneless, lip off, separable lean and fat, trimmed to 0" fat, select, cooked, grilled	26.29	15.9	0	248	0	58	77	0
Beef, rib eye steak, boneless, lip off, separable lean and fat, trimmed to 0" fat, all grades, raw	19.26	16.71	0.12	228	0	52	68	0.12
Beef, rib eye steak, boneless, lip off, separable lean and fat, trimmed to 0" fat, choice, raw	18.69	18.43	0.2	241	0	51	66	0.2
Beef, rib eye steak, boneless, lip off, separable lean and fat, trimmed to 0" fat, select, raw	20.12	14.14	0	208	0	52	61	0
Beef, rib, back ribs, bone-in, separable lean and fat, trimmed to 0" fat, all grades, cooked, braised	24.23	29.21	0	360	0	63	87	0
Beef, rib, back ribs, bone-in, separable lean and fat, trimmed to 0" fat, choice, cooked, braised	23.34	30.95	0	372	0	61	88	0
Beef, rib, back ribs, bone-in, separable lean and fat, trimmed to 0" fat, select, cooked, braised	25.56	26.59	0	341	0	64	85	0
Beef, rib, back ribs, bone-in, separable lean and fat, trimmed to 0" fat, all grades, raw	16.15	28.42	0.78	324	0	53	75	0.78
Beef, rib, back ribs, bone-in, separable lean and fat, trimmed to 0" fat, choice, raw	15.75	29.89	0.9	336	0	53	76	0.9
Beef, rib, back ribs, bone-in, separable lean and fat, trimmed to 0" fat, select, raw	16.75	26.23	0.6	305	0	52	73	0.6
Beef, loin, top sirloin petite roast, boneless, separable lean only, trimmed to 0" fat, choice, cooked, roasted	28.97	6.37	0	173	0	57	88	0
Beef, loin, top sirloin petite roast/filet, boneless, separable lean only, trimmed to 0" fat, choice, raw	23.03	4.4	0	132	0	65	68	0

Food Name ---> per 100 g	Protein (g)	Fat (g)	Carb (g)	Calories	Fiber (g)	Sodium (mg)	Cholesterol (mg)	Net Carb (g)
Beef, loin, top sirloin cap steak, boneless, separable lean only, trimmed to 1/8" fat, all grades, cooked, grilled	28.26	7.23	0.73	181	0	62	84	0.73
Beef, loin, top sirloin cap steak, boneless, separable lean only, trimmed to 1/8" fat, choice, cooked, grilled	28.19	7.96	1.07	189	0	62	83	1.07
Beef, loin, top sirloin cap steak, boneless, separable lean only, trimmed to 1/8" fat, select, cooked, grilled	28.36	6.14	0.22	170	0	63	85	0.22
Beef, loin, top sirloin cap steak, boneless, separable lean only, trimmed to 1/8" fat, all grades, raw	21.38	5.36	0	134	0	55	67	0
Beef, loin, top sirloin cap steak, boneless, separable lean only, trimmed to 1/8" fat, choice, raw	21.34	5.82	0	138	0	60	67	0
Beef, loin, top sirloin cap steak, boneless, separable lean only, trimmed to 1/8" fat, select, raw	21.44	4.68	0	128	0	52	67	0
Beef, top loin filet, boneless, separable lean only, trimmed to 1/8" fat, all grades, cooked, grilled	29.33	8.54	0.3	195	0	63	86	0.3
Beef, top loin filet, boneless, separable lean only, trimmed to 1/8" fat, choice, cooked, grilled	28.99	9.48	0.36	203	0	62	85	0.36
Beef, top loin filet, boneless, separable lean only, trimmed to 1/8" fat, select, cooked, grilled	29.85	7.12	0.2	184	0	65	87	0.2
Beef, top loin petite roast, boneless, separable lean only, trimmed to 1/8" fat, all grades, cooked, roasted	28.33	8.76	0.82	195	0	62	81	0.82
Beef, top loin petite roast, boneless, separable lean only, trimmed to 1/8" fat, choice, cooked, roasted	28.24	9.97	0.88	206	0	62	79	0.88
Beef, top loin petite roast, boneless, separable lean only, trimmed to 1/8" fat, select, cooked, roasted	28.48	6.95	0.74	179	0	64	85	0.74
Beef, top loin petite roast/filet, boneless, separable lean only, trimmed to 1/8" fat, all grades, raw	22.61	5.84	0	143	0	60	69	0
Beef, top loin petite roast/filet, boneless, separable lean only, trimmed to 1/8" fat, choice, raw	22.5	6.48	0.23	149	0	66	65	0.23
Beef, top loin petite roast/filet, boneless, separable lean only, trimmed to 1/8" fat, select, raw	22.77	4.88	0	135	0	57	76	0
Beef, loin, top sirloin filet, boneless, separable lean only, trimmed to 0" fat, all grades, cooked, grilled	30.58	5.37	0	171	0	59	79	0
Beef, loin, top sirloin filet, boneless, separable lean only, trimmed to 0" fat, choice, cooked, grilled	30.45	5.83	0	174	0	59	81	0
Beef, loin, top sirloin filet, boneless, separable lean only, trimmed to 0" fat, select, cooked, grilled	30.78	4.68	0	165	0	56	74	0
Beef, loin, top sirloin petite roast, boneless, separable lean only, trimmed to 0" fat, all grades, cooked, roasted	29.12	5.92	0	170	0	57	86	0
Beef, loin, top sirloin petite roast, boneless, separable lean only, trimmed to 0" fat, select, cooked, roasted	29.35	5.25	0	165	0	58	84	0
Beef, loin, top sirloin petite roast/filet, boneless, separable lean only, trimmed to 0" fat, all grades, raw	23.04	3.98	0	128	0	65	69	0
Beef, loin, top sirloin petite roast/filet, boneless, separable lean only, trimmed to 0" fat, select, raw	23.05	3.35	0	122	0	58	69	0
Beef, ribeye petite roast/filet, boneless, separable	22.66	4.66	0.04	133	0	66	65	0.04

Food Name ---> per 100 g	Protein (g)	Fat (g)	Carb (g)	Calories	Fiber (g)	Sodium (mg)	Cholesterol (mg)	Net Carb (g)
lean only, trimmed to 0" fat, all grades, raw								
Beef, ribeye petite roast/filet, boneless, separable lean only, trimmed to 0" fat, choice, raw	22.52	5.29	0.18	138	0	66	65	0.18
Beef, ribeye petite roast/filet, boneless, separable lean only, trimmed to 0" fat, select, raw	22.89	3.72	0	125	0	57	65	0
Beef, ribeye cap steak, boneless, separable lean only, trimmed to 0" fat, all grades, cooked, grilled	24.66	15.7	1.53	246	0	86	76	1.53
Beef, ribeye cap steak, boneless, separable lean only, trimmed to 0" fat, choice, cooked, grilled	24.24	17.21	1.81	259	0	86	78	1.81
Beef, ribeye cap steak, boneless, separable lean only, trimmed to 0" fat, select, cooked, grilled	25.28	13.43	1.1	226	0	79	73	1.1
Beef, ribeye cap steak, boneless, separable lean only, trimmed to 0" fat, all grades, raw	19.7	10.6	1.51	180	0	88	64	1.51
Beef, ribeye cap steak, boneless, separable lean only, trimmed to 0" fat, choice, raw	19.46	11.4	1.75	187	0	88	64	1.75
Beef, ribeye cap steak, boneless, separable lean only, trimmed to 0" fat, select, raw	20.05	9.39	1.15	169	0	84	63	1.15
Beef, ribeye filet, boneless, separable lean only, trimmed to 0" fat, all grades, cooked, grilled	28.77	9.2	0.17	199	0	56	82	0.17
Beef, ribeye filet, boneless, separable lean only, trimmed to 0" fat, choice, cooked, grilled	28.35	10.26	0.51	208	0	56	82	0.51
Beef, ribeye filet, boneless, separable lean only, trimmed to 0" fat, select, cooked, grilled	29.39	7.61	0	186	0	87	82	0
Beef, ribeye petite roast, boneless, separable lean only, trimmed to 0" fat, all grades, cooked, roasted	28.15	7.31	0	178	0	55	85	0
Beef, ribeye petite roast, boneless, separable lean only, trimmed to 0" fat, choice, cooked, roasted	28	8.42	0	188	0	54	83	0
Beef, ribeye petite roast, boneless, separable lean only, trimmed to 0" fat, select, cooked, roasted	28.37	5.65	0	164	0	84	89	0
Beef, loin, top sirloin cap steak, boneless, separable lean and fat, trimmed to 1/8" fat, all grades, cooked, grilled	26	15	0.8	242	0	89	84	0.8
Beef, loin, top sirloin cap steak, boneless, separable lean and fat, trimmed to 1/8" fat, choice, cooked, grilled	26.3	14.3	1.1	238	0	91	83	1.1
Beef, loin, top sirloin cap steak, boneless, separable lean and fat, trimmed to 1/8" fat, select, cooked, grilled	25.5	16.1	0.4	249	0	78	85	0.4
Beef, loin, top sirloin cap steak, boneless, separable lean and fat, trimmed to 1/8" fat, all grades, raw	19.9	12.4	0	191	0	80	68	0
Beef, loin, top sirloin cap steak, boneless, separable lean and fat, trimmed to 1/8" fat, choice, raw	19.7	13.4	0	199	0	80	68	0
Beef, loin, top sirloin cap steak, boneless, separable lean and fat, trimmed to 1/8" fat, select, raw	20.1	10.9	0	179	0	78	68	0
Beef, top loin filet, boneless, separable lean and fat, trimmed to 1/8" fat, all grades, cooked, grilled	27.4	14.1	0.6	239	0	93	86	0.6
Beef, top loin filet, boneless, separable lean and fat, trimmed to 1/8" fat, choice, cooked, grilled	26.8	15.9	0.6	253	0	91	85	0.6
Beef, top loin filet, boneless, separable lean and fat, trimmed to 1/8" fat, select, cooked, grilled	28.3	11.6	0.4	219	0	86	87	0.4
Beef, top loin petite roast, boneless, separable lean and fat, trimmed to 1/8" fat, all grades, cooked, roasted	27	12.9	1	228	0	93	82	1

Food Name ---> per 100 g	Protein (g)	Fat (g)	Carb (g)	Calories	Fiber (g)	Sodium (mg)	Cholesterol (mg)	Net Carb (g)
Beef, top loin petite roast, boneless, separable lean and fat, trimmed to 1/8" fat, choice, cooked, roasted	26.8	14.1	1.1	239	0	92	80	1.1
Beef, top loin petite roast, boneless, separable lean and fat, trimmed to 1/8" fat, select, cooked, roasted	27.1	11.2	0.9	213	0	84	85	0.9
Beef, top loin petite roast/filet, boneless, separable lean and fat, trimmed to 1/8" fat, all grades, raw	21.1	11.3	0.3	187	0	89	69	0.3
Beef, top loin petite roast/filet, boneless, separable lean and fat, trimmed to 1/8" fat, choice, raw	20.8	12.6	0.6	199	0	89	65	0.6
Beef, top loin petite roast/filet, boneless, separable lean and fat, trimmed to 1/8" fat, select, raw	21.6	9.3	0	170	0	85	76	0
Beef, Australian, imported, grass-fed, ground, 85% lean / 15% fat, raw	17.72	18.12	0	234	0	62	66	0
Beef, Australian, imported, grass-fed, loin, tenderloin steak/roast, boneless, separable lean only, raw	20.85	6.11	0	138	0	63	49	0
Beef, Australian, imported, Wagyu, loin, tenderloin steak/roast, boneless, separable lean only, Aust. marble score 4/5, raw	20.19	12.3	0	191	0	64	59	0
Beef, Australian, imported, grass-fed, external fat, raw	11.32	51.36	0.39	509	0	36	66	0.39
Beef, Australian, imported, grass-fed, seam fat, raw	9.58	57.73	1.06	562	0	34	65	1.06
Beef, Australian, imported, Wagyu, external fat, Aust. marble score 4/5, raw	6.54	63.27	0	596	0	37	73	0
Beef, Australian, imported, Wagyu, seam fat, Aust. marble score 4/5, raw	6	63.3	0	594	0	32	95	0
Beef, Australian, imported, Wagyu, external fat, Aust. marble score 9, raw	5.54	68.07	0.97	639	0	43	95	0.97
Beef, Australian, imported, Wagyu, seam fat, Aust. marble score 9, raw	5.16	67.33	0	627	0	27	96	0
Beef, Australian, imported, grass-fed, loin, tenderloin steak/roast, boneless, separable lean and fat, raw	20.53	7.63	0.01	151	0	62	50	0.01
Beef, Australian, imported, grass-fed, loin, top loin steak/roast, boneless, separable lean only, raw	21.79	4.87	0	131	0	66	41	0
Beef, Australian, imported, Wagyu, loin, tenderloin steak/roast, boneless, separable lean and fat, Aust. marble score 4/5, raw	19.71	14.09	0	206	0	63	60	0
Beef, Australian, imported, grass-fed, loin, top loin steak/roast, boneless, separable lean and fat, raw	19.9	13.17	0.11	199	0	60	46	0.11
Beef, Australian, imported, grass-fed, loin, top sirloin cap-off steak/roast, boneless, separable lean only, raw	21.9	3.87	0	122	0	60	54	0
Beef, Australian, imported, grass-fed, rib, ribeye steak/roast lip-on, boneless, separable lean only, raw	21.47	8.2	0	160	0	65	50	0
Beef, Australian, imported, grass-fed, round, bottom round steak/roast, boneless, separable lean only, raw	21.4	4.93	0	130	0	71	54	0
Beef, Australian, imported, grass-fed, round, top round cap-off steak/roast, boneless, separable lean only, raw	22.41	4.43	0	129	0	60	48	0
Beef, Australian, imported, Wagyu, loin, tenderloin steak/roast, boneless, separable lean	18.87	17.73	0.57	237	0	62	74	0.57

only, Aust. marble score 9, raw

Food Name ---> per 100 g	Protein (g)	Fat (g)	Carb (g)	Calories	Fiber (g)	Sodium (mg)	Cholesterol (mg)	Net Carb (g)
Beef, Australian, imported, Wagyu, loin, top loin steak/roast, boneless, separable lean only, Aust. marble score 4/5, raw	20.15	15.69	0.2	223	0	61	58	0.2
Beef, Australian, imported, Wagyu, loin, top loin steak/roast, boneless, separable lean only, Aust. marble score 9, raw	16.92	29.15	0.13	331	0	68	61	0.13
Beef, Australian, imported, Wagyu, rib, small end rib steak/roast, boneless, separable lean only, Aust. marble score 4/5, raw	20.35	16.93	0	234	0	58	72	0
Beef, Australian, imported, Wagyu, rib, small end rib steak/roast, boneless, separable lean only, Aust. marble score 9, raw	17.61	28.61	0.46	330	0	65	77	0.46
Beef, Australian, imported, grass-fed, loin, top sirloin cap-off steak/roast, boneless, separable lean and fat, raw	21.77	4.45	0.01	127	0	59	55	0.01
Beef, Australian, imported, grass-fed, rib, ribeye steak/roast lip-on, boneless, separable lean and fat, raw	19.8	15.21	0.11	217	0	60	52	0.11
Beef, Australian, imported, grass-fed, round, bottom round steak/roast, boneless, separable lean and fat, raw	21.13	6.16	0.01	140	0	70	55	0.01
Beef, Australian, imported, grass-fed, round, top round cap-off steak/roast, boneless, separable lean and fat, raw	22.24	4.4	0	129	0	59	47	0
Beef, Australian, imported, Wagyu, loin, top loin steak/roast, boneless, separable lean and fat, Aust. marble score 4/5, raw	17.67	24.2	0.17	289	0	56	63	0.17
Beef, Australian, imported, Wagyu, loin, top loin steak/roast, separable lean and fat, Aust. marble score 9, raw	14.58	36.98	0.22	392	0	61	68	0.22
Beef, Australian, imported, Wagyu, rib, small end rib steak/roast, boneless, separable lean and fat, Aust. marble score 4/5, raw	17.07	27.64	0	317	0	52	76	0
Beef, Australian, imported, Wagyu, rib, small end rib steak/roast, boneless, separable lean and fat, Aust. marble score 9, raw	14.54	38.3	0.42	405	0	57	82	0.42
Beef, Australian, imported, Wagyu, loin, tenderloin steak/roast, boneless, separable lean and fat, Aust. marble score 9, raw	18.5	19.11	0.58	248	0	61	74	0.58
Beef, round, top round steak, boneless, separable lean and fat, trimmed to 0" fat, all grades, raw	23.49	3.34	0	124	0	54	62	0
Beef, round, top round steak, boneless, separable lean and fat, trimmed to 0" fat, choice, raw	23.49	3.66	0	127	0	56	62	0
Beef, round, top round steak, boneless, separable lean and fat, trimmed to 0" fat, select, raw	23.49	2.85	0	120	0	54	63	0
Beef, round, top round roast, boneless, separable lean and fat, trimmed to 0" fat, all grades, raw	23.45	3.5	0	125	0	54	62	0
Beef, round, top round roast, boneless, separable lean and fat, trimmed to 0" fat, choice, raw	23.46	3.81	0	128	0	56	62	0
Beef, round, top round roast, boneless, separable lean and fat, trimmed to 0" fat, select, raw	23.44	3.04	0	121	0	54	63	0
Beef, round, eye of round roast, boneless, separable lean and fat, trimmed to 0" fat, all grades, raw	23.27	3.44	0	124	0	53	60	0
Beef, round, eye of round roast, boneless, separable lean and fat, trimmed to 0" fat, choice,	23.26	3.74	0	127	0	52	58	0

raw

Food Name ---> per 100 g	Protein (g)	Fat (g)	Carb (g)	Calories	Fiber (g)	Sodium (mg)	Cholesterol (mg)	Net Carb (g)
Beef, round, eye of round roast, boneless, separable lean and fat, trimmed to 0" fat, select, raw	23.28	3	0	120	0	50	62	0
Beef, round, eye of round steak, boneless, separable lean and fat, trimmed to 0" fat, all grades, raw	23.26	3.48	0	124	0	53	60	0
Beef, round, eye of round steak, boneless separable lean and fat, trimmed to 0" fat, choice, raw	23.24	3.83	0	127	0	52	58	0
Beef, round, eye of round steak, boneless, separable lean and fat, trimmed to 0" fat, select, raw	23.3	2.95	0	120	0	50	62	0
Beef, loin, tenderloin roast, boneless, separable lean and fat, trimmed to 0" fat, all grades, raw	21.67	6.93	0	149	0	44	61	0
Beef, loin, tenderloin roast, boneless, separable lean and fat, trimmed to 0" fat, choice, raw	21.5	7.4	0	153	0	44	61	0
Beef, loin, tenderloin roast, boneless, separable lean and fat, trimmed to 0" fat, select, raw	21.91	6.21	0	144	0	42	62	0
Beef, loin, top loin steak, boneless, lip off, separable lean and fat, trimmed to 0" fat, all grades, raw	22.43	8.17	0	163	0	45	61	0
Beef, loin, top loin steak, boneless, lip off, separable lean and fat, trimmed to 0" fat, choice, raw	22.19	9.16	0	171	0	45	59	0
Beef, loin, top loin steak, boneless, lip off, separable lean and fat, trimmed to 0" fat, select, raw	22.79	6.67	0	151	0	46	63	0
Beef, loin, tenderloin steak, boneless, separable lean and fat, trimmed to 0" fat, all grades, raw	21.72	6.67	0	147	0	44	61	0
Beef, loin, tenderloin steak, boneless, separable lean and fat, trimmed to 0" fat, choice, raw	21.57	7.1	0	150	0	44	60	0
Beef, loin, tenderloin steak, boneless, separable lean and fat, trimmed to 0" fat, select, raw	21.95	6.02	0	142	0	42	62	0
Beef, loin, tenderloin roast, boneless, separable lean and fat, trimmed to 0" fat, all grades, cooked, roasted	27.31	8.14	0	183	0	56	84	0
Beef, loin, tenderloin roast, boneless, separable lean and fat, trimmed to 0" fat, choice, cooked, roasted	27.26	8.82	0	188	0	56	82	0
Beef, loin, tenderloin roast, boneless, separable lean and fat, trimmed to 0" fat, select, cooked, roasted	27.38	7.12	0	174	0	54	85	0
Beef, round, top round roast, boneless, separable lean and fat, trimmed to 0" fat, all grades, cooked, roasted	29.9	4.49	0	160	0	67	77	0
Beef, round, top round roast, boneless, separable lean and fat, trimmed to 0" fat, choice, cooked, roasted	30.08	4.79	0	163	0	69	76	0
Beef, round, top round roast, boneless, separable lean and fat, trimmed to 0" fat, select, cooked, roasted	30.97	3.72	0	157	0	67	78	0
Beef, round, eye of round steak, boneless, separable lean and fat, trimmed to 0" fat, all grades, cooked, grilled	29.66	4.47	0	159	0	68	78	0
Beef, round, eye of round steak, boneless, separable lean and fat, trimmed to 0" fat, choice,	29.79	4.83	0	163	0	67	76	0

Food Name ---> per 100 g	Protein (g)	Fat (g)	Carb (g)	Calories	Fiber (g)	Sodium (mg)	Cholesterol (mg)	Net Carb (g)
cooked, grilled								
Beef, round, eye of round steak, boneless, separable lean and fat, trimmed to 0" fat, select, cooked, grilled	29.47	3.98	0	154	0	65	81	0
Beef, round, top round steak, boneless, separable lean only, trimmed to 0" fat, all grades, raw	23.59	2.94	0	121	0	54	62	0
Beef, round, top round steak, boneless, separable lean only, trimmed to 0" fat, choice, raw	23.59	3.26	0	124	0	56	61	0
Beef, round, top round steak, boneless, separable lean only, trimmed to 0" fat, select, raw	23.59	2.45	0	116	0	55	63	0
Beef, round, top round roast, boneless, separable lean only, trimmed to 0" fat, all grades, raw	23.59	2.94	0	121	0	54	62	0
Beef, round, top round roast, boneless, separable lean only, trimmed to 0" fat, choice, raw	23.59	3.26	0	124	0	56	61	0
Beef, round, top round roast, boneless, separable lean only, trimmed to 0" fat, select, raw	23.59	2.45	0	116	0	55	63	0
Beef, round, eye of round roast, boneless, separable lean only, trimmed to 0" fat, all grades, raw	23.37	3.04	0	121	0	53	60	0
Beef, round, eye of round roast, boneless, separable lean only, trimmed to 0" fat, choice, raw	23.35	3.38	0	124	0	52	58	0
Beef, round, eye of round roast, boneless, separable lean only, trimmed to 0" fat, select, raw	23.41	2.52	0	116	0	50	62	0
Beef, round, eye of round steak, boneless, separable lean only, trimmed to 0" fat, all grades, raw	23.37	3.04	0	121	0	53	60	0
Beef, round, eye of round steak, boneless, separable lean only, trimmed to 0" fat, choice, raw	23.35	3.38	0	124	0	52	58	0
Beef, round, eye of round steak, boneless, separable lean only, trimmed to 0" fat, select, raw	23.41	2.52	0	116	0	50	62	0
Beef, loin, tenderloin roast, boneless, separable lean only, trimmed to 0" fat, all grades, raw	21.94	5.74	0	139	0	44	61	0
Beef, loin, tenderloin roast, boneless, separable lean only, trimmed to 0" fat, choice, raw	21.78	6.16	0	143	0	45	60	0
Beef, loin, tenderloin roast, boneless, separable lean only, trimmed to 0" fat, select, raw	22.16	5.1	0	135	0	42	62	0
Beef, loin, top loin steak, boneless, lip off, separable lean only, trimmed to 0" fat, all grades, raw	23.07	5.67	0	143	0	46	60	0
Beef, loin, top loin steak, boneless, lip off, separable lean only, trimmed to 0" fat, choice, raw	22.93	6.34	0	149	0	46	58	0
Beef, loin, top loin steak, boneless, lip off, separable lean only, trimmed to 0" fat, select, raw	23.3	4.66	0	135	0	47	62	0
Beef, loin, tenderloin steak, boneless, separable lean only, trimmed to 0" fat, all grades, raw	21.94	5.74	0	139	0	44	61	0
Beef, loin, tenderloin steak, boneless, separable lean only, trimmed to 0" fat, choice, raw	21.78	6.16	0	143	0	45	60	0
Beef, loin, tenderloin steak, boneless, separable lean only, trimmed to 0" fat, select, raw	22.16	5.1	0	135	0	42	62	0
Beef, loin, tenderloin roast, boneless, separable lean only, trimmed to 0" fat, all grades, cooked, roasted	27.51	7.49	0	177	0	56	84	0
Beef, loin, tenderloin roast, boneless, separable lean only, trimmed to 0" fat, choice, cooked, roasted	27.48	8.13	0	183	0	56	82	0
Beef, loin, tenderloin roast, separable lean only, boneless, trimmed to 0" fat, select, cooked,	27.55	6.54	0	169	0	54	85	0

roasted

Food Name ---> per 100 g	Protein (g)	Fat (g)	Carb (g)	Calories	Fiber (g)	Sodium (mg)	Cholesterol (mg)	Net Carb (g)
Beef, round, top round roast, boneless, separable lean only, trimmed to 0" fat, all grades, cooked, roasted	30.09	3.77	0	162	0	67	77	0
Beef, round, top round roast, boneless, separable lean only, trimmed to 0" fat, choice, cooked, roasted	30.24	4.11	0.06	158	0	69	76	0.06
Beef, round, top round roast, boneless, separable lean only, trimmed to 0" fat, select, cooked, roasted	29.81	3.37	0	150	0	67	78	0
Beef, round, eye of round steak, boneless, separable lean only, trimmed to 0" fat, all grades, cooked, grilled	29.85	3.9	0	155	0	68	78	0
Beef, round, eye of round steak, boneless, separable lean only, trimmed to 0" fat, choice, cooked, grilled	29.94	4.26	0	158	0	68	76	0
Beef, round, eye of round steak, boneless, separable lean only, trimmed to 0" fat, select, cooked, grilled	29.52	3.43	0	149	0	65	81	0
Beef, loin, top loin steak, boneless, lip-on, separable lean only, trimmed to 1/8" fat, select, raw	23.3	4.66	0	135	0	47	62	0
Beef, loin, top loin steak, boneless, lip-on, separable lean only, trimmed to 1/8" fat, choice, raw	22.93	6.34	0	149	0	46	58	0
Beef, loin, top loin steak, boneless, lip-on, separable lean only, trimmed to 1/8" fat, all grades, raw	23.07	5.67	0	143	0	46	60	0
Beef, loin, top loin steak, boneless, lip-on, separable lean and fat, trimmed to 1/8" fat, select, raw	21.54	11.65	0	191	0	45	64	0
Beef, loin, top loin steak, boneless, lip-on, separable lean and fat, trimmed to 1/8" fat, all grades, raw	21.29	12.68	0	199	0	44	62	0
Beef, loin, top loin steak, boneless, lip-on, separable lean and fat, trimmed to 1/8" fat, choice, cooked, grilled	25.69	19.19	0	275	0	54	81	0
Beef, loin, top loin steak, boneless, lip-on, separable lean and fat, trimmed to 1/8" fat, select, cooked, grilled	26.92	15.44	0	247	0	50	81	0
Beef, loin, top loin steak, boneless, lip-on, separable lean and fat, trimmed to 1/8" fat, all grades, cooked, grilled	26.18	17.69	0	264	0	52	81	0
Beef, loin, top loin steak, boneless, lip-on, separable lean only, trimmed to 1/8" fat, choice, cooked, grilled	28.66	10.34	0	208	0	56	80	0
Beef, loin, top loin steak, boneless, lip-on, separable lean only, trimmed to 1/8" fat, select, cooked, grilled	29.67	7.26	0	184	0	51	80	0
Beef, loin, top loin steak, boneless, lip-on, separable lean only, trimmed to 1/8" fat, all grades, cooked, grilled	29.06	9.11	0	198	0	54	80	0
Beef, loin, top loin steak, boneless, lip-on, separable lean and fat, trimmed to 1/8" fat, choice, raw	21.13	13.36	0	205	0	44	61	0
Beef, New Zealand, imported, bolar blade, separable lean only, cooked, fast roasted	33.53	6.57	0	193	0	33	91	0

Food Name ---> per 100 g	Protein (g)	Fat (g)	Carb (g)	Calories	Fiber (g)	Sodium (mg)	Cholesterol (mg)	Net Carb (g)
Beef, New Zealand, imported, bolar blade, separable lean only, raw	22.09	4.49	0	129	0	55	56	0
Beef, New Zealand, imported, brisket navel end, separable lean only, cooked, braised	29.35	16.37	0	265	0	39	79	0
Beef, New Zealand, imported, brisket navel end, separable lean only, raw	19.74	12.75	0	194	0	66	53	0
Beef, New Zealand, imported, brisket point end, separable lean only, cooked, braised	34.51	7.05	0	202	0	30	95	0
Beef, New Zealand, imported, brisket point end, separable lean only, raw	20.92	4.62	0	125	0	51	54	0
Beef, New Zealand, imported, chuck eye roll, separable lean only, raw	20.46	5.41	0	131	0	56	61	0
Beef, New Zealand, imported, chuck eye roll, separable lean only, cooked, braised	32.08	8.89	0	208	0	38	98	0
Beef, New Zealand, imported, cube roll, separable lean only, cooked, fast roasted	30.09	13.22	0	239	0	52	94	0
Beef, New Zealand, imported, cube roll, separable lean only, raw	19.77	8.51	1.38	161	0	45	59	1.38
Beef, New Zealand, imported, eye round, separable lean only, cooked, slow roasted	29.68	4.98	0	164	0	43	67	0
Beef, New Zealand, imported, eye round, separable lean only, raw	20.15	3.35	1.35	116	0	40	47	1.35
Beef, New Zealand, imported, flank, separable lean only, cooked, braised	30.75	7.92	0	194	0	28	78	0
Beef, New Zealand, imported, flank, separable lean only, raw	20.53	6.67	0	142	0	47	49	0
Beef, New Zealand, imported, flat, separable lean only, cooked, braised	33.22	10.3	0	226	0	30	94	0
Beef, New Zealand, imported, flat, separable lean only, raw	21.3	7.69	0	154	0	50	55	0
Beef, New Zealand, imported, variety meats and by-products, heart, cooked, boiled	31.29	6	0	179	0	59	201	0
Beef, New Zealand, imported, variety meats and by-products, heart, raw	18.52	3.4	0	105	0	86	124	0
Beef, New Zealand, imported, hind shin, separable lean only, cooked, braised	31.23	4.64	0	167	0	44	89	0
Beef, New Zealand, imported, hind shin, separable lean only, raw	21.46	3.12	0	114	0	63	56	0
Beef, New Zealand, imported, inside, raw	22.16	4.36	0.1	128	0	40	55	0.1
Beef, New Zealand, imported, intermuscular fat, cooked	7.9	57.22	3.39	560	0	25	87	3.39
Beef, New Zealand, imported, intermuscular fat, raw	6.97	63.78	0.01	602	0	32	104	0.01
Beef, New Zealand, imported, variety meats and by-products, kidney, cooked, boiled	27.28	5.27	0	157	0	123	1002	0
Beef, New Zealand, imported, knuckle, cooked, fast fried	27.51	7.58	0	178	0	49	76	0
Beef, New Zealand, imported, variety meats and by-products, kidney, raw	15.68	2.64	0	87	0	175	404	0
Beef, New Zealand, imported, variety meats and by-products liver, cooked, boiled	23.3	4.68	3.78	150	0	55	243	3.78
Beef, New Zealand, imported, variety meats and by-products, liver, raw	20.5	4.05	3.6	133	0	53	254	3.6
Beef, New Zealand, imported, manufacturing beef, cooked, boiled	24.21	3.26	0	126	0	32	67	0
Beef, New Zealand, imported, manufacturing	21.23	3.68	0.23	119	0	55	49	0.23

Food Name ---> per 100 g	Protein (g)	Fat (g)	Carb (g)	Calories	Fiber (g)	Sodium (mg)	Cholesterol (mg)	Net Carb (g)
beef, raw								
Beef, New Zealand, imported, oyster blade, separable lean only, cooked, braised	29.87	8.46	0	196	0	25	87	0
Beef, New Zealand, imported, oyster blade, separable lean only, raw	21.83	7.56	0	155	0	59	56	0
Beef, New Zealand, imported, ribs prepared, cooked, fast roasted	27.23	9.74	0.09	197	0	58	69	0.09
Beef, New Zealand, imported, ribs prepared, raw	21.31	6.78	0	146	0	54	57	0
Beef, New Zealand, imported, rump centre, separable lean only, cooked, fast fried	30.17	7.48	0	188	0	55	78	0
Beef, New Zealand, imported, striploin, separable lean only, cooked, fast fried	28.53	11.4	0	217	0	55	70	0
Beef, New Zealand, imported, striploin, separable lean only, raw	20.93	7	0.74	150	0	47	54	0.74
Beef, New Zealand, imported, subcutaneous fat, cooked	6.5	78.3	0	731	0	25	63	0
Beef, New Zealand, imported, subcutaneous fat, raw	8.5	72.38	0	685	0	26	64	0
Beef, New Zealand, imported, sweetbread, cooked, boiled	12.53	29.79	0	318	0	52	249	0
Beef, New Zealand, imported, sweetbread, raw	11.51	28.6	0	303	0	64	217	0
Beef, New Zealand, imported, tenderloin, separable lean only, cooked, fast fried	29.37	9.01	0.27	200	0	45	81	0.27
Beef, New Zealand, imported, oyster blade, separable lean and fat, raw	21.27	10.31	0	178	0	57	56	0
Beef, New Zealand, imported, tenderloin, separable lean only, raw	21.19	6.1	0	140	0	39	58	0
Beef, New Zealand, imported, variety meats and by-products, tongue, cooked, boiled	18.31	20.34	3.68	271	0	57	105	3.68
Beef, New Zealand, imported, variety meats and by-products, tongue, raw	17.77	19.09	0	243	0	73	81	0
Beef, New Zealand, imported, variety meats and by-products, tripe cooked, boiled	19	2.98	0	103	0	40	199	0
Beef, New Zealand, imported, variety meats and by-products, tripe uncooked, raw	14.86	1.98	0	77	0	81	117	0
Beef, New Zealand, imported, bolar blade, separable lean and fat, cooked, fast roasted	31.3	11.37	0	228	0	33	92	0
Beef, New Zealand, imported, bolar blade, separable lean and fat, raw	21.29	8.22	0	159	0	54	57	0
Beef, New Zealand, imported, brisket navel end, separable lean and fat, cooked, braised	20.14	41.33	0	453	0	33	72	0
Beef, New Zealand, imported, brisket navel end, separable lean and fat, raw	15.81	31.27	0	345	0	54	62	0
Beef, New Zealand, imported, brisket point end, separable lean and fat, cooked, braised	31.94	13.6	0	250	0	29	92	0
Beef, New Zealand, imported, brisket point end, separable lean and fat, raw	20.05	9.23	0	163	0	49	55	0
Beef, New Zealand, imported, chuck eye roll, separable lean and fat, cooked, braised	29.92	14.74	0	252	0	37	95	0
Beef, New Zealand, imported, chuck eye roll, separable lean and fat, raw	19.38	11.45	0	181	0	53	61	0
Beef, New Zealand, imported, cube roll, separable lean and fat, cooked, fast roasted	27.79	19.45	0.03	286	0	49	91	0.03
Beef, New Zealand, imported, cube roll, separable lean and fat, raw	18.22	16.31	1.31	225	0	43	60	1.31
Beef, New Zealand, imported, eye round,	29.49	5.57	0	168	0	43	67	0

Food Name ---> per 100 g	Protein (g)	Fat (g)	Carb (g)	Calories	Fiber (g)	Sodium (mg)	Cholesterol (mg)	Net Carb (g)
separable lean and fat, cooked, slow roasted								
Beef, New Zealand, imported, eye round, separable lean and fat, raw	19.88	4.92	1.32	129	0	39	48	1.32
Beef, New Zealand, imported, flank, separable lean and fat, cooked, braised	30.13	9.73	0	208	0	28	78	0
Beef, New Zealand, imported, flank, separable lean and fat, raw	20.12	8.9	0	161	0	46	49	0
Beef, New Zealand, imported, flat, separable lean and fat, cooked, braised	31.86	13.79	0	252	0	30	92	0
Beef, New Zealand, imported, flat, separable lean and fat, raw	20.57	10.55	0	177	0	49	58	0
Beef, New Zealand, imported, hind shin, separable lean and fat, cooked, braised	29.82	8.5	0.07	196	0	43	88	0.07
Beef, New Zealand, imported, hind shin, separable lean and fat, raw	20.61	7.2	0	147	0	61	57	0
Beef, New Zealand, imported, oyster blade, separable lean and fat, cooked, braised	29.79	8.68	0	197	0	25	87	0
Beef, New Zealand, imported, rump centre, separable lean and fat, cooked, fast fried	30.01	7.96	0	192	0	55	78	0
Beef, New Zealand, imported, rump centre, separable lean only, raw	21.74	6.05	0	141	0	49	55	0
Beef, New Zealand, imported, rump centre, separable lean and fat, raw	21.65	6.5	0	145	0	49	55	0
Beef, New Zealand, imported, striploin, separable lean and fat, cooked, fast fried	24.89	22.33	0.02	301	0	50	69	0.02
Beef, New Zealand, imported, striploin, separable lean and fat, raw	18.49	19.53	0.6	252	0	43	57	0.6
Beef, New Zealand, imported, tenderloin, separable lean and fat, cooked, fast fried	29.26	9.35	0.27	202	0	45	81	0.27
Beef, New Zealand, imported, tenderloin, separable lean and fat, raw	21.04	6.88	0	146	0	39	58	0
Beef, ground, 93% lean meat / 7% fat, raw	20.85	7	0	152	0	66	63	0
Beef, ground, 93% lean meat / 7% fat, patty, cooked, broiled	26.22	8.94	0	193	0	66	88	0
Beef, ground, 93% lean meat /7% fat, patty, cooked, pan-broiled	25.56	8.01	0.06	182	0	72	84	0.06
Beef, ground, 93% lean meat / 7% fat, loaf, cooked, baked	27.03	8.43	0	192	0	59	88	0
Beef, ground, 93% lean meat / 7% fat, crumbles, cooked, pan-browned	28.88	9.51	0	209	0	86	89	0
Beef, ground, 97% lean meat / 3% fat, raw	21.98	3	0	121	0	66	60	0
Beef, ground, 97% lean meat / 3% fat, patty, cooked, broiled	26.36	4.46	0	153	0	64	88	0
Beef, ground, 97% lean meat /3% fat, patty, cooked, pan-broiled	26.03	3.65	0	144	0	69	84	0
Beef, ground, 97% lean meat / 3% fat, loaf, cooked, baked	27.58	4.06	0	154	0	56	88	0
Beef, ground, 97% lean meat / 3% fat, crumbles, cooked, pan-browned	29.46	5.46	0	175	0	84	89	0
Beef, composite of trimmed retail cuts, separable lean and fat, trimmed to 0" fat, all grades, raw	20.95	9.3	0.05	169	0	61	65	0.05
Beef, composite of trimmed retail cuts, separable lean only, trimmed to 1/8" fat, all grades, raw	22.15	5.38	0	140	0	56	62	0
Beef, composite of trimmed retail cuts, separable lean only, trimmed to 1/8" fat, all grades, cooked	28.95	8.15	0	194	0	54	80	0
Beef, composite of trimmed retail cuts, separable	22.15	5.54	0.08	139	0	60	63	0.08

lean only, trimmed to 0" fat, all grades, raw

Food Name ---> per 100 g	Protein (g)	Fat (g)	Carb (g)	Calories	Fiber (g)	Sodium (mg)	Cholesterol (mg)	Net Carb (g)
Beef, composite of trimmed retail cuts, separable lean only, trimmed to 1/8" fat, choice, raw	22.01	6.05	0	147	0	55	62	0
Beef composite, separable lean only, trimmed to 1/8" fat, choice, cooked	28.73	9.16	0	203	0	53	82	0
Beef, composite of trimmed retail cuts, separable lean and fat, trimmed to 0" fat, choice, raw	21.34	10.08	0.06	176	0	61	66	0.06
Beef, composite of trimmed retail cuts, separable lean only, trimmed to 0" fat, choice, raw	21.55	7.24	0	151	0	66	66	0
Beef, composite of trimmed retail cuts, separable lean only, trimmed to 0" fat, select, raw	22.03	4.99	0.05	133	0	63	64	0.05
Beef, composite of trimmed retail cuts, separable lean and fat, trimmed to 0" fat, select, raw	21.2	8	0.04	157	0	61	64	0.04
Beef, composite of trimmed retail cuts, separable lean only, trimmed to 1/8" fat, select, cooked	27.51	6.37	0	167	0	51	74	0
Beef, composite of trimmed retail cuts, separable lean only, trimmed to 1/8" fat, select, raw	22.37	4.55	0	130	0	58	62	0
USDA Commodity, beef patties with VPP, frozen, cooked	15.64	16.94	7.89	247	1.4	66	38	6.49
USDA Commodity, beef, ground bulk/coarse ground, frozen, cooked	26.06	16.34	0	259	0	95	89	0
USDA Commodity, beef, patties (100%), frozen, cooked	22.98	16.37	0.91	249	0	66	86	0.91
USDA Commodity, beef patties with VPP, frozen, raw	15.21	16.48	3.84	225	1.3	55	33	2.54
USDA Commodity, beef, patties (100%), frozen, raw	14.63	15.69	0	204	0	74	53	0
USDA Commodity, beef, ground, bulk/coarse ground, frozen, raw	17.37	17.07	0	228	0	57	69	0
Beef, chuck, mock tender steak, separable lean only, trimmed to 0" fat, all grades, cooked, broiled	25.9	5.42	0	159	0	71	63	0
Beef, chuck, top blade, separable lean only, trimmed to 0" fat, all grades, cooked, broiled	26.13	10.16	0	203	0	68	60	0
Beef, chuck, clod roast, separable lean only, trimmed to 1/4" fat, all grades, raw	19.63	5.02	0	129	0	64	59	0
Beef, chuck, clod roast, separable lean only, trimmed to 0" fat, all grades, cooked, roasted	26.82	6.34	0	172	0	74	67	0
Beef, chuck, clod roast, separable lean only, trimmed to 1/4" fat, all grades, cooked, roasted	26.36	6.75	0	173	0	71	71	0
Beef, shoulder steak, boneless, separable lean only, trimmed to 0" fat, all grades, cooked, grilled	28.6	5.82	0	175	0	68	82	0
Beef, chuck, clod steak, separable lean only, trimmed to 1/4" fat, all grades, cooked, braised	29.34	7.04	0	189	0	60	94	0
Beef, chuck, mock tender steak, separable lean and fat, trimmed to 0" fat, USDA choice, cooked, broiled	25.73	5.72	0	161	0	73	65	0
Beef, chuck, mock tender steak, separable lean and fat, trimmed to 0" fat, USDA select, cooked, broiled	26.08	5.24	0	159	0	68	60	0
Beef, chuck, top blade, separable lean and fat, trimmed to 0" fat, choice, cooked, broiled	25.77	12.93	0	227	0	68	58	0
Beef, chuck, top blade, separable lean and fat, trimmed to 0" fat, select, cooked, broiled	25.67	9.99	0	200	0	67	67	0
Beef, chuck, clod roast, separable lean and fat, trimmed to 0" fat, choice, cooked, roasted	24.61	12.26	0	216	0	71	67	0
Beef, chuck, clod roast, separable lean and fat,	27.3	8.76	0	196	0	72	73	0

Food Name ---> per 100 g	Protein (g)	Fat (g)	Carb (g)	Calories	Fiber (g)	Sodium (mg)	Cholesterol (mg)	Net Carb (g)
trimmed to 0" fat, select, cooked, roasted								
Beef, shoulder steak, boneless, separable lean and fat, trimmed to 0" fat, choice, cooked, grilled	28.22	7.25	0	186	0	67	81	0
Beef, shoulder steak, boneless, separable lean and fat, trimmed to 0" fat, select, cooked, grilled	28.41	6.14	0	177	0	67	83	0
Beef, plate, inside skirt steak, separable lean and fat, trimmed to 0" fat, all grades, cooked, broiled	26.13	12.05	0	220	0	75	60	0
Beef, plate, outside skirt steak, separable lean and fat, trimmed to 0" fat, all grades, cooked, broiled	23.51	17.13	0	255	0	92	59	0
Beef, loin, bottom sirloin butt, tri-tip steak, separable lean and fat, trimmed to 0" fat, all grades, cooked, broiled	29.97	15.18	0	265	0	72	68	0
Beef, chuck, mock tender steak, separable lean and fat, trimmed to 0" fat, all grades, cooked, broiled	25.87	5.52	0	160	0	71	63	0
Beef, chuck, top blade, separable lean and fat, trimmed to 0" fat, all grades, cooked, broiled	25.73	11.73	0	216	0	67	61	0
Beef, chuck, clod roast, separable lean and fat, trimmed to 0" fat, all grades, cooked, roasted	25.7	10.84	0	207	0	71	69	0
Beef, shoulder steak, boneless, separable lean and fat, trimmed to 0" fat, all grades, cooked, grilled	28.29	6.8	0	182	0	67	81	0
Beef, ground, 95% lean meat / 5% fat, raw	21.41	5	0	137	0	66	62	0
Beef, ground, 95% lean meat / 5% fat, patty, cooked, broiled	26.29	6.8	0	174	0	65	88	0
Beef, ground, 95% lean meat / 5% fat, patty, cooked, pan-broiled	25.8	5.94	0	164	0	71	84	0
Beef, ground, 95% lean meat / 5% fat, crumbles, cooked, pan-browned	29.17	7.58	0	193	0	85	89	0
Beef, ground, 95% lean meat / 5% fat, loaf, cooked, baked	27.31	6.37	0	174	0	58	88	0
Beef, ground, 90% lean meat / 10% fat, raw	20	10	0	176	0	66	65	0
Beef, ground, 90% lean meat / 10% fat, patty, cooked, broiled	26.11	11.75	0	217	0	68	88	0
Beef, ground, 90% lean meat / 10% fat, patty, cooked, pan-broiled	25.21	10.68	0	204	0	75	84	0
Beef, ground, 90% lean meat / 10% fat, crumbles, cooked, pan-browned	28.45	12.04	0	230	0	87	89	0
Beef, ground, 90% lean meat / 10% fat, loaf, cooked, baked	26.62	11.1	0	214	0	61	88	0
Beef, ground, 85% lean meat / 15% fat, raw	18.59	15	0	215	0	66	68	0
Beef, ground, 85% lean meat / 15% fat, patty, cooked, broiled	25.93	15.41	0	250	0	72	88	0
Beef, ground, 85% lean meat / 15% fat, patty, cooked, pan-broiled	24.62	14.02	0	232	0	79	84	0
Beef, ground, 85% lean meat / 15% fat, crumbles, cooked, pan-browned	27.73	15.3	0	256	0	89	89	0
Beef, ground, 85% lean meat / 15% fat, loaf, cooked, baked	25.93	14.36	0	240	0	64	88	0
Beef, ground, 80% lean meat / 20% fat, raw	17.17	20	0	254	0	66	71	0
Beef, ground, 80% lean meat / 20% fat, patty, cooked, broiled	25.75	17.78	0	270	0	75	88	0
Beef, ground, 80% lean meat / 20% fat, patty, cooked, pan-broiled	24.04	15.94	0	246	0	83	84	0
Beef, ground, 80% lean meat / 20% fat, crumbles, cooked, pan-browned	27	17.36	0	272	0	91	89	0
Beef, ground, 80% lean meat / 20% fat, loaf,	25.25	16.17	0	254	0	67	88	0

cooked, baked

Food Name ---> per 100 g	Protein (g)	Fat (g)	Carb (g)	Calories	Fiber (g)	Sodium (mg)	Cholesterol (mg)	Net Carb (g)
Beef, ground, 75% lean meat / 25% fat, raw	15.76	25	0	293	0	66	75	0
Beef, ground, 75% lean meat / 25% fat, patty, cooked, broiled	25.56	18.87	0	279	0	78	88	0
Beef, ground, 75% lean meat / 25% fat, patty, cooked, pan-broiled	23.45	16.44	0	248	0	87	84	0
Beef, ground, 75% lean meat / 25% fat, crumbles, cooked, pan-browned	26.28	18.21	0	277	0	93	89	0
Beef, ground, 75% lean meat / 25% fat, loaf, cooked, baked	24.56	16.5	0	254	0	70	88	0
Beef, rib, small end (ribs 10-12), separable lean only, trimmed to 1/8" fat, select, raw	22.53	4.2	0	134	0	55	73	0
Beef, tenderloin, steak, separable lean only, trimmed to 1/8" fat, select, raw	22.06	5.93	0	148	0	55	64	0
Beef, top sirloin, steak, separable lean only, trimmed to 1/8" fat, select, raw	22.27	3.54	0	127	0	56	59	0
Beef, short loin, top loin, steak, separable lean only, trimmed to 1/8" fat, select, raw	23.07	3.88	0	133	0	57	40	0
Beef, rib, small end (ribs 10-12), separable lean only, trimmed to 1/8" fat, select, cooked, broiled	30.87	6.22	0	188	0	66	98	0
Beef, tenderloin, steak, separable lean only, trimmed to 1/8" fat, select, cooked, broiled	29.07	7.76	0	194	0	62	83	0
Beef, top sirloin, steak, separable lean only, trimmed to 1/8" fat, select, cooked, broiled	29.34	4.96	0	170	0	62	77	0
Beef, short loin, top loin, steak, separable lean only, trimmed to 1/8" fat, select, cooked, grilled	29.44	5.73	0	177	0	62	78	0
Beef, round, bottom round , roast, separable lean only, trimmed to 1/8" fat, select, cooked, roasted	28.45	4.67	0	164	0	38	74	0
Beef, round, eye of round, roast, separable lean only, trimmed to 1/8" fat, select, cooked, roasted	29.59	4.11	0	163	0	39	75	0
Beef, round, top round, steak, separable lean only, trimmed to 1/8" fat, select, cooked, broiled	31.61	4.65	0	177	0	43	82	0
Beef, round, bottom round, steak, separable lean only, trimmed to 1/8" fat, select, cooked, braised	34.46	6.43	0	205	0	46	92	0
Beef, round, bottom round, roast, separable lean only, trimmed to 1/8" fat, all grades, raw	22.19	4.31	0	128	0	59	61	0
Beef, brisket, flat half, separable lean only, trimmed to 1/8" fat, all grades, cooked, braised	33.15	6	0	196	0	54	97	0
Beef, brisket, flat half, separable lean only, trimmed to 1/8" fat, all grades, raw	21.57	3.84	0	127	0	74	65	0
Beef, round, eye of round, roast, separable lean only, trimmed to 1/8" fat, all grades, raw	22.6	3	0	124	0	60	59	0
Beef, round, eye of round, roast, separable lean only, trimmed to 1/8" fat, all grades, cooked, roasted	29.73	4.71	0	169	0	38	76	0
Beef, rib, small end (ribs 10-12), separable lean only, trimmed to 1/8" fat, all grades, raw	22.33	5.04	0	141	0	56	75	0
Beef, tenderloin, steak, separable lean only, trimmed to 1/8" fat, all grades, cooked, broiled	29.04	8.39	0	200	0	60	82	0
Beef, tenderloin, steak, separable lean only, trimmed to 1/8" fat, all grades, raw	22.12	6.52	0	153	0	56	65	0
Beef, chuck, arm pot roast, separable lean only, trimmed to 1/8" fat, all grades, cooked, braised	34.66	7.36	0	214	0	56	104	0
Beef, chuck, arm pot roast, separable lean only, trimmed to 1/8" fat, all grades, raw	22.11	4.19	0	132	0	74	65	0
Beef, round, bottom round, roast, separable lean	28	5.72	0	163	0	37	76	0

Food Name ---> per 100 g	Protein (g)	Fat (g)	Carb (g)	Calories	Fiber (g)	Sodium (mg)	Cholesterol (mg)	Net Carb (g)
only, trimmed to 1/8" fat, all grades, cooked								
Beef, round, bottom round, steak, separable lean only, trimmed to 1/8" fat, all grades, cooked, braised	34.34	7.73	0	216	0	45	94	0
Beef, short loin, top loin, steak, separable lean only, trimmed to 1/8" fat, all grades, cooked, broiled	29.3	7.09	0	189	0	61	81	0
Beef, short loin, top loin steak, separable lean only, trimmed to 1/8" fat, all grades, raw	22.93	5.15	0	138	0	57	53	0
Beef, round, top round, steak, separable lean only, trimmed to 1/8" fat, all grades, cooked, broiled	31.82	5.45	0	185	0	42	84	0
Beef, round, top round, steak, separable lean only, trimmed to 1/8" fat, all grades, raw	22.91	4.09	0	135	0	61	55	0
Beef, top sirloin, steak, separable lean only, trimmed to 1/8" fat, all grades, cooked, broiled	29.42	5.84	0	178	0	61	79	0
Beef, top sirloin, steak, separable lean only, trimmed to 1/8" fat, all grades, raw	22.09	4.08	0	131	0	56	60	0
Beef, chuck, arm pot roast, separable lean only, trimmed to 1/8" fat, choice, raw	21.96	5.05	0	139	0	74	65	0
Beef, brisket, flat half, separable lean only, trimmed to 1/8" fat, choice, raw	21.69	4.06	0	129	0	75	65	0
Beef, chuck, arm pot roast, separable lean only, trimmed to 1/8" fat, choice, cooked, braised	34.72	8.37	0	224	0	56	106	0
Beef, brisket, flat half, separable lean only, trimmed to 1/8" fat, choice, cooked, braised	33.13	6.79	0	203	0	53	97	0
Beef, round, eye of round, roast, separable lean only, trimmed to 1/8" fat, choice, raw	22.88	3.38	0	128	0	57	60	0
Beef, round, top round, steak, separable lean only, trimmed to 1/8" fat, choice, raw	22.69	4.78	0	140	0	57	63	0
Beef, round, bottom round, roast, separable lean only, trimmed to 1/8" fat, choice, raw	22.22	4.96	0	140	0	56	62	0
Beef, round, bottom round, roast, separable lean only, trimmed to 1/8" fat, choice, cooked, roasted	27.56	6.77	0	179	0	36	77	0
Beef, round, eye of round, roast, separable lean only, trimmed to 1/8" fat, choice, cooked, roasted	29.87	5.3	0	175	0	39	78	0
Beef, round, top round, steak, separable lean only, trimmed to 1/8" fat, choice, cooked, broiled	32.04	6.25	0	193	0	42	86	0
Beef, round, bottom round, steak, separable lean only, trimmed to 1/8" fat, choice, cooked, braised	34.22	9.02	0	228	0	45	97	0
Beef, rib, small end (ribs 10-12), separable lean only, trimmed to 1/8" fat, choice, raw	22.12	5.91	0	148	0	57	68	0
Beef, tenderloin, steak, separable lean only, trimmed to 1/8" fat, choice, raw	22.17	7.07	0	158	0	57	66	0
Beef, top sirloin, steak, separable lean only, trimmed to 1/8" fat, choice, raw	21.91	4.62	0	135	0	57	61	0
Beef, rib, small end (ribs 10-12), separable lean only, trimmed to 1/8"fat, choice, cooked, broiled	28.29	9.05	0	202	0	58	88	0
Beef, short loin, top loin, steak, separable lean only, trimmed to 1/8" fat, choice, raw	22.78	6.43	0	155	0	58	66	0
Beef, tenderloin, steak, separable lean only, trimmed to 1/8" fat, choice, cooked, broiled	29.01	9.1	0	206	0	59	85	0
Beef, top sirloin, steak, separable lean only, trimmed to 1/8" fat, choice, cooked, broiled	29.51	6.72	0	187	0	61	81	0
Beef, short loin, top loin, steak, separable lean only, trimmed to 1/8" fat, choice, cooked, broiled	29.16	8.45	0	201	0	60	84	0
Beef, chuck, arm pot roast, separable lean only,	22.26	3.32	0	125	0	77	66	0

Food Name ---> per 100 g	Protein (g)	Fat (g)	Carb (g)	Calories	Fiber (g)	Sodium (mg)	Cholesterol (mg)	Net Carb (g)
trimmed to 1/8" fat, select, raw								
Beef, brisket, flat half, separable lean only, trimmed to 1/8" fat, select, raw	21.45	3.61	0	124	0	76	66	0
Beef, chuck, arm pot roast, separable lean only, trimmed to 1/8" fat, select, cooked, braised	34.6	6.35	0	205	0	57	103	0
Beef, brisket, flat half, separable lean only, trimmed to 1/8" fat, select, cooked, braised	33.18	5.21	0	189	0	55	98	0
Beef, round, eye of round, roast, separable lean only, trimmed to 1/8" fat, select, raw	22.31	2.62	0	119	0	62	58	0
Beef, round, top round, steak, separable lean only, trimmed to 1/8" fat, select, raw	23.13	3.37	0	129	0	64	61	0
Beef, round, bottom round, roast, separable lean only, trimmed to 1/8" fat, select, raw	22.18	3.66	0	128	0	62	59	0
Beef, rib, small end (ribs 10-12), separable lean only, trimmed to 1/8" fat, all grades, cooked, broiled	29.58	7.63	0	195	0	62	87	0
Beef, variety meats and by-products, tripe, cooked, simmered	11.71	4.05	1.99	94	0	68	157	1.99
Beef, bottom sirloin, tri-tip roast, separable lean only, trimmed to 0" fat, all grades, raw	21.26	5.63	0	142	0	54	61	0
Beef, bottom sirloin, tri-tip roast, separable lean only, trimmed to 0" fat, choice, cooked, roasted	26.34	9.73	0	193	0	54	80	0
Beef, bottom sirloin, tri-tip roast, separable lean only, trimmed to 0" fat, choice, raw	21.17	7.06	0	154	0	54	64	0
Beef, bottom sirloin, tri-tip roast, separable lean only, trimmed to 0" fat, select, cooked, roasted	27.17	6.95	0	179	0	58	76	0
Beef, bottom sirloin, tri-tip roast, separable lean only, trimmed to 0" fat, select, raw	21.34	4.21	0	129	0	54	59	0
Beef, round, tip round, roast, separable lean only, trimmed to 0" fat, all grades, raw	21.07	3.95	0	126	0	54	57	0
Beef, round, tip round, roast, separable lean only, trimmed to 0" fat, choice, raw	20.76	4.55	0	130	0	52	58	0
Beef, round, tip round, roast, separable lean only, trimmed to 0" fat, select, raw	21.38	3.35	0	122	0	58	55	0
Beef, flank, steak, separable lean only, trimmed to 0" fat, all grades, cooked, broiled	27.89	7.4	0	186	0	57	78	0
Beef, flank, steak, separable lean only, trimmed to 0" fat, select, cooked, broiled	27.96	6.48	0	178	0	59	76	0
Beef, flank, steak, separable lean only, trimmed to 0" fat, all grades, raw	21.57	5.47	0	141	0	55	62	0
Beef, flank, steak, separable lean only, trimmed to 0" fat, select, raw	21.43	5	0	137	0	53	60	0
Beef, brisket, flat half, separable lean and fat, trimmed to 1/8" fat, choice, raw	18.12	22.15	0.12	278	0	61	91	0.12
Beef, brisket, flat half, separable lean and fat, trimmed to 1/8" fat, select, raw	17.77	22.21	0	276	0	58	94	0
Beef, brisket, flat half, separable lean and fat, trimmed to 1/8" fat, choice, cooked, braised	28.66	19.47	0	298	0	46	107	0

Cereal Grains and Pasta

Food Name ---> per 100 g	Protein (g)	Fat (g)	Carbohydrates (g)	Calories	Fiber (g)	Sodium (mg)	Cholesterol (mg)	Net Carb (g)
Amaranth grain, uncooked	13.56	7.02	65.25	371	6.7	4	0	58.55
Amaranth grain, cooked	3.8	1.58	18.69	102	2.1	6	0	16.59
Arrowroot flour	0.3	0.1	88.15	357	3.4	2	0	84.75
Barley, hulled	12.48	2.3	73.48	354	17.3	12	0	56.18
Barley, pearled, raw	9.91	1.16	77.72	352	15.6	9	0	62.12
Barley, pearled, cooked	2.26	0.44	28.22	123	3.8	3	0	24.42
Buckwheat	13.25	3.4	71.5	343	10	1	0	61.5
Buckwheat groats, roasted, dry	11.73	2.71	74.95	346	10.3	11	0	64.65
Buckwheat groats, roasted, cooked	3.38	0.62	19.94	92	2.7	4	0	17.24
Buckwheat flour, whole-groat	12.62	3.1	70.59	335	10	11	0	60.59
Bulgur, dry	12.29	1.33	75.87	342	12.5	17	0	63.37
Bulgur, cooked	3.08	0.24	18.58	83	4.5	5	0	14.08
Corn grain, yellow	9.42	4.74	74.26	365	7.3	35	0	66.96
Corn bran, crude	8.36	0.92	85.64	224	79	7	0	6.64
Corn flour, whole-grain, yellow	6.93	3.86	76.85	361	7.3	5	0	69.55
Corn flour, masa, enriched, white	8.46	3.69	76.59	363	6.4	5	0	70.19
Corn flour, yellow, degermed, unenriched	5.59	1.39	82.75	375	1.9	1	0	80.85
Corn flour, masa, unenriched, white	8.46	3.69	76.59	363	6.4	5	0	70.19
Cornmeal, whole-grain, yellow	8.12	3.59	76.89	362	7.3	35	0	69.59
Cornmeal, degermed, enriched, yellow	7.11	1.75	79.45	370	3.9	7	0	75.55
Cornmeal, yellow, self-rising, bolted, plain, enriched	8.28	3.4	70.28	334	6.7	1247	0	63.58
Cornmeal, yellow, self-rising, bolted, with wheat flour added, enriched	8.41	2.85	73.43	348	6.3	1319	0	67.13
Cornmeal, yellow, self-rising, degermed, enriched	8.41	1.72	74.79	355	7.1	1348	0	67.69
Cornstarch	0.26	0.05	91.27	381	0.9	9	0	90.37
Couscous, dry	12.76	0.64	77.43	376	5	10	0	72.43
Couscous, cooked	3.79	0.16	23.22	112	1.4	5	0	21.82
Hominy, canned, white	1.48	0.88	14.26	72	2.5	345	0	11.76
Millet, raw	11.02	4.22	72.85	378	8.5	5	0	64.35
Millet, cooked	3.51	1	23.67	119	1.3	2	0	22.37
Oat bran, raw	17.3	7.03	66.22	246	15.4	4	0	50.82
Oat bran, cooked	3.21	0.86	11.44	40	2.6	1	0	8.84
Quinoa, uncooked	14.12	6.07	64.16	368	7	5	0	57.16
Rice, brown, long-grain, raw	7.54	3.2	76.25	367	3.6	5	0	72.65
Rice, brown, long-grain, cooked	2.74	0.97	25.58	123	1.6	4	0	23.98
Oats	16.89	6.9	66.27	389	10.6	2	0	55.67
Rice, brown, medium-grain, raw	7.5	2.68	76.17	362	3.4	4	0	72.77
Rice, brown, medium-grain, cooked	2.32	0.83	23.51	112	1.8	1	0	21.71
Rice, brown, parboiled, dry, UNCLE BEN'S	7.6	2.75	78.68	370	3.5	6	0	75.18
Rice, white, long-grain, regular, raw, enriched	7.13	0.66	79.95	365	1.3	5	0	78.65
Rice, white, long-grain, regular, enriched, cooked	2.69	0.28	28.17	130	0.4	1	0	27.77
Rice, white, long-grain, parboiled, enriched, dry	7.51	1.03	80.89	374	1.8	2	0	79.09
Rice, white, long-grain, parboiled, enriched, cooked	2.91	0.37	26.05	123	0.9	2	0	25.15
Rice, white, long-grain, precooked or instant, enriched, dry	7.82	0.94	82.32	380	1.9	10	0	80.42

Food Name ---> per 100 g	Protein (g)	Fat (g)	Carbohydrates (g)	Calories	Fiber (g)	Sodium (mg)	Cholesterol (mg)	Net Carb (g)
Rice, white, long-grain, precooked or instant, enriched, prepared	2.18	0.5	26.76	124	0.6	4	0	26.16
Rice, white, medium-grain, raw, enriched	6.61	0.58	79.34	360	1.4	1	0	77.94
Rice, white, medium-grain, enriched, cooked	2.38	0.21	28.59	130	0.3	0	0	28.29
Rice, white, short-grain, enriched, uncooked	6.5	0.52	79.15	358	2.8	1	0	76.35
Rice, white, short-grain, enriched, cooked	2.36	0.19	28.73	130	0	0	0	28.73
Rice, white, glutinous, unenriched, uncooked	6.81	0.55	81.68	370	2.8	7	0	78.88
Rice, white, glutinous, unenriched, cooked	2.02	0.19	21.09	97	1	5	0	20.09
Rice, white, steamed, Chinese restaurant	3.2	0.27	33.88	151	0.9	5	0	32.98
Rice bran, crude	13.35	20.85	49.69	316	21	5	0	28.69
Rice flour, white, unenriched	5.95	1.42	80.13	366	2.4	0	0	77.73
Rye grain	10.34	1.63	75.86	338	15.1	2	0	60.76
Rye flour, dark	15.91	2.22	68.63	325	23.8	2	0	44.83
Rye flour, medium	10.88	1.52	75.43	349	11.8	2	0	63.63
Rye flour, light	9.82	1.33	76.68	357	8	2	0	68.68
Semolina, enriched	12.68	1.05	72.83	360	3.9	1	0	68.93
Sorghum grain	10.62	3.46	72.09	329	6.7	2	0	65.39
Tapioca, pearl, dry	0.19	0.02	88.69	358	0.9	1	0	87.79
Triticale	13.05	2.09	72.13	336	0	5	0	72.13
Triticale flour, whole-grain	13.18	1.81	73.14	338	14.6	2	0	58.54
Wheat, hard red spring	15.4	1.92	68.03	329	12.2	2	0	55.83
Wheat, hard red winter	12.61	1.54	71.18	327	12.2	2	0	58.98
Wheat, soft red winter	10.35	1.56	74.24	331	12.5	2	0	61.74
Wheat, hard white	11.31	1.71	75.9	342	12.2	2	0	63.7
Wheat, soft white	10.69	1.99	75.36	340	12.7	2	0	62.66
Wheat, durum	13.68	2.47	71.13	339	0	2	0	71.13
Wheat bran, crude	15.55	4.25	64.51	216	42.8	2	0	21.71
Wheat germ, crude	23.15	9.72	51.8	360	13.2	12	0	38.6
Wheat flour, whole-grain	13.21	2.5	71.97	340	10.7	2	0	61.27
Wheat flour, white, all-purpose, enriched, bleached	10.33	0.98	76.31	364	2.7	2	0	73.61
Wheat flour, white, all-purpose, self-rising, enriched	9.89	0.97	74.22	354	2.7	1193	0	71.52
Wheat flour, white, bread, enriched	11.98	1.66	72.53	361	2.4	2	0	70.13
Wheat flour, white, cake, enriched	8.2	0.86	78.03	362	1.7	2	0	76.33
Wheat flour, white, tortilla mix, enriched	9.66	10.63	67.14	405	0	677	0	67.14
Wheat, sprouted	7.49	1.27	42.53	198	1.1	16	0	41.43
Wild rice, raw	14.73	1.08	74.9	357	6.2	7	0	68.7
Wild rice, cooked	3.99	0.34	21.34	101	1.8	3	0	19.54
Rice flour, brown	7.23	2.78	76.48	363	4.6	8	0	71.88
Pasta, gluten-free, corn, dry	7.46	2.08	79.26	357	11	3	0	68.26
Pasta, gluten-free, corn, cooked	2.63	0.73	27.91	126	4.8	0	0	23.11
Pasta, fresh-refrigerated, plain, as purchased	11.31	2.3	54.73	288	0	26	73	54.73
Pasta, fresh-refrigerated, plain, cooked	5.15	1.05	24.93	131	0	6	33	24.93
Pasta, fresh-refrigerated, spinach, as purchased	11.26	2.1	55.72	289	0	27	73	55.72
Pasta, fresh-refrigerated, spinach, cooked	5.06	0.94	25.04	130	0	6	33	25.04
Pasta, homemade, made with egg, cooked	5.28	1.74	23.54	130	0	83	41	23.54
Pasta, homemade, made without egg, cooked	4.37	0.98	25.12	124	0	74	0	25.12
Macaroni, vegetable, enriched, dry	13.14	1.04	74.88	367	4.3	43	0	70.58
Macaroni, vegetable, enriched, cooked	4.53	0.11	26.61	128	4.3	6	0	22.31
Noodles, egg, dry, enriched	14.16	4.44	71.27	384	3.3	21	84	67.97
Noodles, egg, enriched, cooked	4.54	2.07	25.16	138	1.2	5	29	23.96

Food Name ---> per 100 g	Protein (g)	Fat (g)	Carbohydrates (g)	Calories	Fiber (g)	Sodium (mg)	Cholesterol (mg)	Net Carb (g)
Noodles, egg, spinach, enriched, dry	14.61	4.55	70.32	382	6.8	72	95	63.52
Noodles, egg, spinach, enriched, cooked	5.04	1.57	24.25	132	2.3	12	33	21.95
Noodles, chinese, chow mein	8.11	15.43	72.8	475	3.7	1174	0	69.1
Noodles, japanese, soba, dry	14.38	0.71	74.62	336	0	792	0	74.62
Noodles, japanese, soba, cooked	5.06	0.1	21.44	99	0	60	0	21.44
Noodles, japanese, somen, dry	11.35	0.81	74.1	356	4.3	1840	0	69.8
Noodles, japanese, somen, cooked	4	0.18	27.54	131	0	161	0	27.54
Noodles, flat, crunchy, Chinese restaurant	10.33	31.72	51.9	521	1.9	378	0	50
Pasta, dry, enriched	13.04	1.51	74.67	371	3.2	6	0	71.47
Pasta, cooked, enriched, without added salt	5.8	0.93	30.86	158	1.8	1	0	29.06
Pasta, whole-wheat, dry	13.87	2.93	73.37	352	9.2	6	0	64.17
Pasta, whole-wheat, cooked	5.99	1.71	30.07	149	3.9	4	0	26.17
Spaghetti, spinach, dry	13.35	1.57	74.81	372	10.6	36	0	64.21
Spaghetti, spinach, cooked	4.58	0.63	26.15	130	0	14	0	26.15
Wheat flours, bread, unenriched	11.98	1.66	72.53	361	2.4	2	0	70.13
Barley flour or meal	10.5	1.6	74.52	345	10.1	4	0	64.42
Barley malt flour	10.28	1.84	78.3	361	7.1	11	0	71.2
Oat flour, partially debranned	14.66	9.12	65.7	404	6.5	19	0	59.2
Rice noodles, dry	5.95	0.56	80.18	364	1.6	182	0	78.58
Rice noodles, cooked	1.79	0.2	24.01	108	1	19	0	23.01
Pasta, whole grain, 51% whole wheat, remaining unenriched semolina, dry	13.51	2.68	73.1	362	10.1	11	0	63
Pasta, whole grain, 51% whole wheat, remaining unenriched semolina, cooked	5.82	1.5	31.51	159	4.6	6	0	26.91
Quinoa, cooked	4.4	1.92	21.3	120	2.8	7	0	18.5
Wheat, KAMUT khorasan, uncooked	14.54	2.13	70.58	337	11.1	5	0	59.48
Wheat, KAMUT khorasan, cooked	5.71	0.83	27.6	132	4.3	8	0	23.3
Spelt, uncooked	14.57	2.43	70.19	338	10.7	8	0	59.49
Spelt, cooked	5.5	0.85	26.44	127	3.9	5	0	22.54
Teff, uncooked	13.3	2.38	73.13	367	8	12	0	65.13
Teff, cooked	3.87	0.65	19.86	101	2.8	8	0	17.06
Noodles, egg, cooked, enriched, with added salt	4.54	2.07	25.16	138	1.2	165	29	23.96
Corn grain, white	9.42	4.74	74.26	365	0	35	0	74.26
Corn flour, whole-grain, blue (harina de maiz morado)	8.75	5.09	73.89	364	8.4	5	0	65.49
Corn flour, whole-grain, white	6.93	3.86	76.85	361	7.3	5	0	69.55
Corn flour, yellow, masa, enriched	8.46	3.69	76.59	363	6.4	5	0	70.19
Cornmeal, whole-grain, white	8.12	3.59	76.89	362	7.3	35	0	69.59
Pasta, cooked, enriched, with added salt	5.8	0.93	30.59	157	1.8	131	0	28.79
Cornmeal, degermed, enriched, white	7.11	1.75	79.45	370	3.9	7	0	75.55
Cornmeal, white, self-rising, bolted, plain, enriched	8.28	3.4	70.28	334	6.7	1247	0	63.58
Cornmeal, white, self-rising, bolted, with wheat flour added, enriched	8.41	2.85	73.43	348	6.3	1319	0	67.13
Cornmeal, white, self-rising, degermed, enriched	8.41	1.72	74.79	355	7.1	1348	0	67.69
Hominy, canned, yellow	1.48	0.88	14.26	72	2.5	345	0	11.76
Rice, white, long-grain, regular, cooked, enriched, with salt	2.69	0.28	28.17	130	0.4	382	0	27.77
Wheat flour, white, all-purpose, enriched, calcium-fortified	10.33	0.98	76.31	364	2.7	2	0	73.61
Noodles, egg, dry, unenriched	14.16	4.44	71.27	384	3.3	21	84	67.97
Noodles, egg, unenriched, cooked, without	4.54	2.07	25.16	138	1.2	5	29	23.96

Food Name ---> per 100 g	Protein (g)	Fat (g)	Carbohydrates (g)	Calories	Fiber (g)	Sodium (mg)	Cholesterol (mg)	Net Carb (g)
added salt								
Pasta, dry, unenriched	13.04	1.51	74.67	371	3.2	6	0	71.47
Pasta, cooked, unenriched, without added salt	5.8	0.93	30.86	158	1.8	1	0	29.06
Cornmeal, degermed, unenriched, yellow	7.11	1.75	79.45	370	3.9	7	0	75.55
Rice, white, long-grain, regular, raw, unenriched	7.13	0.66	79.95	365	1.3	5	0	78.65
Rice, white, long-grain, regular, unenriched, cooked without salt	2.69	0.28	28.17	130	0.4	1	0	27.77
Rice, white, long-grain, parboiled, unenriched, dry	7.51	1.03	80.89	374	1.8	2	0	79.09
Rice, white, long-grain, parboiled, unenriched, cooked	2.91	0.37	26.05	123	0.9	2	0	25.15
Rice, white, medium-grain, raw, unenriched	6.61	0.58	79.34	360	0	1	0	79.34
Rice, white, medium-grain, cooked, unenriched	2.38	0.21	28.59	130	0	0	0	28.59
Rice, white, short-grain, raw, unenriched	6.5	0.52	79.15	358	0	1	0	79.15
Rice, white, short-grain, cooked, unenriched	2.36	0.19	28.73	130	0	0	0	28.73
Semolina, unenriched	12.68	1.05	72.83	360	3.9	1	0	68.93
Wheat flour, white, all-purpose, unenriched	10.33	0.98	76.31	364	2.7	2	0	73.61
Noodles, egg, cooked, unenriched, with added salt	4.54	2.07	25.16	138	1.2	165	29	23.96
Pasta, cooked, unenriched, with added salt	5.8	0.93	30.59	157	1.8	131	0	28.79
Cornmeal, degermed, unenriched, white	7.11	1.75	79.45	370	3.9	7	0	75.55
Spaghetti, protein-fortified, cooked, enriched (n x 6.25)	8.86	0.21	30.88	164	2	5	0	28.88
Rice, white, long-grain, regular, cooked, unenriched, with salt	2.69	0.28	28.17	130	0.4	382	0	27.77
Wheat flour, white, all-purpose, enriched, unbleached	10.33	0.98	76.31	364	2.7	2	0	73.61
Spaghetti, protein-fortified, dry, enriched (n x 6.25)	21.78	2.23	65.65	374	2.4	8	0	63.25
Wheat flour, white (industrial), 9% protein, bleached, enriched	8.89	1.43	77.32	367	0	2	0	77.32
Wheat flour, white (industrial), 9% protein, bleached, unenriched	8.89	1.43	77.32	367	2.4	2	0	74.92
Wheat flour, white (industrial), 10% protein, bleached, enriched	9.71	1.48	76.22	366	2.4	2	0	73.82
Wheat flour, white (industrial), 10% protein, bleached, unenriched	9.71	1.48	76.22	366	2.4	2	0	73.82
Wheat flour, white (industrial), 10% protein, unbleached, enriched	9.71	1.48	76.22	366	2.4	2	0	73.82
Wheat flour, white (industrial), 11.5% protein, bleached, enriched	11.5	1.45	73.81	363	2.4	2	0	71.41
Wheat flour, white (industrial), 11.5% protein, bleached, unenriched	11.5	1.45	73.81	363	2.4	2	0	71.41
Wheat flour, white (industrial), 11.5% protein, unbleached, enriched	11.5	1.45	73.81	363	2.4	2	0	71.41
Wheat flour, white (industrial), 13% protein, bleached, enriched	13.07	1.38	72.2	362	2.4	2	0	69.8
Wheat flour, white (industrial), 13% protein, bleached, unenriched	13.07	1.38	72.2	362	2.4	2	0	69.8
Wheat flour, white (industrial), 15% protein, bleached, enriched	15.33	1.41	69.88	362	2.4	2	0	67.48
Wheat flour, white (industrial), 15% protein, bleached, unenriched	15.33	1.41	69.88	362	2.4	2	0	67.48
Millet flour	10.75	4.25	75.12	382	3.5	4	0	71.62
Sorghum flour, whole-grain	8.43	3.34	76.64	359	6.6	3	0	70.04

Food Name ---> per 100 g	Protein (g)	Fat (g)	Carbohydrates (g)	Calories	Fiber (g)	Sodium (mg)	Cholesterol (mg)	Net Carb (g)
Vital wheat gluten	75.16	1.85	13.79	370	0.6	29	0	13.19

Dairy and Egg Products

Food Name ---> per 100 g	Protein (g)	Fat (g)	Carb (g)	Calories	Fiber (g)	Sodium (mg)	Cholesterol (mg)	Net Carb (g)
Butter, salted	0.85	81.11	0.06	717	0	643	215	0.06
Butter, whipped, with salt	0.49	78.3	2.87	718	0	583	225	2.87
Butter oil, anhydrous	0.28	99.48	0	876	0	2	256	0
Cheese, blue	21.4	28.74	2.34	353	0	1146	75	2.34
Cheese, brick	23.24	29.68	2.79	371	0	560	94	2.79
Cheese, brie	20.75	27.68	0.45	334	0	629	100	0.45
Cheese, camembert	19.8	24.26	0.46	300	0	842	72	0.46
Cheese, caraway	25.18	29.2	3.06	376	0	690	93	3.06
Cheese, cheddar	22.87	33.31	3.09	404	0	653	99	3.09
Cheese, cheshire	23.37	30.6	4.78	387	0	700	103	4.78
Cheese, colby	23.76	32.11	2.57	394	0	604	95	2.57
Cheese, cottage, creamed, large or small curd	11.12	4.3	3.38	98	0	364	17	3.38
Cheese, cottage, creamed, with fruit	10.69	3.85	4.61	97	0.2	344	13	4.41
Cheese, cottage, nonfat, uncreamed, dry, large or small curd	10.34	0.29	6.66	72	0	372	7	6.66
Cheese, cottage, lowfat, 2% milkfat	10.45	2.27	4.76	81	0	308	12	4.76
Cheese, cottage, lowfat, 1% milkfat	12.39	1.02	2.72	72	0	406	4	2.72
Cheese, cream	6.15	34.44	5.52	350	0	314	101	5.52
Cheese, edam	24.99	27.8	1.43	357	0	812	89	1.43
Cheese, feta	14.21	21.28	4.09	264	0	917	89	4.09
Cheese, fontina	25.6	31.14	1.55	389	0	800	116	1.55
Cheese, gjetost	9.65	29.51	42.65	466	0	600	94	42.65
Cheese, gouda	24.94	27.44	2.22	356	0	819	114	2.22
Cheese, gruyere	29.81	32.34	0.36	413	0	714	110	0.36
Cheese, limburger	20.05	27.25	0.49	327	0	800	90	0.49
Cheese, monterey	24.48	30.28	0.68	373	0	600	89	0.68
Cheese, mozzarella, whole milk	22.17	22.35	2.19	300	0	627	79	2.19
Cheese, mozzarella, whole milk, low moisture	21.6	24.64	2.47	318	0	710	89	2.47
Cheese, mozzarella, part skim milk	24.26	15.92	2.77	254	0	619	64	2.77
Cheese, mozzarella, low moisture, part-skim	23.75	19.78	5.58	295	0	666	64	5.58
Cheese, muenster	23.41	30.04	1.12	368	0	628	96	1.12
Cheese, neufchatel	9.15	22.78	3.59	253	0	334	74	3.59
Cheese, parmesan, grated	28.42	27.84	13.91	420	0	1804	86	13.91
Cheese, parmesan, hard	35.75	25.83	3.22	392	0	1376	68	3.22
Cheese, port de salut	23.78	28.2	0.57	352	0	534	123	0.57
Cheese, provolone	25.58	26.62	2.14	351	0	876	69	2.14
Cheese, ricotta, whole milk	11.26	12.98	3.04	174	0	84	51	3.04
Cheese, ricotta, part skim milk	11.39	7.91	5.14	138	0	99	31	5.14
Cheese, romano	31.8	26.94	3.63	387	0	1433	104	3.63
Cheese, roquefort	21.54	30.64	2	369	0	1809	90	2
Cheese, swiss	26.96	30.99	1.44	393	0	187	93	1.44
Cheese, tilsit	24.41	25.98	1.88	340	0	753	102	1.88
Cheese, pasteurized process, American, fortified with vitamin D	18.13	30.71	4.78	366	0	1671	100	4.78
Cheese, pasteurized process, pimento	22.13	31.2	1.73	375	0.1	915	94	1.63
Cheese, pasteurized process, swiss	24.73	25.01	2.1	334	0	1370	85	2.1
Cheese food, cold pack, American	19.66	24.46	8.32	331	0	966	64	8.32

Food Name ---> per 100 g	Protein (g)	Fat (g)	Carb (g)	Calories	Fiber (g)	Sodium (mg)	Cholesterol (mg)	Net Carb (g)
Cheese food, pasteurized process, American, vitamin D fortified	16.86	25.63	8.56	330	0	1284	98	8.56
Cheese food, pasteurized process, swiss	21.92	24.14	4.5	323	0	1552	82	4.5
Cheese spread, pasteurized process, American	16.41	21.23	8.73	290	0	1625	55	8.73
Cream, fluid, half and half	3.13	10.39	4.73	123	0	61	35	4.73
Cream, fluid, light (coffee cream or table cream)	2.96	19.1	2.82	191	0	72	59	2.82
Cream, fluid, light whipping	2.17	30.91	2.96	292	0	34	111	2.96
Cream, fluid, heavy whipping	2.84	36.08	2.74	340	0	27	113	2.74
Cream, whipped, cream topping, pressurized	3.2	22.22	12.49	257	0	8	76	12.49
Cream, sour, reduced fat, cultured	2.94	12	4.26	135	0	89	39	4.26
Cream, sour, cultured	2.44	19.35	4.63	198	0	31	59	4.63
Eggnog	4.55	4.19	8.05	88	0	54	59	8.05
Sour dressing, non-butterfat, cultured, filled cream-type	3.25	16.57	4.68	178	0	48	5	4.68
Milk, filled, fluid, with blend of hydrogenated vegetable oils	3.33	3.46	4.74	63	0	57	2	4.74
Milk, filled, fluid, with lauric acid oil	3.33	3.4	4.74	63	0	57	2	4.74
Cheese, American, nonfat or fat free	21.05	0	10.53	126	0	1316	26	10.53
Cream substitute, liquid, with hydrogenated vegetable oil and soy protein	1	9.97	11.38	136	0	67	0	11.38
Cream substitute, liquid, with lauric acid oil and sodium caseinate	1	9.97	11.38	136	0	79	0	11.38
Cream substitute, powdered	2.48	32.92	59.29	529	0	124	0	59.29
Dessert topping, powdered	4.9	39.92	52.54	577	0	122	0	52.54
Dessert topping, powdered, 1.5 ounce prepared with 1/2 cup milk	3.61	12.72	17.13	194	0	66	10	17.13
Dessert topping, pressurized	0.98	22.3	16.07	264	0	62	0	16.07
Dessert topping, semi solid, frozen	1.25	25.31	23.05	318	0	25	0	23.05
Sour cream, imitation, cultured	2.4	19.52	6.63	208	0	102	0	6.63
Milk substitutes, fluid, with lauric acid oil	1.75	3.41	6.16	61	0	78	0	6.16
Milk, whole, 3.25% milkfat, with added vitamin D	3.15	3.25	4.8	61	0	43	10	4.8
Milk, producer, fluid, 3.7% milkfat	3.28	3.66	4.65	64	0	49	14	4.65
Milk, reduced fat, fluid, 2% milkfat, with added vitamin A and vitamin D	3.3	1.98	4.8	50	0	47	8	4.8
Milk, reduced fat, fluid, 2% milkfat, with added nonfat milk solids and vitamin A and vitamin D	3.48	1.92	4.97	51	0	52	8	4.97
Milk, reduced fat, fluid, 2% milkfat, protein fortified, with added vitamin A and vitamin D	3.95	1.98	5.49	56	0	59	8	5.49
Milk, lowfat, fluid, 1% milkfat, with added vitamin A and vitamin D	3.37	0.97	4.99	42	0	44	5	4.99
Milk, lowfat, fluid, 1% milkfat, with added nonfat milk solids, vitamin A and vitamin D	3.48	0.97	4.97	43	0	52	4	4.97
Milk, lowfat, fluid, 1% milkfat, protein fortified, with added vitamin A and vitamin D	3.93	1.17	5.52	48	0	58	4	5.52
Milk, nonfat, fluid, with added vitamin A and vitamin D (fat free or skim)	3.37	0.08	4.96	34	0	42	2	4.96
Milk, nonfat, fluid, with added nonfat milk solids, vitamin A and vitamin D (fat free or skim)	3.57	0.25	5.02	37	0	53	2	5.02
Milk, nonfat, fluid, protein fortified, with added vitamin A and vitamin D (fat free and skim)	3.96	0.25	5.56	41	0	59	2	5.56
Milk, buttermilk, fluid, cultured, lowfat	3.31	0.88	4.79	40	0	190	4	4.79
Milk, low sodium, fluid	3.1	3.46	4.46	61	0	3	14	4.46

Food Name ---> per 100 g	Protein (g)	Fat (g)	Carb (g)	Calories	Fiber (g)	Sodium (mg)	Cholesterol (mg)	Net Carb (g)
Milk, dry, whole, with added vitamin D	26.32	26.71	38.42	496	0	371	97	38.42
Milk, dry, nonfat, regular, without added vitamin A and vitamin D	36.16	0.77	51.98	362	0	535	20	51.98
Milk, dry, nonfat, instant, with added vitamin A and vitamin D	35.1	0.72	52.19	358	0	549	18	52.19
Milk, dry, nonfat, calcium reduced	35.5	0.2	51.8	354	0	2280	2	51.8
Milk, buttermilk, dried	34.3	5.78	49	387	0	517	69	49
Milk, chocolate, fluid, commercial, whole, with added vitamin A and vitamin D	3.17	3.39	10.34	83	0.8	60	12	9.54
Milk, chocolate, fluid, commercial, reduced fat, with added vitamin A and vitamin D	2.99	1.9	12.13	76	0.7	66	8	11.43
Milk, chocolate, lowfat, with added vitamin A and vitamin D	3.46	1	9.86	62	0.1	65	5	9.76
Milk, chocolate beverage, hot cocoa, homemade	3.52	2.34	10.74	77	1	44	8	9.74
Milk, goat, fluid, with added vitamin D	3.56	4.14	4.45	69	0	50	11	4.45
Milk, human, mature, fluid	1.03	4.38	6.89	70	0	17	14	6.89
Milk, indian buffalo, fluid	3.75	6.89	5.18	97	0	52	19	5.18
Milk, sheep, fluid	5.98	7	5.36	108	0	44	27	5.36
Milk shakes, thick chocolate	3.05	2.7	21.15	119	0.3	111	11	20.85
Milk shakes, thick vanilla	3.86	3.03	17.75	112	0	95	12	17.75
Whey, acid, fluid	0.76	0.09	5.12	24	0	48	1	5.12
Whey, acid, dried	11.73	0.54	73.45	339	0	968	3	73.45
Whey, sweet, fluid	0.85	0.36	5.14	27	0	54	2	5.14
Whey, sweet, dried	12.93	1.07	74.46	353	0	1079	6	74.46
Yogurt, plain, whole milk, 8 grams protein per 8 ounce	3.47	3.25	4.66	61	0	46	13	4.66
Yogurt, plain, low fat, 12 grams protein per 8 ounce	5.25	1.55	7.04	63	0	70	6	7.04
Yogurt, plain, skim milk, 13 grams protein per 8 ounce	5.73	0.18	7.68	56	0	77	2	7.68
Yogurt, vanilla, low fat, 11 grams protein per 8 ounce	4.93	1.25	13.8	85	0	66	5	13.8
Yogurt, fruit, low fat, 9 grams protein per 8 ounce	3.98	1.15	18.64	99	0	53	5	18.64
Yogurt, fruit, low fat, 10 grams protein per 8 ounce	4.37	1.08	19.05	102	0	58	4	19.05
Yogurt, fruit, low fat, 11 grams protein per 8 ounce	4.86	1.41	18.6	105	0	65	6	18.6
Egg, whole, raw, fresh	12.56	9.51	0.72	143	0	142	372	0.72
Egg, white, raw, fresh	10.9	0.17	0.73	52	0	166	0	0.73
Egg, yolk, raw, fresh	15.86	26.54	3.59	322	0	48	1085	3.59
Egg, whole, cooked, fried	13.61	14.84	0.83	196	0	207	401	0.83
Egg, whole, cooked, hard-boiled	12.58	10.61	1.12	155	0	124	373	1.12
Egg, whole, cooked, poached	12.51	9.47	0.71	143	0	297	370	0.71
Egg, yolk, dried	33.63	59.13	0.66	669	0	149	2307	0.66
Egg, duck, whole, fresh, raw	12.81	13.77	1.45	185	0	146	884	1.45
Egg, goose, whole, fresh, raw	13.87	13.27	1.35	185	0	138	852	1.35
Egg, quail, whole, fresh, raw	13.05	11.09	0.41	158	0	141	844	0.41
Egg, turkey, whole, fresh, raw	13.68	11.88	1.15	171	0	151	933	1.15
Egg substitute, powder	55.5	13	21.8	444	0	800	572	21.8
Butter, without salt	0.85	81.11	0.06	717	0	11	215	0.06
Cheese, parmesan, shredded	37.86	27.34	3.41	415	0	1696	72	3.41
Milk, nonfat, fluid, without added vitamin A and vitamin D (fat free or skim)	3.37	0.08	4.96	34	0	42	2	4.96

Food Name ---> per 100 g	Protein (g)	Fat (g)	Carb (g)	Calories	Fiber (g)	Sodium (mg)	Cholesterol (mg)	Net Carb (g)
Milk, reduced fat, fluid, 2% milkfat, with added nonfat milk solids, without added vitamin A	3.95	1.98	5.49	56	0	59	8	5.49
Milk, canned, evaporated, with added vitamin A	6.81	7.56	10.04	134	0	106	29	10.04
Milk, dry, nonfat, regular, with added vitamin A and vitamin D	36.16	0.77	51.98	362	0	535	20	51.98
Milk, dry, nonfat, instant, without added vitamin A and vitamin D	35.1	0.72	52.19	358	0	549	18	52.19
Cheese, goat, hard type	30.52	35.59	2.17	452	0	423	105	2.17
Cheese, goat, semisoft type	21.58	29.84	0.12	364	0	415	79	0.12
Cheese, goat, soft type	18.52	21.08	0	264	0	459	46	0
Egg, yolk, raw, frozen, salted, pasteurized	14.07	22.93	1.77	275	0	3487	912	1.77
Cheese substitute, mozzarella	11.47	12.22	23.67	248	0	685	0	23.67
Cheese sauce, prepared from recipe	10.33	14.92	5.48	197	0.1	493	38	5.38
Cheese, mexican, queso anejo	21.44	29.98	4.63	373	0	1131	105	4.63
Cheese, mexican, queso asadero	22.6	28.26	2.87	356	0	705	105	2.87
Cheese, mexican, queso chihuahua	21.56	29.68	5.56	374	0	617	105	5.56
Cheese, low fat, cheddar or colby	24.35	7	1.91	173	0	873	21	1.91
Cheese, low-sodium, cheddar or colby	24.35	32.62	1.91	398	0	21	100	1.91
Egg, whole, raw, frozen, pasteurized	12.33	9.95	1.01	147	0	128	372	1.01
Egg, white, raw, frozen, pasteurized	10.2	0	1.04	48	0	169	0	1.04
Egg, white, dried	81.1	0	7.8	382	0	1280	0	7.8
Milk, reduced fat, fluid, 2% milkfat, without added vitamin A and vitamin D	3.3	1.98	4.8	50	0	47	8	4.8
Milk, fluid, 1% fat, without added vitamin A and vitamin D	3.37	0.97	4.99	42	0	44	5	4.99
Sour cream, reduced fat	7	14.1	7	181	0	70	35	7
Sour cream, light	3.5	10.6	7.1	136	0	83	35	7.1
Sour cream, fat free	3.1	0	15.6	74	0	141	9	15.6
USDA Commodity, cheese, cheddar, reduced fat	27.2	18.3	2	282	0	725	56	2
Yogurt, vanilla or lemon flavor, nonfat milk, sweetened with low-calorie sweetener	3.86	0.18	7.5	43	0	59	2	7.5
Parmesan cheese topping, fat free	40	5	40	370	0	1150	20	40
Cheese, cream, fat free	15.69	1	7.66	105	0	702	12	7.66
Yogurt, chocolate, nonfat milk	3.53	0	23.53	112	1.2	135	1	22.33
KRAFT CHEEZ WHIZ Pasteurized Process Cheese Sauce	12	21	9.2	276	0.3	1638	75	8.9
KRAFT CHEEZ WHIZ LIGHT Pasteurized Process Cheese Product	16.3	9.5	16.2	215	0.2	1705	35	16
KRAFT FREE Singles American Nonfat Pasteurized Process Cheese Product	22.7	1	11.7	148	0.2	1298	16	11.5
KRAFT VELVEETA Pasteurized Process Cheese Spread	16.3	22	9.8	303	0	1499	80	9.8
KRAFT VELVEETA LIGHT Reduced Fat Pasteurized Process Cheese Product	19.6	10.6	11.8	222	0	1586	42	11.8
KRAFT BREAKSTONE'S Reduced Fat Sour Cream	4.5	12	6.5	152	0.1	59	50	6.4
KRAFT BREAKSTONE'S FREE Fat Free Sour Cream	4.7	1.3	15.1	91	0	72	9	15.1
Cream, half and half, fat free	2.6	1.4	9	59	0	100	5	9
Reddi Wip Fat Free Whipped Topping	3	5	25	149	0.4	72	16	24.6
Milk, chocolate, fluid, commercial, reduced fat, with added calcium	2.99	1.9	12.13	78	0.7	66	8	11.43
Yogurt, fruit, lowfat, with low calorie sweetener	4.86	1.41	18.6	105	0	58	6	18.6
Cheese, parmesan, dry grated, reduced fat	20	20	1.37	265	0	1529	88	1.37

Food Name ---> per 100 g	Protein (g)	Fat (g)	Carb (g)	Calories	Fiber (g)	Sodium (mg)	Cholesterol (mg)	Net Carb (g)
Cream substitute, flavored, liquid	0.69	13.5	35.07	251	1.1	67	0	33.97
Cream substitute, flavored, powdered	0.68	21.47	75.42	482	1.2	123	0	74.22
Cheese, provolone, reduced fat	24.7	17.6	3.5	274	0	615	55	3.5
Cheese, Mexican, blend, reduced fat	24.69	19.4	3.41	282	0	776	62	3.41
Egg Mix, USDA Commodity	35.6	34.5	23.97	555	0	576	975	23.97
Milk, whole, 3.25% milkfat, without added vitamin A and vitamin D	3.15	3.27	4.78	61	0	43	10	4.78
Milk, dry, whole, without added vitamin D	26.32	26.71	38.42	496	0	371	97	38.42
Milk, canned, evaporated, without added vitamin A and vitamin D	6.81	7.56	10.04	135	0	106	29	10.04
Cheese product, pasteurized process, American, reduced fat, fortified with vitamin D	17.6	14.1	10.6	240	0	1201	53	10.6
Yogurt, fruit, low fat, 9 grams protein per 8 ounce, fortified with vitamin D	3.98	1.15	18.64	99	0	53	5	18.64
Yogurt, fruit, low fat, 10 grams protein per 8 ounce, fortified with vitamin D	4.37	1.08	19.05	102	0	58	4	19.05
Yogurt, fruit variety, nonfat, fortified with vitamin D	4.4	0.2	19	95	0	58	2	19
Yogurt, fruit, lowfat, with low calorie sweetener, fortified with vitamin D	4.86	1.41	18.6	105	0	58	6	18.6
Yogurt, vanilla, low fat, 11 grams protein per 8 ounce, fortified with vitamin D	4.93	1.25	13.8	85	0	66	5	13.8
Yogurt, vanilla or lemon flavor, nonfat milk, sweetened with low-calorie sweetener, fortified with vitamin D	3.86	0.18	7.5	43	0	59	2	7.5
Yogurt, chocolate, nonfat milk, fortified with vitamin D	3.53	0	23.53	112	1.2	135	1	22.33
Protein supplement, milk based, Muscle Milk, powder	45.71	17.14	18.5	411	7.1	329	21	11.4
Protein supplement, milk based, Muscle Milk Light, powder	50	12	22	396	2	250	10	20
Dulce de Leche	6.84	7.35	55.35	315	0	129	29	55.35
Egg substitute, liquid or frozen, fat free	10	0	2	48	0	199	0	2
Cheese, dry white, queso seco	24.51	24.35	2.04	325	0	1808	78	2.04
Cheese, fresh, queso fresco	18.09	23.82	2.98	299	0	751	69	2.98
Cheese, white, queso blanco	20.38	24.31	2.53	310	0	704	70	2.53
Milk, buttermilk, fluid, whole	3.21	3.31	4.88	62	0	105	11	4.88
Yogurt, vanilla flavor, lowfat milk, sweetened with low calorie sweetener	4.93	1.25	13.8	86	0	66	5	13.8
Yogurt, frozen, flavors not chocolate, nonfat milk, with low-calorie sweetener	4.4	0.8	19.7	104	2	81	4	17.7
Ice cream, soft serve, chocolate	4.1	13	22.2	222	0.7	61	91	21.5
Ice cream, bar or stick, chocolate covered	4.1	24.1	24.5	331	0.8	68	28	23.7
Ice cream sandwich	4.29	8.57	37.14	237	0	129	21	37.14
Ice cream cookie sandwich	3.7	7.4	39.6	240	1.2	162	6	38.4
Ice cream cone, chocolate covered, with nuts, flavors other than chocolate	5.21	21.88	34.38	354	1	94	21	33.38
Ice cream sandwich, made with light ice cream, vanilla	4.29	3.04	39.64	186	0	146	7	39.64
Ice cream sandwich, vanilla, light, no sugar added	5.71	2.86	42.86	200	7.1	164	21	35.76
Fat free ice cream, no sugar added, flavors other than chocolate	4.41	0	27.94	129	7.4	110	0	20.54
Milk dessert bar, frozen, made from lowfat milk	4.41	1.47	33.09	147	6.6	92	7	26.49
Nutritional supplement for people with diabetes,	4.4	3.08	11.88	88	2.2	92	2	9.68

Food Name ---> per 100 g	Protein (g)	Fat (g)	Carb (g)	Calories	Fiber (g)	Sodium (mg)	Cholesterol (mg)	Net Carb (g)
liquid								
Cheese, Mexican blend	23.54	28.51	1.75	358	0	338	95	1.75
Cheese product, pasteurized process, American, vitamin D fortified	17.12	23.11	8.8	312	0	1309	78	8.8
Cheese, pasteurized process, American, without added vitamin D	18.13	31.79	3.7	371	0	1671	100	3.7
Cheese food, pasteurized process, American, without added vitamin D	16.86	25.63	8.56	330	0	1441	98	8.56
Egg, whole, raw, frozen, salted, pasteurized	10.97	10.07	0.83	138	0	3663	387	0.83
Yogurt, Greek, plain, nonfat	10.19	0.39	3.6	59	0	36	5	3.6
Egg, white, dried, stabilized, glucose reduced	84.08	0.32	4.51	357	0	1299	0	4.51
Cheese spread, American or Cheddar cheese base, reduced fat	13.41	8.88	10.71	176	0	1102	38	10.71
Cheese, cheddar, reduced fat	27.35	20.41	4.06	309	0	628	76	4.06
Ice cream, light, soft serve, chocolate	3.36	3.69	23.15	141	0	64	15	23.15
Ice cream bar, stick or nugget, with crunch coating	2.11	25.26	37.12	358	1.1	84	16	36.02
Cheese, cheddar, nonfat or fat free	32.14	0	7.14	157	0	1000	18	7.14
Cheese, Swiss, nonfat or fat free	28.4	0	3.4	127	0	1000	18	3.4
Cheese, mexican, queso cotija	20	30	3.97	366	0	1400	100	3.97
Cheese, cheddar, sharp, sliced	24.25	33.82	2.13	410	0	644	99	2.13
Cheese, mozzarella, low moisture, part-skim, shredded	23.63	19.72	8.06	304	0	682	65	8.06
Yogurt, Greek, nonfat, vanilla, CHOBANI	9.07	0.22	8.09	71	0.3	36	0	7.79
Yogurt, Greek, strawberry, DANNON OIKOS	8.25	2.92	11.67	106	1	34	13	10.67
Yogurt, Greek, nonfat, vanilla, DANNON OIKOS	8.12	0.14	12.72	85	0.5	32	0	12.22
Yogurt, Greek, nonfat, strawberry, DANNON OIKOS	8.03	0.22	12.53	84	0.4	33	0	12.13
Yogurt, Greek, nonfat, strawberry, CHOBANI	8.03	0.12	11.62	80	0.7	33	0	10.92
Yogurt, Greek, strawberry, lowfat	8.17	2.57	11.89	103	1	33	12	10.89
Yogurt, Greek, strawberry, nonfat	8.05	0.15	12.07	82	0.6	33	4	11.47
Yogurt, Greek, vanilla, nonfat	8.64	0.18	10.37	78	0.5	34	3	9.87
Yogurt, Greek, plain, lowfat	9.95	1.92	3.94	73	0	34	10	3.94
Kefir, lowfat, plain, LIFEWAY	3.79	0.93	4.48	41	0	40	5	4.48
Kefir, lowfat, strawberry, LIFEWAY	3.39	0.9	10.2	62	0	37	5	10.2
Milk, evaporated, 2% fat, with added vitamin A and vitamin D	6.67	2	15.74	107	0	100	0	15.74
Milk, chocolate, fat free, with added vitamin A and vitamin D	3.39	0	13.46	67	0	110	2	13.46
Yogurt, Greek, plain, whole milk	9	5	3.98	97	0	35	13	3.98
Yogurt, Greek, fruit, whole milk	7.33	3	12.29	106	0	37	10	12.29
Yogurt, vanilla, non-fat	2.94	0	17.04	78	0	47	3	17.04
Yogurt, Greek, vanilla, lowfat	8.64	2.5	9.54	95	0	40	5	9.54
Yogurt, frozen, flavors other than chocolate, lowfat	8	2.5	21	139	0	45	45	21
Ice cream bar, covered with chocolate and nuts	5.62	25.84	11.89	303	1.1	56	56	10.79
Ice cream sundae cone	3	14	28.89	254	1	115	15	27.89
Light ice cream, Creamsicle	1.54	3.08	32.75	165	0	46	8	32.75
Cream, half and half, lowfat	3.33	5	3.33	72	0	50	17	3.33
Milk, chocolate, lowfat, reduced sugar	3.43	1.04	7.68	54	0	66	5	7.68
Ice cream, lowfat, no sugar added, cone, added peanuts and chocolate sauce	5.33	9.33	40.01	265	9.3	113	7	30.71
Imitation cheese, american or cheddar, low	25	32	1	390	0	670	15	1

Food Name ---> per 100 g	Protein (g)	Fat (g)	Carb (g)	Calories	Fiber (g)	Sodium (mg)	Cholesterol (mg)	Net Carb (g)
cholesterol								
Whipped topping, frozen, low fat	3	13.1	23.6	224	0	72	2	23.6
Cream substitute, powdered, light	1.9	15.7	73.4	431	0	229	0	73.4
Cream substitute, liquid, light	0.8	3.5	9.1	71	0	60	0	9.1
Cheese, monterey, low fat	28.2	21.6	0.7	313	0	781	65	0.7
Milk, buttermilk, fluid, cultured, reduced fat	4.1	2	5.3	56	0	105	8	5.3
Cheese, pasteurized process, cheddar or American, fat-free	22.5	0.8	13.4	148	0	1528	11	13.4
Cheese, cottage, lowfat, 1% milkfat, lactose reduced	12.4	1	3.2	74	0.6	220	4	2.6
Cheese product, pasteurized process, cheddar, reduced fat	17.6	14.1	10.6	240	0	1587	53	10.6
Milk, fluid, nonfat, calcium fortified (fat free or skim)	3.4	0.18	4.85	35	0	52	2	4.85
Cheese, muenster, low fat	24.7	17.6	3.5	271	0	600	63	3.5
Cheese, mozzarella, nonfat	31.7	0	3.5	141	1.8	743	18	1.7
Beverage, milkshake mix, dry, not chocolate	23.5	2.6	52.9	329	1.6	780	14	51.3
Beverage, instant breakfast powder, chocolate, not reconstituted	19.9	1.4	66.2	353	0.4	385	12	65.8
Beverage, instant breakfast powder, chocolate, sugar-free, not reconstituted	35.8	5.1	41	358	2	717	44	39
Yogurt, fruit variety, nonfat	4.4	0.2	19	95	0	58	2	19
Whipped cream substitute, dietetic, made from powdered mix	0.9	6	10.6	100	0	106	0	10.6
Cheese, cottage, with vegetables	10.9	4.2	3	95	0.1	403	14	2.9
Cheese, cream, low fat	7.85	15.28	8.13	201	0	359	54	8.13
Cheese, pasteurized process, American, low fat	24.6	7	3.5	180	0	1789	35	3.5
Cheese spread, cream cheese base	7.1	28.6	3.5	295	0	436	90	3.5
Cheese, american cheddar, imitation	16.7	14	11.6	239	0	1345	36	11.6
Eggs, scrambled, frozen mixture	13.1	5.6	7.5	131	0	162	277	7.5
Cheese, parmesan, low sodium	41.6	29.99	3.7	451	0	63	79	3.7
Cheese, cottage, lowfat, 1% milkfat, no sodium added	12.4	1	2.7	72	0	13	4	2.7
Cheese, pasteurized process, swiss, low fat	25.5	5.1	4.3	165	0	1430	35	4.3
Cheese, cottage, lowfat, 1% milkfat, with vegetables	10.9	1	3	67	0	403	3	3
Cheese, pasteurized process, cheddar or American, low sodium	22.2	31.19	1.6	376	0	7	94	1.6
Cheese, swiss, low sodium	28.4	27.4	3.4	374	0	14	92	3.4
Milk, imitation, non-soy	1.6	2	5.3	46	0	55	0	5.3
Cheese, swiss, low fat	28.4	5.1	3.4	179	0	199	35	3.4
Cheese, mozzarella, low sodium	27.5	17.1	3.1	280	0	16	54	3.1
Cheese food, pasteurized process, American, imitation, without added vitamin D	4.08	19.5	16.18	257	0	1297	6	16.18

Fats and Oils

Food Name ---> per 100 g	Protein (g)	Fat (g)	Carb (g)	Calories	Fiber (g)	Sodium (mg)	Cholesterol (mg)	Net Carb(g)

Food Name ---> per 100 g	Protein (g)	Fat (g)	Carb (g)	Calories	Fiber (g)	Sodium (mg)	Cholesterol (mg)	Net Carb(g)
Fat, beef tallow	0	100	0	902	0	0	109	0
Lard	0	100	0	902	0	0	95	0
Salad dressing, russian dressing	0.69	26.18	31.9	355	0.7	1133	0	31.2
Salad dressing, sesame seed dressing, regular	3.1	45.2	8.6	443	1	1000	0	7.6
Salad dressing, thousand island, commercial, regular	1.09	35.06	14.64	379	0.8	962	26	13.84
Salad dressing, mayonnaise type, regular, with salt	0.65	21.6	14.78	250	0	653	19	14.78
Salad dressing, french dressing, reduced fat	0.58	11.52	31.22	222	1.5	838	0	29.72
Salad dressing, italian dressing, commercial, reduced fat	0.39	6.68	9.99	102	0	891	0	9.99
Salad dressing, russian dressing, low calorie	0.5	4	27.6	141	0.3	868	6	27.3
Salad dressing, thousand island dressing, reduced fat	0.83	11.32	24.06	195	1.2	955	11	22.86
Salad dressing, mayonnaise, regular	0.96	74.85	0.57	680	0	635	42	0.57
Salad dressing, mayonnaise, soybean and safflower oil, with salt	1.1	79.4	2.7	717	0	568	59	2.7
Salad dressing, mayonnaise, imitation, soybean	0.3	19.2	16	232	0	497	24	16
Salad dressing, mayonnaise, imitation, milk cream	2.1	5.1	11.1	97	0	504	43	11.1
Salad dressing, mayonnaise, imitation, soybean without cholesterol	0.1	47.7	15.8	482	0	353	0	15.8
Sandwich spread, with chopped pickle, regular, unspecified oils	0.9	34	22.4	389	0.4	1000	76	22
Shortening, household, soybean (partially hydrogenated)-cottonseed (partially hydrogenated)	0	100	0	884	0	0	0	0
Oil, soybean, salad or cooking, (partially hydrogenated)	0	100	0	884	0	0	0	0
Oil, rice bran	0	100	0	884	0	0	0	0
Oil, wheat germ	0	100	0	884	0	0	0	0
Oil, peanut, salad or cooking	0	100	0	884	0	0	0	0
Oil, soybean, salad or cooking	0	100	0	884	0	0	0	0
Oil, coconut	0	99.06	0	892	0	0	0	0
Oil, olive, salad or cooking	0	100	0	884	0	2	0	0
Oil, palm	0	100	0	884	0	0	0	0
Oil, sesame, salad or cooking	0	100	0	884	0	0	0	0
Salad dressing, french, home recipe	0.1	70.2	3.4	631	0	658	0	3.4
Salad dressing, home recipe, vinegar and oil	0	50.1	2.5	449	0	1	0	2.5
Salad dressing, french dressing, commercial, regular, without salt	0.77	44.81	15.58	459	0	0	0	15.58
Salad dressing, french dressing, reduced fat, without salt	0.58	13.46	29.28	233	1.1	30	0	28.18
Salad dressing, italian dressing, commercial, regular, without salt	0.38	28.37	10.43	292	0	30	67	10.43
Salad dressing, italian dressing, reduced fat, without salt	0.47	6.38	4.57	76	0	30	6	4.57
Salad dressing, mayonnaise, soybean oil, without salt	1.1	79.4	2.7	717	0	30	59	2.7
Salad dressing, french, cottonseed, oil, home recipe	0.1	70.2	3.4	631	0	658	0	3.4
Salad dressing, french dressing, fat-free	0.2	0.27	32.14	132	2.2	853	0	29.94
Oil, cocoa butter	0	100	0	884	0	0	0	0
Oil, cottonseed, salad or cooking	0	100	0	884	0	0	0	0
Oil, sunflower, linoleic, (approx. 65%)	0	100	0	884	0	0	0	0
Oil, safflower, salad or cooking, linoleic, (over 70%)	0	100	0	884	0	0	0	0
Oil, safflower, salad or cooking, high oleic	0	100	0	884	0	0	0	0

Food Name ---> per 100 g	Protein (g)	Fat (g)	Carb (g)	Calories	Fiber (g)	Sodium (mg)	Cholesterol (mg)	Net Carb(g)
(primary safflower oil of commerce)								
Vegetable oil, palm kernel	0	100	0	862	0	0	0	0
Oil, poppyseed	0	100	0	884	0	0	0	0
Oil, tomatoseed	0	100	0	884	0	0	0	0
Oil, teaseed	0	100	0	884	0	0	0	0
Oil, grapeseed	0	100	0	884	0	0	0	0
Oil, corn, industrial and retail, all purpose salad or cooking	0	100	0	900	0	0	0	0
Fat, mutton tallow	0	100	0	902	0	0	102	0
Oil, walnut	0	100	0	884	0	0	0	0
Oil, almond	0	100	0	884	0	0	0	0
Oil, apricot kernel	0	100	0	884	0	0	0	0
Oil, soybean lecithin	0	100	0	763	0	0	0	0
Oil, hazelnut	0	100	0	884	0	0	0	0
Oil, babassu	0	100	0	884	0	0	0	0
Oil, sheanut	0	100	0	884	0	0	0	0
Salad dressing, blue or roquefort cheese dressing, commercial, regular	1.37	51.1	4.77	484	0.4	642	31	4.37
Oil, cupu assu	0	100	0	884	0	0	0	0
Fat, chicken	0	99.8	0	900	0	0	85	0
Oil, soybean, salad or cooking, (partially hydrogenated) and cottonseed	0	100	0	884	0	0	0	0
Shortening, household, lard and vegetable oil	0	100	0	900	0	0	56	0
Oil, sunflower, linoleic, (partially hydrogenated)	0	100	0	884	0	0	0	0
Shortening bread, soybean (hydrogenated) and cottonseed	0	100	0	884	0	0	0	0
Shortening cake mix, soybean (hydrogenated) and cottonseed (hydrogenated)	0	100	0	884	0	0	0	0
Shortening industrial, lard and vegetable oil	0	100	0	900	0	0	56	0
Shortening frying (heavy duty), beef tallow and cottonseed	0	100	0	900	0	0	100	0
Shortening confectionery, coconut (hydrogenated) and or palm kernel (hydrogenated)	0	100	0	884	0	0	0	0
Shortening industrial, soybean (hydrogenated) and cottonseed	0	100	0	884	0	0	0	0
Shortening frying (heavy duty), palm (hydrogenated)	0	100	0	884	0	0	0	0
Shortening household soybean (hydrogenated) and palm	0	100	0	884	0	0	0	0
Shortening frying (heavy duty), soybean (hydrogenated), linoleic (less than 1%)	0	100	0	884	0	0	0	0
Shortening, confectionery, fractionated palm	0	100	0	884	0	0	0	0
Oil, nutmeg butter	0	100	0	884	0	0	0	0
Oil, ucuhuba butter	0	100	0	884	0	0	0	0
Fat, duck	0	99.8	0	882	0	0	100	0
Fat, turkey	0	99.8	0	900	0	0	102	0
Fat, goose	0	99.8	0	900	0	0	100	0
Oil, avocado	0	100	0	884	0	0	0	0
Oil, canola	0	100	0	884	0	0	0	0
Oil, mustard	0	100	0	884	0	0	0	0
Oil, sunflower, high oleic (70% and over)	0	100	0	884	0	0	0	0
Margarine-like, margarine-butter blend, soybean oil and butter	0.31	80.32	0.77	727	0	719	12	0.77
Shortening, special purpose for cakes and	0	100	0	884	0	0	0	0

Food Name ---> per 100 g	Protein (g)	Fat (g)	Carb (g)	Calories	Fiber (g)	Sodium (mg)	Cholesterol (mg)	Net Carb(g)
frostings, soybean (hydrogenated)								
Shortening, special purpose for baking, soybean (hydrogenated) palm and cottonseed	0	100	0	884	0	0	0	0
Oil, oat	0	100	0	884	0	0	0	0
Fish oil, cod liver	0	100	0	902	0	0	570	0
Fish oil, herring	0	100	0	902	0	0	766	0
Fish oil, menhaden	0	100	0	902	0	0	521	0
Fish oil, menhaden, fully hydrogenated	0	100	0	902	0	0	500	0
Fish oil, salmon	0	100	0	902	0	0	485	0
Fish oil, sardine	0	100	0	902	0	0	710	0
Shortening, multipurpose, soybean (hydrogenated) and palm (hydrogenated)	0	100	0	884	0	0	0	0
Margarine-like, vegetable oil-butter spread, tub, with salt	1	40	1	362	0	786	0	1
Butter, light, stick, with salt	3.3	55.1	0	499	0	450	106	0
Butter, light, stick, without salt	3.3	55.1	0	499	0	36	106	0
Meat drippings (lard, beef tallow, mutton tallow)	0	98.59	0	889	0	545	101	0
Animal fat, bacon grease	0	99.5	0	897	0	150	95	0
Oil, industrial, soy (partially hydrogenated), palm, principal uses icings and fillings	0	100	0	884	0	0	0	0
Margarine, industrial, non-dairy, cottonseed, soy oil (partially hydrogenated), for flaky pastries	1.9	80.2	0	714	0	879	0	0
Shortening, industrial, soy (partially hydrogenated) and corn for frying	0	100	0	884	0	0	0	0
Shortening, industrial, soy (partially hydrogenated) for baking and confections	0	100	0	884	0	0	0	0
Margarine, industrial, soy and partially hydrogenated soy oil, use for baking, sauces and candy	0.18	80	0.71	714	0	886	0	0.71
USDA Commodity Food, oil, vegetable, soybean, refined	0	100	0	884	0	0	0	0
USDA Commodity Food, oil, vegetable, low saturated fat	0	100	0	884	0	0	0	0
Margarine, margarine-like vegetable oil spread, 67-70% fat, tub	0.07	68.29	0.59	606	0	536	0	0.59
Margarine, 80% fat, tub, CANOLA HARVEST Soft Spread (canola, palm and palm kernel oils)	0.41	80.32	1.39	730	0	714	0	1.39
Oil, cooking and salad, ENOVA, 80% diglycerides	0	100	0	884	0	0	0	0
Salad dressing, honey mustard dressing, reduced calorie	0.98	10	28.26	207	0.8	701	0	27.46
Margarine-like spread, BENECOL Light Spread	0	38.71	5.71	357	0	670	0	5.71
Salad dressing, spray-style dressing, assorted flavors	0.16	10.75	16.6	165	0.3	1102	0	16.3
Salad Dressing, mayonnaise, light, SMART BALANCE, Omega Plus light	1.53	34.18	9.39	333	0.2	848	33	9.19
Oil, industrial, canola, high oleic	0	100	0	900	0	0	0	0
Oil, industrial, soy, low linolenic	0	100	0	900	0	0	0	0
Oil, industrial, soy, ultra low linolenic	0	100	0	884	0	0	0	0
Oil, industrial, soy, fully hydrogenated	0	100	0	884	0	0	0	0
Oil, industrial, cottonseed, fully hydrogenated	0	100	0	884	0	0	0	0
Salad dressing, honey mustard, regular	0.87	40.83	23.33	464	0.4	512	29	22.93
Salad dressing, poppyseed, creamy	0.92	33.33	23.73	399	0.3	933	15	23.43
Salad dressing, caesar, fat-free	1.47	0.23	30.73	131	0.2	1265	1	30.53
Dressing, honey mustard, fat-free	1.07	1.47	38.43	169	1.2	1004	1	37.23

Food Name ---> per 100 g	Protein (g)	Fat (g)	Carb (g)	Calories	Fiber (g)	Sodium (mg)	Cholesterol (mg)	Net Carb(g)
Oil, flaxseed, contains added sliced flaxseed	0.37	99.01	0.39	878	0	6	0	0.39
Mayonnaise, reduced fat, with olive oil	0.37	40	0	361	0	800	33	0
Salad dressing, mayonnaise-type, light	0.65	10	16.4	158	0	833	0	16.4
Creamy dressing, made with sour cream and/or buttermilk and oil, reduced calorie	1.5	14	7	160	0	833	0	7
Salad dressing, peppercorn dressing, commercial, regular	1.2	61.4	3.5	564	0	1103	49	3.5
Mayonnaise, reduced-calorie or diet, cholesterol-free	0.9	33.3	6.7	333	0	733	0	6.7
Salad dressing, italian dressing, reduced calorie	0.3	20	6.7	200	0.2	1074	0	6.5
Vegetable oil-butter spread, reduced calorie	0	53	0	465	0	581	54	0
Salad dressing, blue or roquefort cheese dressing, light	2.1	2.7	13.2	86	0	939	10	13.2
Creamy dressing, made with sour cream and/or buttermilk and oil, reduced calorie, fat-free	1.4	2.7	20	107	0	897	0	20
Creamy dressing, made with sour cream and/or buttermilk and oil, reduced calorie, cholesterol-free	1	8	16	140	0	932	0	16
Salad dressing, french dressing, reduced calorie	0.4	13	27	227	0	804	0	27
Mayonnaise, made with tofu	5.95	31.79	3.06	322	1.1	773	0	1.96
Salad dressing, blue or roquefort cheese dressing, fat-free	1.52	1.01	25.6	115	1.8	814	2	23.8
Salad Dressing, mayonnaise-like, fat-free	0.2	2.7	15.5	84	1.9	788	9	13.6
Salad Dressing, coleslaw dressing, reduced fat	0	20	40	329	0.4	1600	25	39.6
Oil, flaxseed, cold pressed	0.11	99.98	0	884	0	0	0	0
Margarine-like, vegetable oil spread, stick or tub, sweetened	0	52	16.7	534	0	542	0	16.7
Oil, corn and canola	0	100	0	884	0	0	0	0
Margarine-like, butter-margarine blend, 80% fat, stick, without salt	0.9	80.7	0.6	718	0	28	88	0.6
Margarine-like, vegetable oil-butter spread, reduced calorie, tub, with salt	1	50	1	450	0	607	71	1
Salad dressing, caesar dressing, regular	2.17	57.85	3.3	542	0.5	1209	39	2.8
Salad dressing, coleslaw	0.9	33.4	23.8	390	0.1	710	26	23.7
Salad dressing, green goddess, regular	1.9	43.33	7.36	427	0.1	867	40	7.26
Salad dressing, sweet and sour	0.1	0	3.7	15	0	208	0	3.7
Salad dressing, blue or roquefort cheese, low calorie	5.1	7.2	2.9	99	0	939	1	2.9
Salad dressing, caesar, low calorie	0.3	4.4	18.6	110	0.1	1148	2	18.5
Butter replacement, without fat, powder	2	1	89	373	0	1200	2	89
Salad dressing, buttermilk, lite	1.25	12.42	21.33	202	1.1	1120	16	20.23
Salad dressing, mayonnaise and mayonnaise-type, low calorie	0.9	19	23.9	263	0	837	26	23.9
Salad dressing, bacon and tomato	1.8	35	2	326	0.2	905	4	1.8
Mayonnaise, low sodium, low calorie or diet	0.3	19.2	16	231	0	110	24	16
Mayonnaise dressing, no cholesterol	0	77.8	0.3	688	0	486	0	0.3
Oil, corn, peanut, and olive	0	100	0	884	0	0	0	0

Finfish and Shellfish Products

Food Name ---> per 100 g	Protein (g)	Fat (g)	Carb (g)	Calories	Fiber (g)	Sodium (mg)	Cholesterol (mg)	Net Carb(g)
Fish, anchovy, european, raw	20.35	4.84	0	131	0	104	60	0
Fish, anchovy, european, canned in oil, drained solids	28.89	9.71	0	210	0	3668	85	0
Fish, bass, fresh water, mixed species, raw	18.86	3.69	0	114	0	70	68	0
Fish, bass, striped, raw	17.73	2.33	0	97	0	69	80	0
Fish, bluefish, raw	20.04	4.24	0	124	0	60	59	0
Fish, burbot, raw	19.31	0.81	0	90	0	97	60	0
Fish, butterfish, raw	17.28	8.02	0	146	0	89	65	0
Fish, carp, raw	17.83	5.6	0	127	0	49	66	0
Fish, carp, cooked, dry heat	22.86	7.17	0	162	0	63	84	0
Fish, catfish, channel, wild, raw	16.38	2.82	0	95	0	43	58	0
Fish, catfish, channel, cooked, breaded and fried	18.09	13.33	8.04	229	0.7	280	71	7.34
Fish, caviar, black and red, granular	24.6	17.9	4	264	0	1500	588	4
Fish, cisco, raw	18.99	1.91	0	98	0	55	50	0
Fish, cisco, smoked	16.36	11.9	0	177	0	481	32	0
Fish, cod, Atlantic, raw	17.81	0.67	0	82	0	54	43	0
Fish, cod, Atlantic, cooked, dry heat	22.83	0.86	0	105	0	78	55	0
Fish, cod, Atlantic, canned, solids and liquid	22.76	0.86	0	105	0	218	55	0
Fish, cod, Atlantic, dried and salted	62.82	2.37	0	290	0	7027	152	0
Fish, cod, Pacific, raw (may have been previously frozen)	15.27	0.41	0	69	0	303	47	0
Fish, croaker, Atlantic, raw	17.78	3.17	0	104	0	56	61	0
Fish, croaker, Atlantic, cooked, breaded and fried	18.2	12.67	7.54	221	0.4	348	84	7.14
Fish, cusk, raw	18.99	0.69	0	87	0	31	41	0
Fish, mahimahi, raw	18.5	0.7	0	85	0	88	73	0
Fish, drum, freshwater, raw	17.54	4.93	0	119	0	75	64	0
Fish, eel, mixed species, raw	18.44	11.66	0	184	0	51	126	0
Fish, eel, mixed species, cooked, dry heat	23.65	14.95	0	236	0	65	161	0
Fish, fish sticks, frozen, prepared	11.01	16.23	21.66	277	1.5	402	28	20.16
Fish, flatfish (flounder and sole species), raw	12.41	1.93	0	70	0	296	45	0
Fish, flatfish (flounder and sole species), cooked, dry heat	15.24	2.37	0	86	0	363	56	0
Fish, gefiltefish, commercial, sweet recipe	9.07	1.73	7.41	84	0	524	30	7.41
Fish, grouper, mixed species, raw	19.38	1.02	0	92	0	53	37	0
Fish, grouper, mixed species, cooked, dry heat	24.84	1.3	0	118	0	53	47	0
Fish, haddock, raw	16.32	0.45	0	74	0	213	54	0
Fish, haddock, cooked, dry heat	19.99	0.55	0	90	0	261	66	0
Fish, haddock, smoked	25.23	0.96	0	116	0	763	77	0
Fish, halibut, Atlantic and Pacific, raw	18.56	1.33	0	91	0	68	49	0
Fish, halibut, Atlantic and Pacific, cooked, dry heat	22.54	1.61	0	111	0	82	60	0
Fish, halibut, Greenland, raw	14.37	13.84	0	186	0	80	46	0
Fish, herring, Atlantic, raw	17.96	9.04	0	158	0	90	60	0
Fish, herring, Atlantic, cooked, dry heat	23.03	11.59	0	203	0	115	77	0
Fish, herring, Atlantic, pickled	14.19	18	9.64	262	0	870	13	9.64
Fish, herring, Atlantic, kippered	24.58	12.37	0	217	0	918	82	0
Fish, herring, Pacific, raw	16.39	13.88	0	195	0	74	77	0
Fish, ling, raw	18.99	0.64	0	87	0	135	40	0
Fish, lingcod, raw	17.66	1.06	0	85	0	59	52	0

Food Name ---> per 100 g	Protein (g)	Fat (g)	Carb (g)	Calories	Fiber (g)	Sodium (mg)	Cholesterol (mg)	Net Carb (g)
Fish, mackerel, Atlantic, raw	18.6	13.89	0	205	0	90	70	0
Fish, mackerel, Atlantic, cooked, dry heat	23.85	17.81	0	262	0	83	75	0
Fish, mackerel, jack, canned, drained solids	23.19	6.3	0	156	0	379	79	0
Fish, mackerel, king, raw	20.28	2	0	105	0	158	53	0
Fish, mackerel, Pacific and jack, mixed species, raw	20.07	7.89	0	158	0	86	47	0
Fish, mackerel, spanish, raw	19.29	6.3	0	139	0	59	76	0
Fish, mackerel, spanish, cooked, dry heat	23.59	6.32	0	158	0	66	73	0
Fish, milkfish, raw	20.53	6.73	0	148	0	72	52	0
Fish, monkfish, raw	14.48	1.52	0	76	0	18	25	0
Fish, mullet, striped, raw	19.35	3.79	0	117	0	65	49	0
Fish, mullet, striped, cooked, dry heat	24.81	4.86	0	150	0	71	63	0
Fish, ocean perch, Atlantic, raw	15.31	1.54	0	79	0	287	52	0
Fish, ocean perch, Atlantic, cooked, dry heat	18.51	1.87	0	96	0	347	63	0
Fish, pout, ocean, raw	16.64	0.91	0	79	0	61	52	0
Fish, perch, mixed species, raw	19.39	0.92	0	91	0	62	90	0
Fish, perch, mixed species, cooked, dry heat	24.86	1.18	0	117	0	79	115	0
Fish, pike, northern, raw	19.26	0.69	0	88	0	39	39	0
Fish, pike, northern, cooked, dry heat	24.69	0.88	0	113	0	49	50	0
Fish, pike, walleye, raw	19.14	1.22	0	93	0	51	86	0
Fish, pollock, Atlantic, raw	19.44	0.98	0	92	0	86	71	0
Fish, pollock, Alaska, raw (may have been previously frozen)	12.19	0.41	0	56	0	333	46	0
Fish, pollock, Alaska, cooked, dry heat (may have been previously frozen)	23.48	1.18	0	111	0	419	86	0
Fish, pompano, florida, raw	18.48	9.47	0	164	0	65	50	0
Fish, pompano, florida, cooked, dry heat	23.69	12.14	0	211	0	76	64	0
Fish, rockfish, Pacific, mixed species, raw	18.36	1.34	0	90	0	74	50	0
Fish, rockfish, Pacific, mixed species, cooked, dry heat	22.23	1.62	0	109	0	89	61	0
Fish, roe, mixed species, raw	22.32	6.42	1.5	143	0	91	374	1.5
Fish, roughy, orange, raw	16.41	0.7	0	76	0	72	60	0
Fish, sablefish, raw	13.41	15.3	0	195	0	56	49	0
Fish, sablefish, smoked	17.65	20.14	0	257	0	737	64	0
Fish, salmon, Atlantic, wild, raw	19.84	6.34	0	142	0	44	55	0
Fish, salmon, chinook, smoked	18.28	4.32	0	117	0	672	23	0
Fish, salmon, chinook, raw	19.93	10.43	0	179	0	47	50	0
Fish, salmon, chum, raw	20.14	3.77	0	120	0	50	74	0
Fish, salmon, chum, canned, drained solids with bone	21.43	5.5	0	141	0	391	39	0
Fish, salmon, coho, wild, raw	21.62	5.93	0	146	0	46	45	0
Fish, salmon, coho, wild, cooked, moist heat	27.36	7.5	0	184	0	53	57	0
Fish, salmon, pink, raw	20.5	4.4	0	127	0	75	46	0
Fish, salmon, pink, canned, total can contents	19.68	4.97	0	129	0	403	55	0
Fish, salmon, sockeye, raw	22.25	4.69	0	131	0	78	51	0
Fish, salmon, sockeye, cooked, dry heat	26.48	5.57	0	156	0	92	61	0
Fish, salmon, sockeye, canned, drained solids	23.59	7.39	0	167	0	408	79	0
Fish, sardine, Atlantic, canned in oil, drained solids with bone	24.62	11.45	0	208	0	307	142	0
Fish, sardine, Pacific, canned in tomato sauce, drained solids with bone	20.86	10.45	0.54	185	0.1	414	61	0.44
Fish, scup, raw	18.88	2.73	0	105	0	42	52	0
Fish, sea bass, mixed species, raw	18.43	2	0	97	0	68	41	0

Food Name ---> per 100 g	Protein (g)	Fat (g)	Carb (g)	Calories	Fiber (g)	Sodium (mg)	Cholesterol (mg)	Net Carb(g)
Fish, sea bass, mixed species, cooked, dry heat	23.63	2.56	0	124	0	87	53	0
Fish, seatrout, mixed species, raw	16.74	3.61	0	104	0	58	83	0
Fish, shad, american, raw	16.93	13.77	0	197	0	51	75	0
Fish, shark, mixed species, raw	20.98	4.51	0	130	0	79	51	0
Fish, shark, mixed species, cooked, batter-dipped and fried	18.62	13.82	6.39	228	0	122	59	6.39
Fish, sheepshead, raw	20.21	2.41	0	108	0	71	50	0
Fish, sheepshead, cooked, dry heat	26.02	1.63	0	126	0	73	64	0
Fish, smelt, rainbow, raw	17.63	2.42	0	97	0	60	70	0
Fish, smelt, rainbow, cooked, dry heat	22.6	3.1	0	124	0	77	90	0
Fish, snapper, mixed species, raw	20.51	1.34	0	100	0	64	37	0
Fish, snapper, mixed species, cooked, dry heat	26.3	1.72	0	128	0	57	47	0
Fish, spot, raw	18.51	4.9	0	123	0	29	60	0
Fish, sturgeon, mixed species, raw	16.14	4.04	0	105	0	54	60	0
Fish, sturgeon, mixed species, cooked, dry heat	20.7	5.18	0	135	0	69	77	0
Fish, sturgeon, mixed species, smoked	31.2	4.4	0	173	0	739	80	0
Fish, sucker, white, raw	16.76	2.32	0	92	0	40	41	0
Fish, sunfish, pumpkin seed, raw	19.4	0.7	0	89	0	80	67	0
Fish, surimi	15.18	0.9	6.85	99	0	143	30	6.85
Fish, swordfish, raw	19.66	6.65	0	144	0	81	66	0
Fish, swordfish, cooked, dry heat	23.45	7.93	0	172	0	97	78	0
Fish, tilefish, raw	17.5	2.31	0	96	0	53	50	0
Fish, tilefish, cooked, dry heat	24.49	4.69	0	147	0	59	64	0
Fish, trout, mixed species, raw	20.77	6.61	0	148	0	52	58	0
Fish, trout, rainbow, wild, raw	20.48	3.46	0	119	0	31	59	0
Fish, trout, rainbow, wild, cooked, dry heat	22.92	5.82	0	150	0	56	69	0
Fish, tuna, fresh, bluefin, raw	23.33	4.9	0	144	0	39	38	0
Fish, tuna, fresh, bluefin, cooked, dry heat	29.91	6.28	0	184	0	50	49	0
Fish, tuna, light, canned in oil, drained solids	29.13	8.21	0	198	0	416	18	0
Fish, tuna, light, canned in water, drained solids	19.44	0.96	0	86	0	247	36	0
Fish, tuna, fresh, skipjack, raw	22	1.01	0	103	0	37	47	0
Fish, tuna, white, canned in oil, drained solids	26.53	8.08	0	186	0	396	31	0
Fish, tuna, white, canned in water, drained solids	23.62	2.97	0	128	0	377	42	0
Fish, tuna, fresh, yellowfin, raw	24.4	0.49	0	109	0	45	39	0
Fish, tuna salad	16.04	9.26	9.41	187	0	402	13	9.41
Fish, turbot, european, raw	16.05	2.95	0	95	0	150	48	0
Fish, whitefish, mixed species, raw	19.09	5.86	0	134	0	51	60	0
Fish, whitefish, mixed species, smoked	23.4	0.93	0	108	0	1019	33	0
Fish, whiting, mixed species, raw	18.31	1.31	0	90	0	72	67	0
Fish, whiting, mixed species, cooked, dry heat	23.48	1.69	0	116	0	132	84	0
Fish, wolffish, Atlantic, raw	17.5	2.39	0	96	0	85	46	0
Fish, yellowtail, mixed species, raw	23.14	5.24	0	146	0	39	55	0
Crustaceans, crab, alaska king, raw	18.29	0.6	0	84	0	836	42	0
Crustaceans, crab, alaska king, cooked, moist heat	19.35	1.54	0	97	0	1072	53	0
Crustaceans, crab, alaska king, imitation, made from surimi	7.62	0.46	15	95	0.5	529	20	14.5
Crustaceans, crab, blue, raw	18.06	1.08	0.04	87	0	293	78	0.04
Crustaceans, crab, blue, cooked, moist heat	17.88	0.74	0	83	0	395	97	0
Crustaceans, crab, blue, canned	17.88	0.74	0	83	0	563	97	0
Crustaceans, crab, blue, crab cakes, home recipe	20.21	7.52	0.48	155	0	330	150	0.48

Food Name ---> per 100 g	Protein (g)	Fat (g)	Carb (g)	Calories	Fiber (g)	Sodium (mg)	Cholesterol (mg)	Net Carb (g)
Crustaceans, crab, dungeness, raw	17.41	0.97	0.74	86	0	295	59	0.74
Crustaceans, crab, queen, raw	18.5	1.18	0	90	0	539	55	0
Crustaceans, crayfish, mixed species, wild, raw	15.97	0.95	0	77	0	58	114	0
Crustaceans, crayfish, mixed species, wild, cooked, moist heat	16.77	1.2	0	82	0	94	133	0
Crustaceans, lobster, northern, raw	16.52	0.75	0	77	0	423	127	0
Crustaceans, lobster, northern, cooked, moist heat	19	0.86	0	89	0	486	146	0
Crustaceans, shrimp, mixed species, raw (may have been previously frozen)	13.61	1.01	0.91	71	0	566	126	0.91
Crustaceans, shrimp, mixed species, cooked, breaded and fried	21.39	12.28	11.47	242	0.4	344	138	11.07
Crustaceans, shrimp, mixed species, cooked, moist heat (may have been previously frozen)	22.78	1.7	1.52	119	0	947	211	1.52
Crustaceans, shrimp, mixed species, canned	20.42	1.36	0	100	0	870	252	0
Crustaceans, shrimp, mixed species, imitation, made from surimi	12.39	1.47	9.13	101	0	705	36	9.13
Crustaceans, spiny lobster, mixed species, raw	20.6	1.51	2.43	112	0	177	70	2.43
Mollusks, abalone, mixed species, raw	17.1	0.76	6.01	105	0	301	85	6.01
Mollusks, abalone, mixed species, cooked, fried	19.63	6.78	11.05	189	0	591	94	11.05
Mollusks, clam, mixed species, raw	14.67	0.96	3.57	86	0	601	30	3.57
Mollusks, clam, mixed species, cooked, breaded and fried	14.24	11.15	10.33	202	-	364	61	10.33
Mollusks, clam, mixed species, cooked, moist heat	25.55	1.95	5.13	148	0	1202	67	5.13
Mollusks, clam, mixed species, canned, drained solids	24.25	1.59	5.9	142	0	112	50	5.9
Mollusks, clam, mixed species, canned, liquid	0.4	0.02	0.1	2	0	215	3	0.1
Mollusks, cuttlefish, mixed species, raw	16.24	0.7	0.82	79	0	372	112	0.82
Mollusks, mussel, blue, raw	11.9	2.24	3.69	86	0	286	28	3.69
Mollusks, mussel, blue, cooked, moist heat	23.8	4.48	7.39	172	0	369	56	7.39
Mollusks, octopus, common, raw	14.91	1.04	2.2	82	0	230	48	2.2
Mollusks, oyster, eastern, wild, raw	5.71	1.71	2.72	51	0	85	40	2.72
Mollusks, oyster, eastern, cooked, breaded and fried	8.77	12.58	11.62	199	-	417	71	11.62
Mollusks, oyster, eastern, wild, cooked, moist heat	11.42	3.42	5.45	102	0	166	79	5.45
Mollusks, oyster, eastern, canned	7.06	2.47	3.91	68	0	112	55	3.91
Mollusks, oyster, Pacific, raw	9.45	2.3	4.95	81	0	106	50	4.95
Mollusks, scallop, mixed species, raw	12.06	0.49	3.18	69	0	392	24	3.18
Mollusks, scallop, mixed species, cooked, breaded and fried	18.07	10.94	10.13	216	-	464	54	10.13
Mollusks, scallop, mixed species, imitation, made from surimi	12.77	0.41	10.62	99	0	795	22	10.62
Mollusks, squid, mixed species, raw	15.58	1.38	3.08	92	0	44	233	3.08
Mollusks, squid, mixed species, cooked, fried	17.94	7.48	7.79	175	0	306	260	7.79
Mollusks, whelk, unspecified, raw	23.84	0.4	7.76	137	0	206	65	7.76
Mollusks, whelk, unspecified, cooked, moist heat	47.68	0.8	15.52	275	0	412	130	15.52
Fish, salmon, chinook, smoked, (lox), regular	18.28	4.32	0	117	0	2000	23	0
Fish, salmon, chum, canned, without salt, drained solids with bone	21.43	5.5	0	141	0	75	39	0
Fish, salmon, pink, canned, without salt, solids with bone and liquid	19.78	6.05	0	139	0	75	55	0

Food Name ---> per 100 g	Protein (g)	Fat (g)	Carb (g)	Calories	Fiber (g)	Sodium (mg)	Cholesterol (mg)	Net Carb(g)
Fish, salmon, sockeye, canned, without salt, drained solids with bone	20.47	7.31	0	153	0	75	44	0
Fish, tuna, light, canned in oil, without salt, drained solids	29.13	8.21	0	198	0	50	18	0
Fish, tuna, light, canned in water, without salt, drained solids	25.51	0.82	0	116	0	50	30	0
Fish, tuna, white, canned in oil, without salt, drained solids	26.53	8.08	0	186	0	50	31	0
Fish, tuna, white, canned in water, without salt, drained solids	23.62	2.97	0	128	0	50	42	0
Fish, bass, freshwater, mixed species, cooked, dry heat	24.18	4.73	0	146	0	90	87	0
Fish, bass, striped, cooked, dry heat	22.73	2.99	0	124	0	88	103	0
Fish, bluefish, cooked, dry heat	25.69	5.44	0	159	0	77	76	0
Fish, burbot, cooked, dry heat	24.76	1.04	0	115	0	124	77	0
Fish, butterfish, cooked, dry heat	22.15	10.28	0	187	0	114	83	0
Fish, cod, Pacific, cooked, dry heat (may have been previously frozen)	18.73	0.5	0	85	0	372	57	0
Fish, cusk, cooked, dry heat	24.35	0.88	0	112	0	40	53	0
Fish, mahimahi, cooked, dry heat	23.72	0.9	0	109	0	113	94	0
Fish, drum, freshwater, cooked, dry heat	22.49	6.32	0	153	0	96	82	0
Fish, halibut, greenland, cooked, dry heat	18.42	17.74	0	239	0	103	59	0
Fish, herring, Pacific, cooked, dry heat	21.01	17.79	0	250	0	95	99	0
Fish, ling, cooked, dry heat	24.35	0.82	0	111	0	173	51	0
Fish, lingcod, cooked, dry heat	22.64	1.36	0	109	0	76	67	0
Fish, mackerel, king, cooked, dry heat	26	2.56	0	134	0	203	68	0
Fish, mackerel, Pacific and jack, mixed species, cooked, dry heat	25.73	10.12	0	201	0	110	60	0
Fish, milkfish, cooked, dry heat	26.32	8.63	0	190	0	92	67	0
Fish, monkfish, cooked, dry heat	18.56	1.95	0	97	0	23	32	0
Fish, pike, walleye, cooked, dry heat	24.54	1.56	0	119	0	65	110	0
Fish, pollock, Atlantic, cooked, dry heat	24.92	1.26	0	118	0	110	91	0
Fish, pout, ocean, cooked, dry heat	21.33	1.17	0	102	0	78	67	0
Fish, roe, mixed species, cooked, dry heat	28.62	8.23	1.92	204	0	117	479	1.92
Fish, sablefish, cooked, dry heat	17.19	19.62	0	250	0	72	63	0
Fish, salmon, Atlantic, wild, cooked, dry heat	25.44	8.13	0	182	0	56	71	0
Fish, salmon, chinook, cooked, dry heat	25.72	13.38	0	231	0	60	85	0
Fish, salmon, chum, cooked, dry heat	25.82	4.83	0	154	0	64	95	0
Fish, salmon, pink, cooked, dry heat	24.58	5.28	0	153	0	90	55	0
Fish, scup, cooked, dry heat	24.21	3.5	0	135	0	54	67	0
Fish, seatrout, mixed species, cooked, dry heat	21.46	4.63	0	133	0	74	106	0
Fish, shad, american, cooked, dry heat	21.71	17.65	0	252	0	65	96	0
Fish, spot, cooked, dry heat	23.73	6.28	0	158	0	37	77	0
Fish, sucker, white, cooked, dry heat	21.49	2.97	0	119	0	51	53	0
Fish, sunfish, pumpkin seed, cooked, dry heat	24.87	0.9	0	114	0	103	86	0
Fish, trout, mixed species, cooked, dry heat	26.63	8.47	0	190	0	67	74	0
Fish, tuna, skipjack, fresh, cooked, dry heat	28.21	1.29	0	132	0	47	60	0
Fish, tuna, yellowfin, fresh, cooked, dry heat	29.15	0.59	0	130	0	54	47	0
Fish, turbot, european, cooked, dry heat	20.58	3.78	0	122	0	192	62	0
Fish, whitefish, mixed species, cooked, dry heat	24.47	7.51	0	172	0	65	77	0
Fish, wolffish, Atlantic, cooked, dry heat	22.44	3.06	0	123	0	109	59	0
Fish, yellowtail, mixed species, cooked, dry heat	29.67	6.72	0	187	0	50	71	0

Food Name ---> per 100 g	Protein (g)	Fat (g)	Carb (g)	Calories	Fiber (g)	Sodium (mg)	Cholesterol (mg)	Net Carb(g)
Crustaceans, crab, dungeness, cooked, moist heat	22.32	1.24	0.95	110	0	378	76	0.95
Crustaceans, crab, queen, cooked, moist heat	23.72	1.51	0	115	0	691	71	0
Crustaceans, spiny lobster, mixed species, cooked, moist heat	26.41	1.94	3.12	143	0	227	90	3.12
Mollusks, cuttlefish, mixed species, cooked, moist heat	32.48	1.4	1.64	158	0	744	224	1.64
Mollusks, octopus, common, cooked, moist heat	29.82	2.08	4.4	164	0	460	96	4.4
Mollusks, oyster, Pacific, cooked, moist heat	18.9	4.6	9.9	163	0	212	100	9.9
Fish, roughy, orange, cooked, dry heat	22.64	0.9	0	105	0	69	80	0
Fish, catfish, channel, wild, cooked, dry heat	18.47	2.85	0	105	0	50	72	0
Fish, catfish, channel, farmed, raw	15.23	5.94	0	119	0	98	55	0
Fish, catfish, channel, farmed, cooked, dry heat	18.44	7.19	0	144	0	119	66	0
Fish, salmon, Atlantic, farmed, raw	20.42	13.42	0	208	0	59	55	0
Fish, salmon, Atlantic, farmed, cooked, dry heat	22.1	12.35	0	206	0	61	63	0
Fish, salmon, coho, farmed, raw	21.27	7.67	0	160	0	47	51	0
Fish, salmon, coho, farmed, cooked, dry heat	24.3	8.23	0	178	0	52	63	0
Fish, trout, rainbow, farmed, raw	19.94	6.18	0	141	0	51	59	0
Fish, trout, rainbow, farmed, cooked, dry heat	23.8	7.38	0	168	0	61	70	0
Crustaceans, crayfish, mixed species, farmed, raw	14.85	0.97	0	72	0	62	107	0
Crustaceans, crayfish, mixed species, farmed, cooked, moist heat	17.52	1.3	0	87	0	97	137	0
Mollusks, oyster, eastern, wild, cooked, dry heat	8.87	2.65	4.23	79	0	132	62	4.23
Mollusks, oyster, eastern, farmed, raw	5.22	1.55	5.53	59	0	178	25	5.53
Mollusks, oyster, eastern, farmed, cooked, dry heat	7	2.12	7.28	79	0	163	38	7.28
Fish, salmon, coho, wild, cooked, dry heat	23.45	4.3	0	139	0	58	55	0
Mollusks, conch, baked or broiled	26.3	1.2	1.7	130	0	153	65	1.7
USDA Commodity, salmon nuggets, breaded, frozen, heated	12.69	11.72	13.96	212	0	173	26	13.96
USDA Commodity, salmon nuggets, cooked as purchased, unheated	11.97	10.43	11.85	189	0	167	27	11.85
Salmon, sockeye, canned, total can contents	20.63	7.17	0	153	0	433	67	0
Fish, salmon, pink, canned, drained solids	23.1	5.02	0	138	0	381	83	0
Fish, tilapia, raw	20.08	1.7	0	96	0	52	50	0
Fish, tilapia, cooked, dry heat	26.15	2.65	0	128	0	56	57	0
Salmon, sockeye, canned, drained solids, without skin and bones	26.33	5.87	0	158	0	386	66	0
Fish, Salmon, pink, canned, drained solids, without skin and bones	24.62	4.21	0	136	0	378	83	0
Fish, pollock, Alaska, raw (not previously frozen)	17.17	0.19	0	70	-	159	61	0
Fish, pollock, Alaska, cooked (not previously frozen)	19.42	0.26	0	80	-	166	74	0
Fish, cod, Pacific, raw (not previously frozen)	17.54	0.2	0	72	-	109	46	0
Fish, cod, Pacific, cooked (not previously frozen)	20.42	0.25	0	84	-	134	61	0
Crustaceans, shrimp, raw (not previously frozen)	20.1	0.51	0	85	-	119	161	0
Crustaceans, shrimp, cooked (not previously frozen)	23.98	0.28	0.2	99	-	111	189	0.2
Fish, trout, brook, raw, New York State	21.23	2.73	0	110	-	45	60	0
Jellyfish, dried, salted	5.5	1.4	0	36	0	9690	5	0

Food Name ---> per 100 g	Protein (g)	Fat (g)	Carb (g)	Calories	Fiber (g)	Sodium (mg)	Cholesterol (mg)	Net Carb(g)
Frog legs, raw	16.4	0.3	0	73	0	58	50	0
Fish, mackerel, salted	18.5	25.1	0	305	0	4450	95	0
Mollusks, scallop, (bay and sea), cooked, steamed	20.54	0.84	5.41	111	0	667	41	5.41
Mollusks, snail, raw	16.1	1.4	2	90	0	70	50	2

Fruits and Fruits Juices

Food Name ---> per 100 g	Protein (g)	Fat (g)	Carb (g)	Calories	Fiber (g)	Sodium (mg)	Cholesterol (mg)	Net Carb (g)
Acerola, (west indian cherry), raw	0.4	0.3	7.69	32	1.1	7	0	6.59
Acerola juice, raw	0.4	0.3	4.8	23	0.3	3	0	4.5
Apples, raw, with skin	0.26	0.17	13.81	52	2.4	1	0	11.41
Apples, raw, without skin	0.27	0.13	12.76	48	1.3	0	0	11.46
Apples, raw, without skin, cooked, boiled	0.26	0.36	13.64	53	2.4	1	0	11.24
Apples, raw, without skin, cooked, microwave	0.28	0.42	14.41	56	2.8	1	0	11.61
Apples, canned, sweetened, sliced, drained, unheated	0.18	0.49	16.7	67	1.7	3	0	15
Apples, canned, sweetened, sliced, drained, heated	0.18	0.43	16.84	67	2	3	0	14.84
Apples, dehydrated (low moisture), sulfured, uncooked	1.32	0.58	93.53	346	12.4	124	0	81.13
Apples, dehydrated (low moisture), sulfured, stewed	0.28	0.12	19.91	74	2.6	26	0	17.31
Apples, dried, sulfured, uncooked	0.93	0.32	65.89	243	8.7	87	0	57.19
Apples, dried, sulfured, stewed, without added sugar	0.22	0.07	15.32	57	2	20	0	13.32
Apples, dried, sulfured, stewed, with added sugar	0.2	0.07	20.73	83	1.9	19	0	18.83
Apples, frozen, unsweetened, unheated	0.28	0.32	12.31	48	1.3	3	0	11.01
Apples, frozen, unsweetened, heated	0.29	0.33	12	47	1.3	3	0	10.7
Apple juice, canned or bottled, unsweetened, without added ascorbic acid	0.1	0.13	11.3	46	0.2	4	0	11.1
Apple juice, frozen concentrate, unsweetened, undiluted, without added ascorbic acid	0.51	0.37	41	166	0.4	25	0	40.6
Apple juice, frozen concentrate, unsweetened, diluted with 3 volume water without added ascorbic acid	0.14	0.1	11.54	47	0.1	7	0	11.44
Applesauce, canned, unsweetened, without added ascorbic acid (includes USDA commodity)	0.17	0.1	11.27	42	1.1	2	0	10.17
Applesauce, canned, sweetened, without salt (includes USDA commodity)	0.16	0.17	17.49	68	1.2	2	0	16.29
Apricots, raw	1.4	0.39	11.12	48	2	1	0	9.12
Apricots, canned, water pack, with skin, solids and liquids	0.71	0.16	6.39	27	1.6	3	0	4.79
Apricots, canned, water pack, without skin, solids and liquids	0.69	0.03	5.48	22	1.1	11	0	4.38
Apricots, canned, juice pack, with skin, solids and liquids	0.63	0.04	12.34	48	1.6	4	0	10.74
Apricots, canned, extra light syrup pack, with skin, solids and liquids	0.6	0.1	12.5	49	1.6	2	0	10.9
Apricots, canned, light syrup pack, with skin, solids and liquids	0.53	0.05	16.49	63	1.6	4	0	14.89
Apricots, canned, heavy syrup pack, with skin, solids and liquids	0.53	0.08	21.47	83	1.6	4	0	19.87
Apricots, canned, heavy syrup pack, without skin, solids and liquids	0.51	0.09	21.45	83	1.6	11	0	19.85
Apricots, canned, extra heavy syrup pack, without skin, solids and liquids	0.55	0.04	24.85	96	1.6	13	0	23.25

Food Name ---> per 100 g	Protein (g)	Fat (g)	Carb (g)	Calories	Fiber (g)	Sodium (mg)	Cholesterol (mg)	Net Carb (g)
Apricots, dehydrated (low-moisture), sulfured, uncooked	4.9	0.62	82.89	320	-	13	0	82.89
Apricots, dehydrated (low-moisture), sulfured, stewed	1.93	0.24	32.62	126	-	5	0	32.62
Apricots, dried, sulfured, uncooked	3.39	0.51	62.64	241	7.3	10	0	55.34
Apricots, dried, sulfured, stewed, without added sugar	1.2	0.18	22.15	85	2.6	4	0	19.55
Apricots, dried, sulfured, stewed, with added sugar	1.17	0.15	29.26	113	4.1	3	0	25.16
Apricots, frozen, sweetened	0.7	0.1	25.1	98	2.2	4	0	22.9
Apricot nectar, canned, without added ascorbic acid	0.37	0.09	14.39	56	0.6	3	0	13.79
Avocados, raw, all commercial varieties	2	14.66	8.53	160	6.7	7	0	1.83
Avocados, raw, California	1.96	15.41	8.64	167	6.8	8	0	1.84
Avocados, raw, Florida	2.23	10.06	7.82	120	5.6	2	0	2.22
Bananas, raw	1.09	0.33	22.84	89	2.6	1	0	20.24
Bananas, dehydrated, or banana powder	3.89	1.81	88.28	346	9.9	3	0	78.38
Blackberries, raw	1.39	0.49	9.61	43	5.3	1	0	4.31
Blackberry juice, canned	0.3	0.6	7.8	38	0.1	1	0	7.7
Cherries, tart, dried, sweetened	1.25	0.73	80.45	333	2.5	13	0	77.95
Blackberries, canned, heavy syrup, solids and liquids	1.31	0.14	23.1	92	3.4	3	0	19.7
Blackberries, frozen, unsweetened	1.18	0.43	15.67	64	5	1	0	10.67
Blueberries, raw	0.74	0.33	14.49	57	2.4	1	0	12.09
Blueberries, canned, heavy syrup, solids and liquids	0.65	0.33	22.06	88	1.6	3	0	20.46
Blueberries, wild, frozen	0	0.16	13.85	57	4.4	3	0	9.45
Blueberries, frozen, unsweetened	0.42	0.64	12.17	51	2.7	1	0	9.47
Blueberries, frozen, sweetened	0.4	0.13	21.95	85	2.2	1	0	19.75
Boysenberries, canned, heavy syrup	0.99	0.12	22.31	88	2.6	3	0	19.71
Boysenberries, frozen, unsweetened	1.1	0.26	12.19	50	5.3	1	0	6.89
Breadfruit, raw	1.07	0.23	27.12	103	4.9	2	0	22.22
Carambola, (starfruit), raw	1.04	0.33	6.73	31	2.8	2	0	3.93
Carissa, (natal-plum), raw	0.5	1.3	13.63	62	-	3	0	13.63
Cherimoya, raw	1.57	0.68	17.71	75	3	7	0	14.71
Cherries, sour, red, raw	1	0.3	12.18	50	1.6	3	0	10.58
Cherries, sour, red, canned, water pack, solids and liquids (includes USDA commodity red tart cherries, canned)	0.77	0.1	8.94	36	1.1	7	0	7.84
Cherries, sour, red, canned, light syrup pack, solids and liquids	0.74	0.1	19.3	75	0.8	7	0	18.5
Cherries, sour, red, canned, heavy syrup pack, solids and liquids	0.73	0.1	23.27	91	1.1	7	0	22.17
Cherries, sour, red, canned, extra heavy syrup pack, solids and liquids	0.71	0.09	29.23	114	0.8	7	0	28.43
Cherries, sour, red, frozen, unsweetened	0.92	0.44	11.02	46	1.6	1	0	9.42
Cherries, sweet, raw	1.06	0.2	16.01	63	2.1	0	0	13.91
Cherries, sweet, canned, water pack, solids and liquids	0.77	0.13	11.76	46	1.5	1	0	10.26
Cherries, sweet, canned, juice pack, solids and liquids	0.91	0.02	13.81	54	1.5	3	0	12.31
Cherries, sweet, canned, light syrup pack, solids and liquids	0.61	0.15	17.29	67	1.5	3	0	15.79
Cherries, sweet, canned, pitted, heavy syrup	0.6	0.15	21.27	83	1.4	3	0	19.87

pack, solids and liquids

Food Name ---> per 100 g	Protein (g)	Fat (g)	Carb (g)	Calories	Fiber (g)	Sodium (mg)	Cholesterol (mg)	Net Carb (g)
Cherries, sweet, canned, extra heavy syrup pack, solids and liquids	0.59	0.15	26.23	102	1.5	3	0	24.73
Cherries, sweet, frozen, sweetened	1.15	0.13	22.36	89	2.1	1	0	20.26
Crabapples, raw	0.4	0.3	19.95	76	-	1	0	19.95
Cranberries, raw	0.46	0.13	11.97	46	3.6	2	0	8.37
Cranberries, dried, sweetened	0.17	1.09	82.8	308	5.3	5	0	77.5
Cranberry sauce, canned, sweetened	0.9	0.15	40.4	159	1.1	5	0	39.3
Cranberry-orange relish, canned	0.3	0.1	46.2	178	0	32	0	46.2
Currants, european black, raw	1.4	0.41	15.38	63	-	2	0	15.38
Currants, red and white, raw	1.4	0.2	13.8	56	4.3	1	0	9.5
Currants, zante, dried	4.08	0.27	74.08	283	6.8	8	0	67.28
Custard-apple, (bullock's-heart), raw	1.7	0.6	25.2	101	2.4	4	0	22.8
Dates, deglet noor	2.45	0.39	75.03	282	8	2	0	67.03
Elderberries, raw	0.66	0.5	18.4	73	7	6	0	11.4
Figs, raw	0.75	0.3	19.18	74	2.9	1	0	16.28
Figs, canned, water pack, solids and liquids	0.4	0.1	13.99	53	2.2	1	0	11.79
Figs, canned, light syrup pack, solids and liquids	0.39	0.1	17.95	69	1.8	1	0	16.15
Figs, canned, heavy syrup pack, solids and liquids	0.38	0.1	22.9	88	2.2	1	0	20.7
Figs, canned, extra heavy syrup pack, solids and liquids	0.38	0.1	27.86	107	-	1	0	27.86
Figs, dried, uncooked	3.3	0.93	63.87	249	9.8	10	0	54.07
Figs, dried, stewed	1.42	0.4	27.57	107	4.2	4	0	23.37
Fruit cocktail, (peach and pineapple and pear and grape and cherry), canned, water pack, solids and liquids	0.42	0.05	8.51	32	1	4	0	7.51
Fruit cocktail, (peach and pineapple and pear and grape and cherry), canned, juice pack, solids and liquids	0.46	0.01	11.86	46	1	4	0	10.86
Fruit cocktail, (peach and pineapple and pear and grape and cherry), canned, extra light syrup, solids and liquids	0.4	0.07	11.63	45	1.1	4	0	10.53
Fruit cocktail, (peach and pineapple and pear and grape and cherry), canned, light syrup, solids and liquids	0.4	0.07	14.93	57	1	6	0	13.93
Fruit cocktail, (peach and pineapple and pear and grape and cherry), canned, heavy syrup, solids and liquids	0.39	0.07	18.91	73	1	6	0	17.91
Fruit cocktail, (peach and pineapple and pear and grape and cherry), canned, extra heavy syrup, solids and liquids	0.39	0.07	22.89	88	1.1	6	0	21.79
Fruit salad, (peach and pear and apricot and pineapple and cherry), canned, water pack, solids and liquids	0.35	0.07	7.87	30	1	3	0	6.87
Fruit salad, (peach and pear and apricot and pineapple and cherry), canned, juice pack, solids and liquids	0.51	0.03	13.05	50	1	5	0	12.05
Fruit salad, (peach and pear and apricot and pineapple and cherry), canned, light syrup, solids and liquids	0.34	0.07	15.14	58	1	6	0	14.14
Fruit salad, (peach and pear and apricot and pineapple and cherry), canned, heavy syrup, solids and liquids	0.34	0.07	19.11	73	1	6	0	18.11
Fruit salad, (peach and pear and apricot and	0.33	0.06	22.77	88	1	5	0	21.77

Food Name ---> per 100 g	Protein (g)	Fat (g)	Carb (g)	Calories	Fiber (g)	Sodium (mg)	Cholesterol (mg)	Net Carb (g)
pineapple and cherry), canned, extra heavy syrup, solids and liquids								
Gooseberries, raw	0.88	0.58	10.18	44	4.3	1	0	5.88
Gooseberries, canned, light syrup pack, solids and liquids	0.65	0.2	18.75	73	2.4	2	0	16.35
Goji berries, dried	14.26	0.39	77.06	349	13	298	0	64.06
Grapefruit, raw, pink and red and white, all areas	0.63	0.1	8.08	32	1.1	0	0	6.98
Grapefruit, raw, pink and red, all areas	0.77	0.14	10.66	42	1.6	0	0	9.06
Grapefruit, raw, pink and red, California and Arizona	0.5	0.1	9.69	37	-	1	0	9.69
Grapefruit, raw, pink and red, Florida	0.55	0.1	7.5	30	1.1	0	0	6.4
Grapefruit, raw, white, all areas	0.69	0.1	8.41	33	1.1	0	0	7.31
Grapefruit, raw, white, California	0.88	0.1	9.09	37	-	0	0	9.09
Grapefruit, raw, white, Florida	0.63	0.1	8.19	32	-	0	0	8.19
Grapefruit, sections, canned, water pack, solids and liquids	0.58	0.1	9.15	36	0.4	2	0	8.75
Grapefruit, sections, canned, juice pack, solids and liquids	0.7	0.09	9.21	37	0.4	7	0	8.81
Grapefruit, sections, canned, light syrup pack, solids and liquids	0.56	0.1	15.44	60	0.4	2	0	15.04
Grapefruit juice, white, canned or bottled, unsweetened	0.58	0.1	7.93	34	0.8	3	0	7.13
Grapefruit juice, white, canned, sweetened	0.58	0.09	11.13	46	0.1	2	0	11.03
Grapefruit juice, white, frozen concentrate, unsweetened, undiluted	1.97	0.48	34.56	146	0.4	3	0	34.16
Grapefruit juice, white, frozen concentrate, unsweetened, diluted with 3 volume water	0.55	0.13	9.73	41	0.1	1	0	9.63
Grapefruit juice, pink or red, with added calcium	0.5	0.1	8.69	38	0	1	0	8.69
Grapefruit juice, white, raw	0.5	0.1	9.2	39	0.1	1	0	9.1
Grapes, muscadine, raw	0.81	0.47	13.93	57	3.9	1	-	10.03
Grape juice, canned or bottled, unsweetened, with added ascorbic acid	0.37	0.13	14.77	60	0.2	5	0	14.57
Grapes, american type (slip skin), raw	0.63	0.35	17.15	67	0.9	2	0	16.25
Grapes, red or green (European type, such as Thompson seedless), raw	0.72	0.16	18.1	69	0.9	2	0	17.2
Grapes, canned, thompson seedless, water pack, solids and liquids	0.5	0.11	10.3	40	0.6	6	0	9.7
Grapes, canned, thompson seedless, heavy syrup pack, solids and liquids	0.48	0.1	19.65	76	0.6	5	0	19.05
Grape juice, canned or bottled, unsweetened, without added ascorbic acid	0.37	0.13	14.77	60	0.2	5	0	14.57
Groundcherries, (cape-gooseberries or poha), raw	1.9	0.7	11.2	53	-	-	0	11.2
Guavas, common, raw	2.55	0.95	14.32	68	5.4	2	0	8.92
Guavas, strawberry, raw	0.58	0.6	17.36	69	5.4	37	0	11.96
Guava sauce, cooked	0.32	0.14	9.48	36	3.6	4	0	5.88
Jackfruit, raw	1.72	0.64	23.25	95	1.5	2	0	21.75
Java-plum, (jambolan), raw	0.72	0.23	15.56	60	-	14	0	15.56
Jujube, raw	1.2	0.2	20.23	79	-	3	0	20.23
Jujube, Chinese, fresh, dried	4.72	0.5	72.52	281	6	5	0	66.52
Kiwifruit, green, raw	1.14	0.52	14.66	61	3	3	0	11.66
Kumquats, raw	1.88	0.86	15.9	71	6.5	10	0	9.4
Lemons, raw, without peel	1.1	0.3	9.32	29	2.8	2	0	6.52
Lemon juice, raw	0.35	0.24	6.9	22	0.3	1	0	6.6

Food Name ---> per 100 g	Protein (g)	Fat (g)	Carb (g)	Calories	Fiber (g)	Sodium (mg)	Cholesterol (mg)	Net Carb (g)
Lemon juice from concentrate, canned or bottled	0.45	0.07	5.62	17	0.7	24	0	4.92
Lemon juice, frozen, unsweetened, single strength	0.46	0.32	6.5	22	0.4	1	0	6.1
Lemon peel, raw	1.5	0.3	16	47	10.6	6	0	5.4
Limes, raw	0.7	0.2	10.54	30	2.8	2	0	7.74
Lime juice, raw	0.42	0.07	8.42	25	0.4	2	0	8.02
Lime juice, canned or bottled, unsweetened	0.25	0.23	6.69	21	0.4	16	0	6.29
Blueberries, dried, sweetened	2.5	2.5	80	317	7.5	3	0	72.5
Litchis, raw	0.83	0.44	16.53	66	1.3	1	0	15.23
Litchis, dried	3.8	1.2	70.7	277	4.6	3'	0	66.1
Loganberries, frozen	1.52	0.31	13.02	55	5.3	1	0	7.72
Longans, raw	1.31	0.1	15.14	60	1.1	0	0	14.04
Longans, dried	4.9	0.4	74	286	-	48	0	74
Loquats, raw	0.43	0.2	12.14	47	1.7	1	0	10.44
Mammy-apple, (mamey), raw	0.5	0.5	12.5	51	3	15	0	9.5
Mangos, raw	0.82	0.38	14.98	60	1.6	1	0	13.38
Mangosteen, canned, syrup pack	0.41	0.58	17.91	73	1.8	7	0	16.11
Mango, dried, sweetened	2.45	1.18	78.58	319	2.4	162	0	76.18
Melons, cantaloupe, raw	0.84	0.19	8.16	34	0.9	16	0	7.26
Melons, casaba, raw	1.11	0.1	6.58	28	0.9	9	0	5.68
Melons, honeydew, raw	0.54	0.14	9.09	36	0.8	18	0	8.29
Melon balls, frozen	0.84	0.25	7.94	33	0.7	31	0	7.24
Mulberries, raw	1.44	0.39	9.8	43	1.7	10	0	8.1
Nectarines, raw	1.06	0.32	10.55	44	1.7	0	0	8.85
Oheloberries, raw	0.38	0.22	6.84	28	-	1	0	6.84
Olives, ripe, canned (small-extra large)	0.84	10.68	6.26	115	3.2	735	0	3.06
Olives, ripe, canned (jumbo-super colossal)	0.97	6.87	5.61	81	2.5	735	0	3.11
Olives, pickled, canned or bottled, green	1.03	15.32	3.84	145	3.3	1556	0	0.54
Oranges, raw, all commercial varieties	0.94	0.12	11.75	47	2.4	0	0	9.35
Oranges, raw, California, valencias	1.04	0.3	11.89	49	2.5	0	0	9.39
Oranges, raw, navels	0.91	0.15	12.54	49	2.2	1	0	10.34
Oranges, raw, Florida	0.7	0.21	11.54	46	2.4	0	0	9.14
Oranges, raw, with peel	1.3	0.3	15.5	63	4.5	2	0	11
Orange juice, raw	0.7	0.2	10.4	45	0.2	1	0	10.2
Orange juice, canned, unsweetened	0.68	0.15	11.01	47	0.3	4	0	10.71
Orange juice, chilled, includes from concentrate	0.68	0.12	11.54	49	0.3	2	0	11.24
Orange juice, chilled, includes from concentrate, with added calcium and vitamin D	0.68	0.12	11.27	47	0.3	2	0	10.97
Orange juice, chilled, includes from concentrate, with added calcium	0.68	0.12	11.27	47	0.3	2	0	10.97
Orange juice, frozen concentrate, unsweetened, diluted with 3 volume water, with added calcium	0.6	0.06	8.47	37	0.2	4	0	8.27
Orange juice, frozen concentrate, unsweetened, undiluted, with added calcium	2.4	0.25	33.86	147	1	7	0	32.86
Orange juice, frozen concentrate, unsweetened, undiluted	2.4	0.25	35.19	148	1	7	0	34.19
Orange juice, frozen concentrate, unsweetened, diluted with 3 volume water	0.6	0.06	8.8	37	0.2	4	0	8.6
Orange peel, raw	1.5	0.2	25	97	10.6	3	0	14.4
Orange-grapefruit juice, canned or bottled, unsweetened	0.6	0.1	10.28	43	0.1	3	0	10.18
Tangerines, (mandarin oranges), raw	0.81	0.31	13.34	53	1.8	2	0	11.54
Tangerines, (mandarin oranges), canned, juice	0.62	0.03	9.57	37	0.7	5	0	8.87

Food Name ---> per 100 g	Protein (g)	Fat (g)	Carb (g)	Calories	Fiber (g)	Sodium (mg)	Cholesterol (mg)	Net Carb (g)
pack								
Tangerines, (mandarin oranges), canned, light syrup pack	0.45	0.1	16.19	61	0.7	6	0	15.49
Tangerine juice, raw	0.5	0.2	10.1	43	0.2	1	0	9.9
Tangerine juice, canned, sweetened	0.5	0.2	12	50	0.2	1	0	11.8
Papayas, raw	0.47	0.26	10.82	43	1.7	8	0	9.12
Papaya, canned, heavy syrup, drained	0.14	0.55	55.83	206	1.5	9	-	54.33
Papaya nectar, canned	0.17	0.15	14.51	57	0.6	5	0	13.91
Passion-fruit, (granadilla), purple, raw	2.2	0.7	23.38	97	10.4	28	0	12.98
Passion-fruit juice, purple, raw	0.39	0.05	13.6	51	0.2	6	0	13.4
Passion-fruit juice, yellow, raw	0.67	0.18	14.45	60	0.2	6	0	14.25
Peaches, yellow, raw	0.91	0.25	9.54	39	1.5	0	0	8.04
Peaches, canned, water pack, solids and liquids	0.44	0.06	6.11	24	1.3	3	0	4.81
Peaches, canned, juice pack, solids and liquids	0.63	0.03	11.57	44	1.3	4	0	10.27
Peaches, canned, extra light syrup, solids and liquids	0.4	0.1	11.1	42	1	5	0	10.1
Peaches, canned, light syrup pack, solids and liquids	0.45	0.03	14.55	54	1.3	5	0	13.25
Peaches, canned, heavy syrup pack, solids and liquids	0.45	0.1	19.94	74	1.3	6	0	18.64
Peaches, canned, extra heavy syrup pack, solids and liquids	0.47	0.03	26.06	96	1	8	0	25.06
Peaches, spiced, canned, heavy syrup pack, solids and liquids	0.41	0.1	20.08	75	1.3	4	0	18.78
Peaches, dehydrated (low-moisture), sulfured, uncooked	4.89	1.03	83.18	325	-	10	0	83.18
Peaches, dehydrated (low-moisture), sulfured, stewed	2.01	0.42	34.14	133	-	4	0	34.14
Peaches, dried, sulfured, uncooked	3.61	0.76	61.33	239	8.2	7	0	53.13
Peaches, dried, sulfured, stewed, without added sugar	1.16	0.25	19.69	77	2.7	2	0	16.99
Peaches, dried, sulfured, stewed, with added sugar	1.06	0.22	26.6	103	2.4	2	0	24.2
Peaches, frozen, sliced, sweetened	0.63	0.13	23.98	94	1.8	6	0	22.18
Peach nectar, canned, without added ascorbic acid	0.27	0.02	13.92	54	0.6	7	0	13.32
Pears, raw	0.36	0.14	15.23	57	3.1	1	0	12.13
Pears, canned, water pack, solids and liquids	0.19	0.03	7.81	29	1.6	2	0	6.21
Pears, canned, juice pack, solids and liquids	0.34	0.07	12.94	50	1.6	4	0	11.34
Pears, canned, extra light syrup pack, solids and liquids	0.3	0.1	12.2	47	1.6	2	0	10.6
Pears, canned, light syrup pack, solids and liquids	0.19	0.03	15.17	57	1.6	5	0	13.57
Pears, canned, heavy syrup pack, solids and liquids	0.2	0.13	19.17	74	1.6	5	0	17.57
Pears, canned, extra heavy syrup pack, solids and liquids	0.19	0.13	25.25	97	1.6	5	0	23.65
Pears, dried, sulfured, uncooked	1.87	0.63	69.7	262	7.5	6	0	62.2
Pears, dried, sulfured, stewed, without added sugar	0.91	0.31	33.81	127	6.4	3	0	27.41
Pears, dried, sulfured, stewed, with added sugar	0.86	0.29	37.14	140	5.8	3	0	31.34
Pear nectar, canned, without added ascorbic acid	0.11	0.01	15.76	60	0.6	4	0	15.16
Persimmons, japanese, raw	0.58	0.19	18.59	70	3.6	1	0	14.99
Persimmons, japanese, dried	1.38	0.59	73.43	274	14.5	2	0	58.93

Food Name ---> per 100 g	Protein (g)	Fat (g)	Carb (g)	Calories	Fiber (g)	Sodium (mg)	Cholesterol (mg)	Net Carb (g)
Persimmons, native, raw	0.8	0.4	33.5	127	-	1	0	33.5
Pineapple, raw, all varieties	0.54	0.12	13.12	50	1.4	1	0	11.72
Pineapple, canned, water pack, solids and liquids	0.43	0.09	8.3	32	0.8	1	0	7.5
Pineapple, canned, juice pack, solids and liquids	0.42	0.08	15.7	60	0.8	1	0	14.9
Pineapple, canned, light syrup pack, solids and liquids	0.36	0.12	13.45	52	0.8	1	0	12.65
Pineapple, canned, heavy syrup pack, solids and liquids	0.35	0.11	20.2	78	0.8	1	0	19.4
Pineapple, canned, extra heavy syrup pack, solids and liquids	0.34	0.11	21.5	83	0.8	1	0	20.7
Pineapple, frozen, chunks, sweetened	0.4	0.1	22.2	86	1.1	2	0	21.1
Pineapple juice, canned or bottled, unsweetened, without added ascorbic acid	0.36	0.12	12.87	53	0.2	2	0	12.67
Pineapple juice, frozen concentrate, unsweetened, undiluted	1.3	0.1	44.3	179	0.7	3	0	43.6
Pineapple juice, frozen concentrate, unsweetened, diluted with 3 volume water	0.4	0.03	12.67	51	0.2	1	0	12.47
Pitanga, (surinam-cherry), raw	0.8	0.4	7.49	33	-	3	0	7.49
Plantains, raw	1.3	0.37	31.89	122	2.3	4	0	29.59
Plantains, cooked	0.79	0.18	31.15	116	2.3	5	0	28.85
Plums, raw	0.7	0.28	11.42	46	1.4	0	0	10.02
Plums, canned, purple, water pack, solids and liquids	0.39	0.01	11.03	41	0.9	1	0	10.13
Plums, canned, purple, juice pack, solids and liquids	0.51	0.02	15.15	58	0.9	1	0	14.25
Plums, canned, purple, light syrup pack, solids and liquids	0.37	0.1	16.28	63	0.9	20	0	15.38
Plums, canned, purple, heavy syrup pack, solids and liquids	0.36	0.1	23.24	89	0.9	19	0	22.34
Plums, canned, purple, extra heavy syrup pack, solids and liquids	0.36	0.1	26.31	101	1	19	0	25.31
Pomegranates, raw	1.67	1.17	18.7	83	4	3	0	14.7
Prickly pears, raw	0.73	0.51	9.57	41	3.6	5	0	5.97
Prunes, canned, heavy syrup pack, solids and liquids	0.87	0.2	27.8	105	3.8	3	0	24
Prunes, dehydrated (low-moisture), uncooked	3.7	0.73	89.07	339	-	5	0	89.07
Prunes, dehydrated (low-moisture), stewed	1.23	0.24	29.7	113	-	2	0	29.7
Plums, dried (prunes), uncooked	2.18	0.38	63.88	240	7.1	2	0	56.78
Plums, dried (prunes), stewed, without added sugar	0.96	0.16	28.08	107	3.1	1	0	24.98
Plums, dried (prunes), stewed, with added sugar	1.09	0.22	32.88	124	3.8	2	0	29.08
Prune juice, canned	0.61	0.03	17.45	71	1	4	0	16.45
Pummelo, raw	0.76	0.04	9.62	38	1	1	0	8.62
Quinces, raw	0.4	0.1	15.3	57	1.9	4	0	13.4
Raisins, golden seedless	3.39	0.46	79.52	302	4	12	0	75.52
Raisins, seedless	3.07	0.46	79.18	299	3.7	11	0	75.48
Raisins, seeded	2.52	0.54	78.47	296	6.8	28	0	71.67
Rambutan, canned, syrup pack	0.65	0.21	20.87	82	0.9	11	0	19.97
Raspberries, raw	1.2	0.65	11.94	52	6.5	1	0	5.44
Raspberries, canned, red, heavy syrup pack, solids and liquids	0.83	0.12	23.36	91	3.3	3	0	20.06
Raspberries, frozen, red, sweetened	0.7	0.16	26.16	103	4.4	1	0	21.76
Rhubarb, raw	0.9	0.2	4.54	21	1.8	4	0	2.74
Rhubarb, frozen, uncooked	0.55	0.11	5.1	21	1.8	2	0	3.3

Food Name ---> per 100 g	Protein (g)	Fat (g)	Carb (g)	Calories	Fiber (g)	Sodium (mg)	Cholesterol (mg)	Net Carb (g)
Rhubarb, frozen, cooked, with sugar	0.39	0.05	31.2	116	2	1	0	29.2
Roselle, raw	0.96	0.64	11.31	49	-	6	0	11.31
Rose-apples, raw	0.6	0.3	5.7	25	-	0	0	5.7
Sapodilla, raw	0.44	1.1	19.96	83	5.3	12	0	14.66
Sapote, mamey, raw	1.45	0.46	32.1	124	5.4	7	0	26.7
Soursop, raw	1	0.3	16.84	66	3.3	14	0	13.54
Strawberries, raw	0.67	0.3	7.68	32	2	1	0	5.68
Strawberries, canned, heavy syrup pack, solids and liquids	0.56	0.26	23.53	92	1.7	4	0	21.83
Strawberries, frozen, unsweetened	0.43	0.11	9.13	35	2.1	2	0	7.03
Strawberries, frozen, sweetened, whole	0.52	0.14	21	78	1.9	1	0	19.1
Strawberries, frozen, sweetened, sliced	0.53	0.13	25.92	96	1.9	3	0	24.02
Sugar-apples, (sweetsop), raw	2.06	0.29	23.64	94	4.4	9	0	19.24
Tamarinds, raw	2.8	0.6	62.5	239	5.1	28	0	57.4
Fruit salad, (pineapple and papaya and banana and guava), tropical, canned, heavy syrup, solids and liquids	0.41	0.1	22.36	86	1.3	2	0	21.06
Watermelon, raw	0.61	0.15	7.55	30	0.4	1	0	7.15
Maraschino cherries, canned, drained	0.22	0.21	41.97	165	3.2	4	0	38.77
Feijoa, raw	0.71	0.42	15.21	61	6.4	3	0	8.81
Pears, asian, raw	0.5	0.23	10.65	42	3.6	0	0	7.05
Fruit cocktail, canned, heavy syrup, drained	0.47	0.1	18.8	70	1.7	6	0	17.1
Blueberries, canned, light syrup, drained	1.04	0.4	22.66	88	2.6	3	0	20.06
Blueberries, wild, canned, heavy syrup, drained	0.56	0.34	28.32	107	4.9	1	-	23.42
Pineapple, canned, juice pack, drained	0.51	0.11	15.56	60	1.3	1	0	14.26
Apricots, canned, heavy syrup, drained	0.64	0.11	21.31	83	2.7	4	0	18.61
Cherries, sour, canned, water pack, drained	0.69	0.21	10.45	42	1.2	4	-	9.25
Cherries, sweet, canned, pitted, heavy syrup, drained	0.73	0.21	21.07	83	2.3	3	0	18.77
Peaches, canned, heavy syrup, drained	0.52	0.18	18.43	72	1.2	6	0	17.23
Pears, canned, heavy syrup, drained	0.24	0.18	19.08	74	2.7	5	0	16.38
Plums, canned, heavy syrup, drained	0.44	0.14	23.12	89	1.5	19	0	21.62
Tangerines, (mandarin oranges), canned, juice pack, drained	0.75	0.04	9.41	38	1.2	5	0	8.21
Apple juice, canned or bottled, unsweetened, with added ascorbic acid	0.1	0.13	11.3	46	0.2	4	0	11.1
Applesauce, canned, unsweetened, with added ascorbic acid	0.17	0.1	11.27	42	1.1	2	0	10.17
Applesauce, canned, sweetened, with salt	0.18	0.18	19.91	76	1.2	28	0	18.71
Apricot nectar, canned, with added ascorbic acid	0.37	0.09	14.39	56	0.6	3	0	13.79
Grapefruit juice, pink, raw	0.5	0.1	9.2	39	-	1	0	9.2
Peach nectar, canned, with added ascorbic acid	0.27	0.02	13.92	54	0.6	7	0	13.32
Pear nectar, canned, with added ascorbic acid	0.11	0.01	15.76	60	0.6	4	0	15.16
Pineapple juice, canned or bottled, unsweetened, with added ascorbic acid	0.36	0.12	12.87	53	0.2	2	0	12.67
Apple juice, frozen concentrate, unsweetened, undiluted, with added ascorbic acid	0.51	0.37	41	166	-	25	0	41
Apple juice, frozen concentrate, unsweetened, diluted with 3 volume water, with added ascorbic acid	0.14	0.1	11.54	47	0.1	7	0	11.44
Pears, raw, bartlett	0.39	0.16	15.01	63	3.1	1	-	11.91
Pears, raw, red anjou	0.33	0.14	14.94	62	3	1	-	11.94
Pears, raw, bosc	0.36	0.09	16.1	67	3.1	1	-	13

Food Name ---> per 100 g	Protein (g)	Fat (g)	Carb (g)	Calories	Fiber (g)	Sodium (mg)	Cholesterol (mg)	Net Carb (g)
Pears, raw, green anjou	0.44	0.1	15.79	66	3.1	1	-	12.69
Grapefruit juice, white, bottled, unsweetened, OCEAN SPRAY	0.58	0.1	7.93	34	0.8	3	0	7.13
Jackfruit, canned, syrup pack	0.36	0.14	23.94	92	0.9	11	0	23.04
Dates, medjool	1.81	0.15	74.97	277	6.7	1	-	68.27
Durian, raw or frozen	1.47	5.33	27.09	147	3.8	2	0	23.29
Prune puree	2.1	0.2	65.1	257	3.3	23	0	61.8
Candied fruit	0.34	0.07	82.74	322	1.6	98	0	81.14
Abiyuch, raw	1.5	0.1	17.6	69	5.3	20	-	12.3
Rowal, raw	2.3	2	23.9	111	6.2	4	-	17.7
Pineapple, raw, traditional varieties	0.55	0.13	11.82	45	-	1	-	11.82
Pineapple, raw, extra sweet variety	0.53	0.11	13.5	51	1.4	1	-	12.1
USDA Commodity, mixed fruit (peaches, pears, grapes), canned, light syrup, drained	0.46	0.1	14.65	57	1.6	5	0	13.05
USDA Commodity, mixed fruit (peaches, pears, grapes), canned, light syrup, solids and liquids	0.41	0.08	14.3	55	1.2	6	0	13.1
Clementines, raw	0.85	0.15	12.02	47	1.7	1	-	10.32
Guanabana nectar, canned	0.11	0.17	14.93	59	0.1	8	0	14.83
Guava nectar, canned, with added ascorbic acid	0.09	0.06	16.25	63	1	6	0	15.25
Mango nectar, canned	0.11	0.06	13.12	51	0.3	5	0	12.82
Tamarind nectar, canned	0.09	0.12	14.73	57	0.5	7	0	14.23
USDA Commodity peaches, canned, light syrup, drained	0.56	0.15	15.65	61	0.7	7	-	14.95
USDA Commodity pears, canned, juice pack, drained	0.34	0.19	12.91	51	2.2	4	-	10.71
USDA Commodity pears, canned, light syrup, drained	0.28	0.15	16.21	62	1.6	5	-	14.61
Pomegranate juice, bottled	0.15	0.29	13.13	54	0.1	9	0	13.03
Juice, apple and grape blend, with added ascorbic acid	0.16	0.12	12.46	50	0.2	7	0	12.26
Juice, apple, grape and pear blend, with added ascorbic acid and calcium	0.17	0.12	12.96	52	0.2	5	0	12.76
Plantains, green, fried	1.5	11.81	49.17	309	3.5	2	-	45.67
Plantains, yellow, fried, Latino restaurant	1.42	7.51	40.77	236	3.2	6	-	37.57
Nance, canned, syrup, drained	0.56	1.28	22.79	95	7	8	-	15.79
Nance, frozen, unsweetened	0.66	1.16	16.97	73	7.5	3	-	9.47
Naranjilla (lulo) pulp, frozen, unsweetened	0.44	0.22	5.9	25	1.1	4	-	4.8
Horned melon (Kiwano)	1.78	1.26	7.56	44	-	2	-	7.56
Orange Pineapple Juice Blend	0.41	0.08	12.2	51	0.2	4	0	12
Apples, raw, red delicious, with skin	0.27	0.2	14.06	59	2.3	1	-	11.76
Apples, raw, golden delicious, with skin	0.28	0.15	13.6	57	2.4	2	-	11.2
Apples, raw, granny smith, with skin	0.44	0.19	13.61	58	2.8	1	-	10.81
Apples, raw, gala, with skin	0.25	0.12	13.68	57	2.3	1	-	11.38
Apples, raw, fuji, with skin	0.2	0.18	15.22	63	2.1	1	-	13.12
Orange juice, chilled, includes from concentrate, with added calcium and vitamins A, D, E	0.68	0.12	11.54	49	0.3	2	0	11.24
Pineapple juice, canned, not from concentrate, unsweetened, with added vitamins A, C and E	0.36	0.14	12.18	50	0.2	3	0	11.98
Grape juice, canned or bottled, unsweetened, with added ascorbic acid and calcium	0.37	0.13	14.77	62	0.2	5	0	14.57
Apple juice, canned or bottled, unsweetened, with added ascorbic acid, calcium, and potassium	0.12	0.17	11.49	48	0.3	5	0	11.19
Raspberries, frozen, unsweetened	1.2	0.65	11.94	52	6.5	1	0	5.44

Food Name ---> per 100 g	Protein (g)	Fat (g)	Carb (g)	Calories	Fiber (g)	Sodium (mg)	Cholesterol (mg)	Net Carb (g)
Guava nectar, with sucralose, canned	0.3	0.07	13.3	48	1.2	6	0	12.1
Kiwifruit, ZESPRI SunGold, raw	1.02	0.28	15.79	63	1.4	3	0	14.39
Cranberry juice blend, 100% juice, bottled, with added vitamin C and calcium	0.27	0.12	10.91	45	0.1	6	0	10.81
Lemon juice from concentrate, bottled, CONCORD	0.4	0.07	5.37	24	-	29	-	5.37
Lemon juice from concentrate, bottled, REAL LEMON	0.47	0.07	5.66	17	0.7	26	-	4.96
Cranberry sauce, whole, canned, OCEAN SPRAY	0.75	0.05	40.4	158	1.2	5	0	39.2
Cranberry sauce, jellied, canned, OCEAN SPRAY	1.05	0.04	40.61	160	1	5	0	39.61
Ruby Red grapefruit juice blend (grapefruit, grape, apple), OCEAN SPRAY, bottled, with added vitamin C	0.5	0.1	10.53	44	0.2	8	0	10.33
Fruit juice smoothie, ODWALLA, strawberry banana	0.5	0.32	11.05	48	0.6	2	0	10.45
Fruit juice smoothie, NAKED JUICE, strawberry banana	0.48	0.27	11.66	50	0.6	2	0	11.06
Cranberry juice, unsweetened	0.39	0.13	12.2	46	0.1	2	0	12.1

Fast food

Food Name ---> per serving	Weight (g)	Measure	Calories	Total Carb (g)	Net Carb (g)	Sodium (mg)
ARBY'S, roast beef sandw., classic	149	1 sand..	*361*	**33.09**	**31.19**	973
BURGER KING, Cheeseburger	133	1 item	*380*	**31.53**	**30.23**	801
BURGER KING, Chicken Strips	36	1strip	*105*	**7.38**	**6.88**	309
BURGER KING, CROISSAN'WICH with Egg and Cheese	110	1 item	*311*	**27.27**	**26.47**	715
BURGER KING, CROISSAN'WICH with Sausage and Cheese	131	1 item	*493*	**30.13**	**29.23**	1024
BURGER KING, CROISSAN'WICH with Sausage, Egg and Cheese	171	1 sand..	*527*	**27.19**	**24.09**	987
BURGER KING, Double Cheeseburger	162	1 sand..	*457*	**28.24**	**28.24**	910
BURGER KING, DOUBLE WHOPPER, no cheese	374	1 item	*942*	**51.39**	**46.19**	1081
BURGER KING, DOUBLE WHOPPER, with cheese	399	1 item	*1061*	**53.94**	**47.54**	1544
BURGER KING, french fries	74	1 small serv	*207*	**28.64**	**26.54**	206
BURGER KING, french toast sticks	21	1 stick	*73*	**8.65**	**8.35**	90
BURGER KING, Hamburger	99	1 sand..	*258*	**26.49**	**25.49**	456
BURGER KING, Hash Brown Rounds	5.6	1 piece	*17*	**1.64**	**1.54**	32
BURGER KING, Onion Rings	91	1 small	*379*	**39.66**	**37.16**	706
BURGER KING, Original Chicken Sandw.	199	1 sand..	*569*	**52.18**	**47.38**	1270
BURGER KING, Premium Fish Sandw.	220	1 sand..	*572*	**58.72**	**56.72**	1324
BURGER KING, Vanilla Shake	24.8	1fl oz	*42*	**4.72**	**4.72**	25
BURGER KING, WHOPPER, no cheese	291	1 item	*678*	**53.98**	**48.78**	911
BURGER KING, WHOPPER, with cheese	316	1 item	*790*	**52.77**	**49.57**	1431
CHICK-FIL-A, Chick-n-Strips	50	1strip	*114*	**5.2**	**4.7**	288
CHICK-FIL-A, chicken sandw.	187	1 sand..	*466*	**39.06**	**36.46**	1408
CHICK-FIL-A, hash browns	5.5	1 piece	*17*	**1.68**	**1.48**	25
DIGIORNO Pizza, cheese topping, cheese stuffed crust, frozen, baked	164	1slice 1/4 of pie	*458*	**48.97**	**45.87**	1322
DIGIORNO Pizza, cheese topping, rising crust, frozen, baked	183	1slice 1/4 of pie	*468*	**58.16**	**53.76**	1274
DIGIORNO Pizza, cheese topping, thin crispy crust, frozen, baked	161	1slice 1/4 of pie	*398*	**42.62**	**37.82**	815
DIGIORNO Pizza, pepperoni topping, cheese stuffed crust, frozen, baked	179	1slice 1/4 of pie	*499*	**52.73**	**48.93**	1348
DIGIORNO Pizza, pepperoni topping, rising crust, frozen, baked	207	1slice 1/4 of pie	*549*	**64.48**	**59.68**	1538
DIGIORNO Pizza, pepperoni topping, thin crispy crust, frozen, baked	145	1slice 1/4 of pie	*410*	**41.57**	**37.47**	961
DIGIORNO Pizza, supreme topping, rising crust, frozen, baked	227	1slice 1/4 of pie	*579*	**63.4**	**58.2**	1616

Food Name ---> per serving	Weight (g)	Measure	Calories	Total Carb (g)	Net Carb (g)	Sodium (mg)
DIGIORNO Pizza, supreme topping, thin crispy crust, frozen, baked	155	1slice 1/4 of pie	395	43.48	39.18	860
DOMINO'S 14" Cheese Pizza, Classic Hand-Tossed Crust	108	1slice	278	35.9	33.5	565
DOMINO'S 14" Cheese Pizza, Crunchy Thin Crust	70	1slice	209	19.73	17.93	440
DOMINO'S 14" Cheese Pizza, Ultimate Deep Dish Crust	118	1slice	313	39.51	36.71	726
DOMINO'S 14" EXTRAVAGANZZA FEAST Pizza, Classic Hand-Tossed Crust	151	1slice	368	38.84	35.84	689
DOMINO'S 14" Pepperoni Pizza, Classic Hand-Tossed Crust	113	1slice	308	36	33.6	690
DOMINO'S 14" Pepperoni Pizza, Crunchy Thin Crust	79	1slice	259	20.03	17.93	619
DOMINO'S 14" Pepperoni Pizza, Ultimate Deep Dish Crust	123	1slice	348	39.22	36.22	852
DOMINO'S 14" Sausage Pizza, Classic Hand-Tossed Crust	114	1slice	311	36.3	33.6	677
DOMINO'S 14" Sausage Pizza, Crunchy Thin Crust	78	1slice	249	19.73	17.73	566
DOMINO'S 14" Sausage Pizza, Ultimate Deep Dish Crust	129	1slice	357	40.21	36.81	873
Fast food, biscuit	55	1biscuit	204	23.55	22.15	538
Fast Food, Pizza Chain, 14" pizza, cheese topping, regular crust	107	1slice	285	35.66	33.16	640
Fast Food, Pizza Chain, 14" pizza, cheese topping, stuffed crust	117	1slice 1/8 pizza	321	35.1	33.1	720
Fast Food, Pizza Chain, 14" pizza, cheese topping, thick crust	115	1slice	312	38.15	35.65	687
Fast Food, Pizza Chain, 14" pizza, cheese topping, thin crust	76	1slice	230	23.71	21.81	564
Fast Food, Pizza Chain, 14" pizza, meat and vegetable topping, regular crust	136	1slice	332	34.52	31.52	801
Fast Food, Pizza Chain, 14" pizza, pepperoni topping, regular crust	111	1slice	313	35.5	32.9	760
Fast Food, Pizza Chain, 14" pizza, pepperoni topping, thick crust	118	1slice	339	37.57	34.97	807
Fast Food, Pizza Chain, 14" pizza, pepperoni topping, thin crust	79	1slice	261	22.91	21.11	691
Fast Food, Pizza Chain, 14" pizza, sausage topping, regular crust	116	1slice	325	35.52	32.82	734
Fast Food, Pizza Chain, 14" pizza, sausage topping, thick crust	127	1slice	358	38.56	35.66	809
Fast Food, Pizza Chain, 14" pizza, sausage topping, thin crust	88	1slice	282	23.76	21.56	688
Fast foods, bagel, with breakfast steak, egg, cheese, and condiments	254	1 item	716	58.39	57.89	1631
Fast foods, bagel, with egg, sausage patty, cheese, and condiments	219	1 item	646	49.58	49.18	1204
Fast foods, biscuit, with crispy chicken fillet	132	1 item	396	40.34	38.54	1146
Fast foods, biscuit, with egg and bacon	150	1biscuit	458	28.59	27.79	1266
Fast foods, biscuit, with egg and ham	182	1biscuit	424	29.79	29.09	1989
Fast Foods, biscuit, with egg and sausage	162	1 item	505	34.1	33.8	1089

Food Name ---> per serving	Weight (g)	Measure	Calories	Total Carb (g)	Net Carb (g)	Sodium (mg)
Fast foods, biscuit, with egg, cheese, and bacon	145	1 item	*436*	**35.44**	**35.14**	1183
Fast foods, biscuit, with ham	162	1biscuit	*554*	**62.77**	**61.67**	1578
Fast foods, biscuit, with sausage	111	1 item	*412*	**33.29**	**32.89**	904
Fast foods, breadstick, soft, prepared with garlic and parmesan cheese	43	1breadstick	*147*	**19.13**	**18.13**	232
Fast foods, breakfast burrito, with egg, cheese, and sausage	109	1burrito	*302*	**25.04**	**23.74**	811
Fast foods, burrito, with beans	217	2.0 pieces	*447*	**71.44**	**71.44**	985
Fast foods, burrito, with beans and beef	241	1 item	*460*	**47.04**	**39.84**	1374
Fast foods, burrito, with beans and cheese	185	1each burrito	*379*	**57.78**	**49.98**	1042
Fast foods, burrito, with beans, cheese, and beef	241	1burrito	*434*	**56.32**	**47.42**	1087
Fast foods, cheeseburger, double, regular patty and bun, with condiments	155	1 sand..	*437*	**27.85**	**26.25**	956
Fast foods, cheeseburger; double, large patty; with condiments	280	1 item	*762*	**40.4**	**37.6**	1344
Fast Foods, cheeseburger; double, large patty; with condiments, vegetables and mayonnaise	355	1 item	*898*	**44.8**	**40.2**	1438
Fast foods, cheeseburger; double, regular patty; double decker bun with condiments and special sauce	219	1 item	*572*	**47.15**	**44.05**	1062
Fast foods, cheeseburger; double, regular patty; with condiments	155	1 sand..	*437*	**27.85**	**26.45**	956
Fast foods, cheeseburger; single, large patty; plain	182	1 sand..	*564*	**43.81**	**40.71**	875
Fast foods, cheeseburger; single, large patty; with condiments	199	1 item	*535*	**39.24**	**36.84**	1176
Fast foods, cheeseburger; single, large patty; with condiments, vegetables and mayonnaise	215	1 sand..	*576*	**38.12**	**35.72**	1017
Fast foods, cheeseburger; single, regular patty, with condiments	127	1 item	*343*	**32.33**	**29.93**	798
Fast foods, cheeseburger; single, regular patty, with condiments and vegetables	115	1 sand..	*292*	**28.72**	**27.12**	628
Fast foods, cheeseburger; single, regular patty; plain	91	1 sand..	*280*	**25.51**	**23.71**	469
Fast foods, chicken fillet sandw., plain with pickles	187	1 sand..	*468*	**39.06**	**36.46**	1408
Fast foods, chicken tenders	30	1strip	*81*	**5.17**	**4.77**	231
Fast foods, chicken, breaded and fried, boneless pieces, plain	96	6.0 pieces	*295*	**14.33**	**13.43**	570
Fast foods, coleslaw	191	1cup	*292*	**28.44**	**24.84**	388
Fast Foods, crispy chicken filet sandw., with lettuce and mayonnaise	152	1 sand..	*420*	**41.65**	**39.55**	938
Fast foods, crispy chicken in tortilla, with lettuce, cheese, and ranch sauce	133	1 item	*366*	**30.88**	**29.18**	807
Fast foods, crispy chicken, bacon, and tomato club sandw., with cheese, lettuce, and mayonnaise	271	1 sand..	*696*	**61.27**	**57.97**	1640
Fast foods, croissant, with egg, cheese, and bacon	128	1 item	*370*	**28.8**	**27.5**	771
Fast foods, croissant, with egg, cheese,	155	1 item	*405*	**29.42**	**28.02**	1102

Food Name ---> per serving	Weight (g)	Measure	Calories	Total Carb (g)	Net Carb (g)	Sodium (mg)
and ham						
Fast foods, croissant, with egg, cheese, and sausage	171	1 sand..	527	27.19	24.09	987
Fast foods, egg, scrambled	96	2.0 eggs	204	2	2	180
Fast foods, english muffin, with cheese and sausage	108	1 item	365	27.3	26.8	721
Fast foods, english muffin, with egg, cheese, and canadian bacon	126	1 sand..	287	27.3	26.8	777
Fast foods, english muffin, with egg, cheese, and sausage	165	1 item	472	28.78	28.48	904
Fast foods, fish sandw., with tartar sauce	220	1 sand..	565	58.72	56.52	1324
Fast foods, fish sandw., with tartar sauce and cheese	134	1 sand..	374	35.36	34.26	582
Fast foods, french toast sticks	65	3.0 pieces	221	26.79	25.89	260
Fast Foods, Fried Chicken, Breast, meat and skin and breading	203	1breast, with skin	467	12.24	12.04	1334
Fast Foods, Fried Chicken, Breast, meat only, skin and breading removed	142	1breast without skin	217	0	0	727
Fast Foods, Fried Chicken, Drumstick, meat and skin with breading	75	1drumsti ck, with skin	200	5.69	5.29	443
Fast Foods, Fried Chicken, Drumstick, meat only, skin and breading removed	40	1drum stick,	69	0	0	197
Fast Foods, Fried Chicken, Thigh, meat and skin and breading	136	1thigh with skin	373	11.8	11.7	1016
Fast Foods, Fried Chicken, Thigh, meat only, skin and breading removed	84	1thigh without skin	150	0.2	0.2	485
Fast Foods, Fried Chicken, Wing, meat and skin and breading	58	1wing, with skin	180	6.49	6.39	503
Fast Foods, Fried Chicken, Wing, meat only, skin and breading removed	37	1wing without skin	80	0.79	0.79	282
Fast foods, griddle cake sandw., egg, cheese, and bacon	174	1 item 6.1 oz	473	45.57	44.17	1249
Fast foods, griddle cake sandw., egg, cheese, and sausage	199	1 item	579	43.86	42.66	1297
Fast foods, griddle cake sandw., sausage	135	1 item	429	42.19	40.79	995
Fast Foods, grilled chicken filet sandw., with lettuce, tomato and spread	230	1 sand..	419	38.59	36.49	982
Fast foods, grilled chicken in tortilla, with lettuce, cheese, and ranch sauce	123	1 item	273	22.67	21.57	710
Fast foods, grilled chicken, bacon and tomato club sandw., with cheese, lettuce, and mayonnaise	268	1 sand..	590	53.25	50.05	1688
Fast foods, hamburger, large, single patty, with condiments	171	1 item	438	37.86	35.96	640
Fast foods, hamburger; double, large patty; with condiments, vegetables and mayonnaise	374	1 item	942	51.39	46.19	1081
Fast foods, hamburger; single, large patty; with condiments, vegetables and mayonnaise	247	1 item	558	42.81	39.11	845
Fast foods, hamburger; single, regular	205	1 item	531	46.51	43.61	791

Food Name ---> per serving	Weight (g)	Measure	Calories	Total Carb (g)	Net Carb (g)	Sodium (mg)
patty; double decker bun with condiments and special sauce						
Fast foods, hamburger; single, regular patty; plain	78	1 sand..	232	24.57	23.27	258
Fast foods, hamburger; single, regular patty; with condiments	97	1 sand..	255	28.68	26.98	472
Fast foods, hush puppies	22	1 piece	65	8.85	8.25	179
Fast foods, miniature cinnamon rolls	25	1each	101	13.35	12.75	138
Fast foods, nachos, with cheese	80	1serv	274	27.93	25.33	250
Fast foods, nachos, with cheese, beans, ground beef, and tomatoes	222	1serv	486	47.49	39.29	773
Fast foods, onion rings, breaded and fried	117	1package (18 onion rings)	481	50.99	47.79	908
Fast foods, potato, french fried in vegetable oil	71	1serv small	222	29.42	26.72	149
Fast foods, potato, mashed	242	1cup	215	35.45	32.35	741
Fast foods, potatoes, hash browns, round pieces or patty	5.5	1round piece	15	1.59	1.49	31
Fast foods, quesadilla, with chicken	180	1each quesadilla	529	43.27	40.17	1341
Fast foods, roast beef sandw., plain	149	1 sand..	364	33.09	31.19	973
Fast foods, shrimp, breaded and fried	39	3.0 pieces shrimp	120	10.92	10.62	350
Fast foods, strawberry banana smoothie made with ice and low-fat yogurt	347	12.0 fl oz	226	52.22	49.12	49
Fast foods, submarine sandw., bacon, lettuce, and tomato on white bread	148	6.0 inch sub	303	39.46	37.06	524
Fast foods, submarine sand., cold cut on white bread, lettuce and tomato	196	6.0 inch sub	417	40.04	37.64	1127
Fast foods, submarine sandw., ham on white bread with lettuce and tomato	184	6.0 inch sub	278	42.15	39.75	729
Fast foods, submarine sandw., meatball marinara on white bread	209	6.0 inch sub	458	54.36	49.96	913
Fast foods, submarine sandw., oven roasted chicken on white bread with lettuce and tomato	198	6.0 inch sub	311	42.27	39.87	531
Fast foods, submarine sandw., roast beef on white bread with lettuce and tomato	190	6.0 inch sub	296	38.65	37.35	625
Fast foods, submarine sandw., steak and cheese on white bread with cheese, lettuce and tomato	201	6.0 inch sub	368	43.19	40.79	892
Fast foods, submarine sandw., sweet onion chicken teriyaki on white bread with lettuce, tomato and sweet onion sauce	228	6.0 inch sub	353	51.39	48.69	695
Fast foods, submarine sandw., tuna on white bread with lettuce and tomato	237	6.0 inch sub	517	37.8	36.1	780
Fast foods, submarine sandw., turkey breast on white bread with lettuce and tomato	184	6.0 inch sub	270	41.25	38.85	583
Fast foods, submarine sandw., turkey, roast beef and ham on white bread with	413	12.0 inch sub	603	84.09	78.29	1437

Food Name ---> per serving	Weight (g)	Measure	Calories	Total Carb (g)	Net Carb (g)	Sodium (mg)
lettuce and tomato						
Fast foods, sundae, caramel	155	1sundae	304	49.31	49.31	195
Fast foods, sundae, hot fudge	158	1sundae	284	47.67	47.67	182
Fast foods, sundae, strawberry	153	1sundae	268	44.65	44.65	92
Fast foods, taco with beef, cheese and lettuce, hard shell	69	1each taco	156	13.7	11	274
Fast foods, taco with beef, cheese and lettuce, soft	102	1each taco	210	20.63	17.63	571
Fast foods, taco with chicken, lettuce and cheese, soft	98	1each taco	185	19.3	18.1	601
Fast foods, vanilla, light, soft-serve ice cream, with cone	120	1 item	196	31.63	31.53	97
KFC, biscuit	49	1biscuit	175	21.34	20.34	524
KFC, Coleslaw	112	1packag e	161	17.53	15.33	212
KFC, Crispy Chicken Strips	47	1strip	129	6.42	5.72	446
KFC, Fried Chicken, EXTRA CRISPY, Breast, meat and skin with breading	212	1breast, with skin	568	17.96	17.96	1287
KFC, Fried Chicken, EXTRA CRISPY, Breast, meat only, skin and breading removed	140	1breast, without skin	214	0.35	0.35	668
KFC, Fried Chicken, EXTRA CRISPY, Drumstick, meat and skin with breading	81	1drumsti ck, with skin	222	6.45	6.45	512
KFC, Fried Chicken, EXTRA CRISPY, Drumstick, meat only, skin and breading removed	41	1drumsti ck	70	0	0	216
KFC, Fried Chicken, EXTRA CRISPY, Thigh, meat and skin with breading	152	1thigh, with skin	470	15.66	15.66	1037
KFC, Fried Chicken, EXTRA CRISPY, Thigh, meat only, skin and breading removed	91	1thigh, without skin	163	0	0	508
KFC, Fried Chicken, EXTRA CRISPY, Wing, meat and skin with breading	68	1wing, with skin	229	7.93	7.93	520
KFC, Fried Chicken, EXTRA CRISPY, Wing, meat only, skin and breading removed	44	1wing, without skin	104	1.31	1.31	314
KFC, Fried Chicken, ORIGINAL RECIPE, Breast, meat and skin with breading	212	1breast, with skin	490	13.31	13.31	1285
KFC, Fried Chicken, ORIGINAL RECIPE, Breast, meat only, skin and breading removed	152	1breast without skin	226	0	0	758
KFC, Fried Chicken, ORIGINAL RECIPE, Drumstick, meat and skin with breading	75	1drumsti ck, with skin	179	4.04	4.04	469
KFC, Fried Chicken, ORIGINAL RECIPE, Drumstick, meat only, skin and breading removed	40	1drumsti ck, bone and skin removed	70	0.04	0.04	210
KFC, Fried Chicken, ORIGINAL RECIPE, Thigh, meat and skin with breading	135	1thigh, with skin	363	11.42	11.42	1054
KFC, Fried Chicken, ORIGINAL RECIPE, Thigh, meat only, skin and breading removed	86	1thigh without skin	150	0.01	0.01	488

Food Name ---> per serving	Weight (g)	Measure	Calories	Total Carb (g)	Net Carb (g)	Sodium (mg)
KFC, Fried Chicken, ORIGINAL RECIPE, Wing, meat and skin with breading	60	1wing, with skin	178	5.96	5.96	530
KFC, Fried Chicken, ORIGINAL RECIPE, Wing, meat only, skin and breading removed	39	1wing wing without skin	84	0.69	0.69	288
KFC, Popcorn Chicken	6.4	1 piece	22	1.36	1.26	73
Light Ice Cream, soft serve, blended with cookie pieces	337	12.0 fl oz cup	570	86.1	85.8	253
Light Ice Cream, soft serve, blended with milk chocolate candies	348	12.0 fl oz cup	633	93.33	92.63	188
LITTLE CAESARS 14" Cheese Pizza, Large Deep Dish Crust	102	1slice	268	30.7	29.4	441
LITTLE CAESARS 14" Cheese Pizza, Thin Crust	48	1slice	148	10.97	10.17	218
LITTLE CAESARS 14" Original Round Cheese Pizza, Regular Crust	89	1slice	236	28.04	26.54	404
LITTLE CAESARS 14" Original Round Meat and Vegetable Pizza, Regular Crust	115	1slice	279	26.57	24.17	665
LITTLE CAESARS 14" Original Round Pepperoni Pizza, Regular Crust	90	1slice	246	27.91	26.41	466
LITTLE CAESARS 14" Pepperoni Pizza, Large Deep Dish Crust	104	1slice	276	30.19	28.59	512
McDONALD'S Bacon Ranch Salad with Crispy Chicken	319	1 item 11.3 oz	389	19.4	16.2	871
McDONALD'S, Bacon Egg & Cheese Biscuit	142	1 item 4.9 oz	432	31.61	30.31	1225
McDONALD'S, Bacon Ranch Salad with Grilled Chicken	305	1 item 10.8 oz	247	11.1	8.1	702
McDONALD'S, Bacon Ranch Salad without chicken	223	1 item 7.8 oz	136	9.37	6.07	294
McDONALD'S, Bacon, Egg & Cheese McGRIDDLES	165	1 item 5.8 oz	449	43.21	41.91	1110
McDONALD'S, BIG BREAKFAST	269	1 item 9.5 oz	767	47.08	44.08	1477
McDONALD'S, BIG MAC	219	1 item 7.6 oz	563	43.98	40.48	1007
McDONALD'S, BIG MAC (without Big Mac Sauce)	200	1 item	468	42.02	38.62	908
McDONALD'S, Cheeseburger	119	1 item 4 oz	313	33.09	31.79	745
McDONALD'S, Chicken McNUGGETS	64	4.0 pieces	193	9.66	9.66	362
McDONALD'S, Deluxe Breakfast, with syrup and margarine	420	1 item 14.8 oz	1197	123.82	119.62	1835
McDONALD'S, Double Cheeseburger	155	1 sand..	437	29.12	27.92	1035
McDONALD'S, DOUBLE QUARTER POUNDER with Cheese	280	1 item	734	40.4	37.6	1333
McDONALD'S, Egg McMUFFIN	126	1 sand..	287	27.3	25.9	777
McDONALD'S, FILET-O-FISH	134	1 sand..	378	35.36	33.46	582
McDONALD'S, FILET-O-FISH (without tartar sauce)	124	1 item	301	38.54	37.34	575
McDONALD'S, french fries	71	1 small serv	229	30.23	27.43	134
McDONALD'S, Fruit 'n Yogurt Parfait	149	1 item	156	30.87	29.37	86

Food Name ---> per serving	Weight (g)	Measure	Calories	Total Carb (g)	Net Carb (g)	Sodium (mg)
		5.2 oz				
McDONALD'S, Fruit 'n Yogurt Parfait (without granola)	142	1 item	*128*	**25.09**	**23.79**	54
McDONALD'S, Hamburger	95	1 sand..	*251*	**28.77**	**27.57**	469
McDONALD'S, Hash Brown	53	1serv 1 patty	*144*	**15.14**	**13.64**	307
McDONALD'S, Hot Caramel Sundae	182	1 item (6.4 oz)	*342*	**60.72**	**60.72**	146
McDONALD'S, Hot Fudge Sundae	179	1 item (6.3 oz)	*333*	**53.79**	**53.09**	168
McDONALD'S, Hotcakes (plain)	149	3.0 hotcakes 5.3 oz	*340*	**57.02**	**54.92**	533
McDONALD'S, Hotcakes (with 2 pats margarine & syrup)	221	1 item	*601*	**101.84**	**99.84**	625
McDONALD'S, Hotcakes and Sausage	192	1 item	*564*	**72.1**	**69**	929
McDONALD'S, McCHICKEN Sandw.	131	1 sand..	*358*	**36.64**	**34.94**	817
McDONALD'S, McCHICKEN Sandw. (without mayonnaise)	138	1 item	*331*	**42.71**	**40.81**	766
McDONALD'S, McFLURRY with M & M'S CANDIES	348	1regular (12 fl oz)	*616*	**93.33**	**92.63**	188
McDONALD'S, McFLURRY with OREO cookies	337	1regular (12 fl oz)	*556*	**86.1**	**85.8**	253
McDONALD'S, QUARTER POUNDER	171	1 item	*417*	**37.91**	**35.21**	730
McDONALD'S, QUARTER POUNDER with Cheese	199	1 item 7.1 oz	*513*	**39.7**	**36.9**	1152
McDONALD'S, RANCH SNACK WRAP, Crispy	133	1wrap	*366*	**30.88**	**29.18**	807
McDONALD'S, RANCH SNACK WRAP, Grilled	123	1wrap	*273*	**22.67**	**21.57**	710
McDONALD'S, Sausage Biscuit	117	1 item 4.1 oz	*440*	**31.82**	**30.42**	1024
McDONALD'S, Sausage Biscuit with Egg	163	1 item 5.7 oz	*507*	**31.43**	**30.13**	1082
McDONALD'S, Sausage Burrito	109	1burrito	*302*	**25.04**	**23.74**	811
McDONALD'S, Sausage McGRIDDLES	135	1 item	*421*	**42.19**	**40.79**	995
McDONALD'S, Sausage McMUFFIN	115	1 item 4 oz	*383*	**28.2**	**26.6**	797
McDONALD'S, Sausage McMUFFIN with Egg	165	1 item 5.8 oz	*452*	**28.51**	**27.01**	944
McDONALD'S, Sausage, Egg & Cheese McGRIDDLES	199	1 item 7 oz	*563*	**43.86**	**42.66**	1297
McDONALD'S, Side Salad	87	1 item 3.1 oz	*17*	**3.74**	**2.34**	10
McDONALD'S, Southern Style Chicken Biscuit	132	1biscuit regular size biscuit	*401*	**40.34**	**38.54**	1146
McDONALD'S, Strawberry Sundae	178	1 item (6.3 oz)	*281*	**50**	**50**	84
McDONALD'S, Vanilla Reduced Fat Ice Cream Cone	90	1 item (3.2 oz)	*146*	**23.72**	**23.62**	60
PAPA JOHN'S 14" Cheese Pizza, Original Crust	117	1slice	*304*	**38.31**	**36.11**	676
PAPA JOHN'S 14" Cheese Pizza, Thin Crust	87	1slice	*257*	**22.85**	**20.85**	459

Food Name ---> per serving	Weight (g)	Measure	Calories	Total Carb (g)	Net Carb (g)	Sodium (mg)
PAPA JOHN'S 14" Pepperoni Pizza, Original Crust	123	1slice	338	36.95	35.45	825
PAPA JOHN'S 14" The Works Pizza, Original Crust	153	1slice	367	40.84	37.04	872
PIZZA HUT 12" Cheese Pizza, Hand-Tossed Crust	96	1slice	260	29.97	28.27	658
PIZZA HUT 12" Cheese Pizza, Pan Crust	100	1slice	280	29.93	28.23	624
PIZZA HUT 12" Cheese Pizza, THIN 'N CRISPY Crust	69	1slice	209	19.76	18.66	541
PIZZA HUT 12" Pepperoni Pizza, Hand-Tossed Crust	96	1slice	269	30.29	28.69	769
PIZZA HUT 12" Pepperoni Pizza, Pan Crust	96	1slice	286	29.27	27.57	664
PIZZA HUT 12" Super Supreme Pizza, Hand-Tossed Crust	127	1slice	309	32.54	30.04	875
PIZZA HUT 14" Cheese Pizza, Hand-Tossed Crust	105	1slice	289	35.09	32.59	708
PIZZA HUT 14" Cheese Pizza, Pan Crust	112	1slice	309	36.79	34.39	650
PIZZA HUT 14" Cheese Pizza, Stuffed Crust	117	1slice	321	35.1	33.1	720
PIZZA HUT 14" Cheese Pizza, THIN 'N CRISPY Crust	79	1slice	242	27.03	25.13	677
PIZZA HUT 14" Pepperoni Pizza, Hand-Tossed Crust	110	1slice	320	35.32	32.42	835
PIZZA HUT 14" Pepperoni Pizza, Pan Crust	113	1slice	329	35.92	33.62	764
PIZZA HUT 14" Pepperoni Pizza, THIN 'N CRISPY Crust	80	1slice	266	26.13	24.43	774
PIZZA HUT 14" Sausage Pizza, Hand-Tossed Crust	119	1slice	342	34.97	32.27	798
PIZZA HUT 14" Sausage Pizza, Pan Crust	125	1slice	359	36.95	34.45	745
PIZZA HUT 14" Sausage Pizza, THIN 'N CRISPY Crust	92	1slice	297	26.4	24.2	772
PIZZA HUT 14" Super Supreme Pizza, Hand-Tossed Crust	123	1slice	305	31.99	29.19	809
PIZZA HUT, breadstick, parmesan garlic	43	1breadstick	147	19.13	18.13	232
Pizza, cheese topping, regular crust, frozen, cooked	81	1serv	217	23.51	21.71	362
Pizza, cheese topping, rising crust, frozen, cooked	139	1serv	361	45.74	42.24	773
Pizza, cheese topping, thin crust, frozen, cooked	69	1slice	181	19.87	17.77	325
Pizza, meat and vegetable topping, regular crust, frozen, cooked	143	1serv	395	35.95	32.85	794
Pizza, meat and vegetable topping, rising crust, frozen, cooked	170	1serv	461	48.93	45.03	1088
Pizza, meat topping, thick crust, frozen, cooked	103	1slice	282	31.68	29.28	711
Pizza, pepperoni topping, regular crust, frozen, cooked	127	0.25 pizza	348	31.36	28.86	749
POPEYES, biscuit	60	1biscuit	241	24.57	22.27	447
POPEYES, Coleslaw	120	1packag	193	16.94	14.94	262
POPEYES, Fried Chicken, Mild, Breast, meat and skin with breading	194	1breast, with skin	532	19.07	18.27	1048

Food Name ---> per serving	Weight (g)	Measure	Calories	Total Carb (g)	Net Carb (g)	Sodium (mg)
POPEYES, Fried Chicken, Mild, Breast, meat only, skin and breading removed	132	1 breast without skin	207	0	0	694
POPEYES, Fried Chicken, Mild, Drumstick, meat and skin with breading	76	1 drumst	223	7.48	7.48	447
POPEYES, Fried Chicken, Mild, Drumstick, meat only, skin and breading removed	44	1 drumsti ck,	75	0.02	0.02	210
POPEYES, Fried Chicken, Mild, Thigh, meat and skin with breading	138	1 thigh with skin	428	15.46	14.76	945
POPEYES, Fried Chicken, Mild, Thigh, meat only, skin and breading removed	83	1 thigh thigh without skin	156	0.71	0.71	499
POPEYES, Fried Chicken, Mild, Wing, meat and skin with breading	57	1 wing, with skin	193	7.71	7.41	449
POPEYES, Fried Chicken, Mild, Wing, meat only, skin and breading removed	16	1 wing	34	0.46	0.46	130
POPEYES, Mild Chicken Strips, analyzed 2006	54	1 strip	146	10.43	10.03	498
POPEYES, Spicy Chicken Strips, analyzed 2006	53	1 strip	134	9.82	9.22	528
School Lunch, chicken nuggets, whole grain breaded	88	5.0 pieces	238	20.12	18.22	450
School Lunch, chicken patty, whole grain breaded	86	1 patty	212	10.75	8.75	402
School Lunch, pizza, BIG DADDY'S LS 16" 51% Whole Grain Rolled Edge Cheese Pizza, frozen	155	1 slice 1/8 per pizza	377	42.01	37.81	620
School Lunch, pizza, BIG DADDY'S LS 16" 51% Whole Grain Rolled Edge Turkey Pepperoni Pizza, frozen	156	1 slice 1/8 per pizza	387	42.67	36.27	702
School Lunch, pizza, cheese topping, thick crust, whole grain, frozen, cooked	124	1 slice per 1/10 pizza	315	34.82	31.22	522
School Lunch, pizza, cheese topping, thin crust, whole grain, frozen, cooked	130	1 piece 4"x6"	321	40.7	35.5	547
School Lunch, pizza, pepperoni topping, thick crust, whole grain, frozen, cooked	124	1 slice per 1/10 pizza	321	35.09	29.79	588
School Lunch, pizza, pepperoni topping, thin crust, whole grain, frozen, cooked	127	1 piece 4"x6"	323	39.67	34.17	629
School Lunch, pizza, sausage topping, thick crust, whole grain, frozen, cooked	129	1/10 pizza	332	39.45	34.25	559
School Lunch, pizza, sausage topping, thin crust, whole grain, frozen, cooked	133	1 piece 4" x 6"	332	42.88	37.68	608
School Lunch, pizza, TONY'S Breakfast Pizza Sausage, frozen	91	1 piece 3.2 oz	218	24.56	22.76	546
School Lunch, pizza, TONY'S SMARTPIZZA Whole Grain 4x6 Cheese Pizza 50/50 Cheese, frozen	130	1 piece 4" x 6"	303	38.05	33.15	520
School Lunch, pizza, TONY'S SMARTPIZZA Whole Grain 4x6 Pepperoni Pizza 50/50 Cheese, frozen	127	1 piece 4"x6"	302	36.63	31.43	597
SUBWAY, B.L.T. sub on white bread with bacon, lettuce and tomato	148	6.0 inch sub	303	39.46	37.06	524

Food Name ---> per serving	Weight (g)	Measure	Calories	Total Carb (g)	Net Carb (g)	Sodium (mg)
SUBWAY, black forest ham sub on white bread with lettuce and tomato	184	6.0 inch sub	278	42.15	39.75	729
SUBWAY, cold cut sub on white bread with lettuce and tomato	196	6.0 inch sub	419	40.04	37.64	1127
SUBWAY, meatball marinara sub on white bread (no toppings)	209	6.0 inch sub	458	54.36	49.96	913
SUBWAY, oven roasted chicken sub on white bread with lettuce and tomato	198	6.0 inch sub	311	42.27	39.87	531
SUBWAY, roast beef sub on white bread with lettuce and tomato	190	6.0 inch sub	294	38.65	37.35	625
SUBWAY, steak & cheese sub on white bread with American cheese, lettuce and tomato	201	6.0 inch sub	368	43.19	40.79	892
SUBWAY, SUBWAY CLUB sub on white bread with lettuce and tomato	207	6.0 inch sub	302	42.15	39.25	720
SUBWAY, sweet onion chicken teriyaki sub on white bread with lettuce, tomato and sweet sauce	228	6.0 inch sub	353	51.39	48.69	695
SUBWAY, tuna sub on white bread with lettuce and tomato	237	6.0 inch sub	524	37.8	36.1	780
SUBWAY, turkey breast sub on white bread with lettuce and tomato	184	6.0 inch sub	270	41.25	38.85	583
TACO BELL, Bean Burrito	185	1each burrito	387	57.78	49.98	1042
TACO BELL, BURRITO SUPREME with beef	241	1burrito	441	56.32	47.42	1087
TACO BELL, BURRITO SUPREME with chicken	248	1 item	444	50.86	44.86	1399
TACO BELL, BURRITO SUPREME with steak	248	1 item	454	50.39	44.39	1324
TACO BELL, Nachos	80	1serv	280	27.93	25.33	250
TACO BELL, Nachos Supreme	222	1serv	495	47.49	39.29	773
TACO BELL, Original Taco with beef, cheese and lettuce	69	1each taco	158	13.7	11	274
TACO BELL, Soft Taco with beef, cheese and lettuce	102	1each taco	210	20.63	17.63	571
TACO BELL, Soft Taco with chicken, cheese and lettuce	98	1each taco	185	19.3	18.1	601
TACO BELL, Soft Taco with steak	127	1 item	286	21.87	19.87	700
TACO BELL, Taco Salad	533	1 item	906	80.48	64.48	1935
WEND'YS, Crispy Chicken Sandw.	126	1 sand..	350	33.21	33.21	713
WENDY'S, Chicken Nuggets	68	5.0 pieces	222	9.73	9.73	481
WENDY'S, CLASSIC DOUBLE, with cheese	310	1 item	747	36.3	32.9	1308
WENDY'S, CLASSIC SINGLE Hamburger, no cheese	218	1 item	464	36.67	33.87	861
WENDY'S, CLASSIC SINGLE Hamburger, with cheese	236	1 item	522	33.51	30.21	1123
WENDY'S, DAVE'S Hot 'N Juicy 1/4 LB, single	215	1 sand..	576	38.12	35.72	1017
WENDY'S, Double Stack, with cheese	146	1 sand..	416	22.41	22.41	696
WENDY'S, french fries	71	1kid's meal Serv	214	28.21	25.41	155
WENDY'S, Frosty Dairy Dessert	113	1junior 6	149	26.69	22.99	111

Food Name ---> per serving	Weight (g)	Measure	Calories	Total Carb (g)	Net Carb (g)	Sodium (mg)
		oz. cup				
WENDY'S, Homestyle Chicken Fillet Sandw.	230	1 item	*492*	**49.56**	**46.56**	922
WENDY'S, Jr. Hamburger, with cheese	129	1 item	*330*	**32.21**	**30.41**	851
WENDY'S, Jr. Hamburger, without cheese	117	1 item	*284*	**33.29**	**31.29**	631
WENDY'S, Ultimate Chicken Grill Sandw.	225	1 item	*403*	**42.48**	**39.98**	961
Yogurt parfait, lowfat, with fruit and granola	149	1 item	*125*	**23.63**	**22.03**	73

Lamb, Veal, and Game Products

Food Name ---> per 100 g	Protein (g)	Fat (g)	Carb (g)	Calories	Fiber (g)	Sodium (mg)	Cholesterol (mg)	Net Carb (g)
Veal, Australian, rib, rib roast, separable lean only, raw	21.7	4.63	1.4	134	0	83	58	1.4
Lamb, domestic, composite of trimmed retail cuts, separable lean and fat, trimmed to 1/4" fat, choice, raw	16.88	21.59	0	267	0	58	72	0
Lamb, domestic, composite of trimmed retail cuts, separable lean and fat, trimmed to 1/4" fat, choice, cooked	24.52	20.94	0	294	0	72	97	0
Lamb, domestic, composite of trimmed retail cuts, separable lean only, trimmed to 1/4" fat, choice, raw	20.29	5.25	0	134	0	66	65	0
Lamb, domestic, composite of trimmed retail cuts, separable lean only, trimmed to 1/4" fat, choice, cooked	28.22	9.52	0	206	0	76	92	0
Lamb, domestic, composite of trimmed retail cuts, separable fat, trimmed to 1/4" fat, choice, raw	6.65	70.61	0	665	0	31	90	0
Lamb, domestic, composite of trimmed retail cuts, separable fat, trimmed to 1/4" fat, choice, cooked	12.16	59.18	0	586	0	58	114	0
Lamb, domestic, foreshank, separable lean and fat, trimmed to 1/4" fat, choice, raw	18.91	13.38	0	201	0	72	72	0
Lamb, domestic, foreshank, separable lean and fat, trimmed to 1/4" fat, choice, cooked, braised	28.37	13.46	0	243	0	72	106	0
Lamb, domestic, foreshank, separable lean only, trimmed to 1/4" fat, choice, raw	21.08	3.29	0	120	0	79	69	0
Lamb, domestic, foreshank, separable lean only, trimmed to 1/4" fat, choice, cooked, braised	31.01	6.02	0	187	0	74	104	0
Lamb, domestic, leg, whole (shank and sirloin), separable lean and fat, trimmed to 1/4" fat, choice, raw	17.91	17.07	0	230	0	56	69	0
Lamb, domestic, leg, whole (shank and sirloin), separable lean and fat, trimmed to 1/4" fat, choice, cooked, roasted	25.55	16.48	0	258	0	66	93	0
Lamb, domestic, leg, whole (shank and sirloin), separable lean only, trimmed to 1/4" fat, choice, raw	20.56	4.51	0	128	0	62	64	0
Lamb, domestic, leg, whole (shank and sirloin), separable lean only, trimmed to 1/4" fat, choice, cooked, roasted	28.3	7.74	0	191	0	68	89	0
Lamb, domestic, leg, shank half, separable lean and fat, trimmed to 1/4" fat, choice, raw	18.58	13.49	0	201	0	57	67	0
Lamb, domestic, leg, shank half, separable lean and fat, trimmed to 1/4" fat, choice, cooked, roasted	26.41	12.45	0	225	0	65	90	0
Lamb, domestic, leg, shank half, separable lean only, trimmed to 1/4" fat, choice, raw	20.52	4.19	0	125	0	61	64	0
Lamb, domestic, leg, shank half, separable lean only, trimmed to 1/4" fat, choice, cooked, roasted	28.17	6.67	0	180	0	66	87	0
Lamb, domestic, leg, sirloin half, separable lean and fat, trimmed to 1/4" fat, choice, raw	16.94	22.11	0	272	0	56	72	0
Lamb, domestic, leg, sirloin half, separable lean and fat, trimmed to 1/4" fat, choice, cooked, roasted	24.63	20.67	0	292	0	68	97	0
Lamb, domestic, leg, sirloin half, separable lean	20.55	5.08	0	134	0	64	66	0

only, trimmed to 1/4" fat, choice, raw

Food Name ---> per 100 g	Protein (g)	Fat (g)	Carb (g)	Calories	Fiber (g)	Sodium (mg)	Cholesterol (mg)	Net Carb (g)
Lamb, domestic, leg, sirloin half, separable lean only, trimmed to 1/4" fat, choice, cooked, roasted	28.35	9.17	0	204	0	71	92	0
Lamb, domestic, loin, separable lean and fat, trimmed to 1/4" fat, choice, raw	16.32	26.63	0	310	0	56	74	0
Lamb, domestic, loin, separable lean and fat, trimmed to 1/4" fat, choice, cooked, broiled	25.17	23.08	0	316	0	77	100	0
Lamb, domestic, loin, separable lean and fat, trimmed to 1/4" fat, choice, cooked, roasted	22.55	23.59	0	309	0	64	95	0
Lamb, domestic, loin, separable lean only, trimmed to 1/4" fat, choice, raw	20.88	5.94	0	143	0	68	66	0
Lamb, domestic, loin, separable lean only, trimmed to 1/4" fat, choice, cooked, broiled	29.99	9.73	0	216	0	84	95	0
Lamb, domestic, loin, separable lean only, trimmed to 1/4" fat, choice, cooked, roasted	26.59	9.76	0	202	0	66	87	0
Lamb, domestic, rib, separable lean and fat, trimmed to 1/4" fat, choice, raw	14.52	34.39	0	372	0	56	76	0
Lamb, domestic, rib, separable lean and fat, trimmed to 1/4" fat, choice, cooked, broiled	22.13	29.59	0	361	0	76	99	0
Lamb, domestic, rib, separable lean and fat, trimmed to 1/4" fat, choice, cooked, roasted	21.12	29.82	0	359	0	73	97	0
Lamb, domestic, rib, separable lean only, trimmed to 1/4" fat, choice, raw	19.98	9.23	0	169	0	72	66	0
Lamb, domestic, rib, separable lean only, trimmed to 1/4" fat, choice, cooked, broiled	27.74	12.95	0	235	0	85	91	0
Lamb, domestic, rib, separable lean only, trimmed to 1/4" fat, choice, cooked, roasted	26.16	13.31	0	232	0	81	88	0
Lamb, domestic, shoulder, whole (arm and blade), separable lean and fat, trimmed to 1/4" fat, choice, raw	16.58	21.45	0	264	0	61	72	0
Lamb, domestic, shoulder, whole (arm and blade), separable lean and fat, trimmed to 1/4" fat, choice, cooked, braised	28.68	24.55	0	344	0	75	116	0
Lamb, domestic, shoulder, whole (arm and blade), separable lean and fat, trimmed to 1/4" fat, choice, cooked, broiled	24.42	19.26	0	278	0	78	97	0
Lamb, domestic, shoulder, whole (arm and blade), separable lean and fat, trimmed to 1/4" fat, choice, cooked, roasted	22.51	19.97	0	276	0	66	92	0
Lamb, domestic, shoulder, whole (arm and blade), separable lean only, trimmed to 1/4" fat, choice, raw	19.55	6.76	0	144	0	70	66	0
Lamb, domestic, shoulder, whole (arm and blade), separable lean only, trimmed to 1/4" fat, choice, cooked, braised	32.81	15.89	0	283	0	79	117	0
Lamb, domestic, shoulder, whole (arm and blade), separable lean only, trimmed to 1/4" fat, choice, cooked, broiled	27.12	10.5	0	210	0	83	93	0
Lamb, domestic, shoulder, whole (arm and blade), separable lean only, trimmed to 1/4" fat, choice, cooked, roasted	24.94	10.77	0	204	0	68	87	0
Lamb, domestic, shoulder, arm, separable lean and fat, trimmed to 1/4" fat, choice, raw	16.79	20.9	0	260	0	60	71	0
Lamb, domestic, shoulder, arm, separable lean and fat, trimmed to 1/4" fat, choice, cooked, braised	30.39	24	0	346	0	72	120	0
Lamb, domestic, shoulder, arm, separable lean	24.44	19.55	0	281	0	77	96	0

Food Name ---> per 100 g	Protein (g)	Fat (g)	Carb (g)	Calories	Fiber (g)	Sodium (mg)	Cholesterol (mg)	Net Carb (g)
and fat, trimmed to 1/4" fat, choice, cooked, broiled								
Lamb, domestic, shoulder, arm, separable lean and fat, trimmed to 1/4" fat, choice, cooked, roasted	22.53	20.24	0	279	0	65	92	0
Lamb, domestic, shoulder, arm, separable lean only, trimmed to 1/4" fat, choice, raw	19.99	5.2	0	132	0	69	64	0
Lamb, domestic, shoulder, arm, separable lean only, trimmed to 1/4" fat, choice, cooked, braised	35.54	14.08	0	279	0	76	121	0
Lamb, domestic, shoulder, arm, separable lean only, trimmed to 1/4" fat, choice, cooked, broiled	27.71	9.02	0	200	0	82	92	0
Lamb, domestic, shoulder, arm, separable lean only, trimmed to 1/4" fat, choice, cooked, roasted	25.46	9.26	0	192	0	67	86	0
Lamb, domestic, shoulder, blade, separable lean and fat, trimmed to 1/4" fat, choice, raw	16.63	20.86	0	259	0	62	72	0
Lamb, domestic, shoulder, blade, separable lean and fat, trimmed to 1/4" fat, choice, cooked, braised	28.51	24.73	0	345	0	75	116	0
Lamb, domestic, shoulder, blade, separable lean and fat, trimmed to 1/4" fat, choice, cooked, broiled	23.08	19.94	0	278	0	82	95	0
Lamb, domestic, shoulder, blade, separable lean and fat, trimmed to 1/4" fat, choice, cooked, roasted	22.25	20.61	0	281	0	66	92	0
Lamb, domestic, shoulder, blade, separable lean only, trimmed to 1/4" fat, choice, raw	19.29	7.63	0	151	0	70	67	0
Lamb, domestic, shoulder, blade, separable lean only, trimmed to 1/4" fat, choice, cooked, braised	32.35	16.64	0	288	0	79	117	0
Lamb, domestic, shoulder, blade, separable lean only, trimmed to 1/4" fat, choice, cooked, broiled	25.48	11.32	0	211	0	88	91	0
Lamb, domestic, shoulder, blade, separable lean only, trimmed to 1/4" fat, choice, cooked, roasted	24.61	11.57	0	209	0	68	87	0
Lamb, domestic, cubed for stew or kabob (leg and shoulder), separable lean only, trimmed to 1/4" fat, raw	20.21	5.28	0	134	0	65	65	0
Lamb, domestic, cubed for stew or kabob (leg and shoulder), separable lean only, trimmed to 1/4" fat, cooked, braised	33.69	8.8	0	223	0	70	108	0
Lamb, domestic, cubed for stew or kabob (leg and shoulder), separable lean only, trimmed to 1/4" fat, cooked, broiled	28.08	7.33	0	186	0	76	90	0
Lamb, New Zealand, imported, frozen, composite of trimmed retail cuts, separable lean and fat, raw	16.74	22.74	0	277	0	39	78	0
Lamb, New Zealand, imported, frozen, composite of trimmed retail cuts, separable lean and fat, cooked	24.42	22.26	0	305	0	46	109	0
Lamb, New Zealand, imported, frozen, composite of trimmed retail cuts, separable lean only, raw	20.75	4.41	0	128	0	46	74	0
Lamb, New Zealand, imported, frozen, composite of trimmed retail cuts, separable lean only, cooked	29.59	8.86	0	206	0	50	109	0
Lamb, New Zealand, imported, frozen, composite of trimmed retail cuts, separable fat, raw	6.92	67.63	0	640	0	22	87	0
Lamb, New Zealand, imported, frozen, composite of trimmed retail cuts, separable fat, cooked	9.72	60.39	0	586	0	35	109	0
Lamb, New Zealand, imported, fore-shank, separable lean and fat, raw	20.09	11.38	0.09	183	0	76	66	0.09
Lamb, New Zealand, imported, fore-shank,	30.35	14.99	0.03	256	0	74	110	0.03

Food Name ---> per 100 g	Protein (g)	Fat (g)	Carb (g)	Calories	Fiber (g)	Sodium (mg)	Cholesterol (mg)	Net Carb (g)
separable lean and fat, cooked, braised								
Lamb, New Zealand, imported, fore-shank, separable lean only, raw	22.05	3.77	0	122	0	82	65	0
Lamb, New Zealand, imported, fore-shank, separable lean only, cooked, braised	33.31	8.4	0	209	0	77	115	0
Lamb, New Zealand, imported, leg chop/steak, bone-in, separable lean and fat, raw	18.64	14.52	0.13	206	0	59	67	0.13
Lamb, New Zealand, imported, frozen, leg, whole (shank and sirloin), separable lean and fat, cooked, roasted	24.81	15.56	0	246	0	43	101	0
Lamb, New Zealand, imported, leg chop/steak, bone-in, separable lean only, raw	21.1	4.64	0	126	0	64	66	0
Lamb, New Zealand, imported, frozen, leg, whole (shank and sirloin), separable lean only, cooked, roasted	27.68	7.01	0	181	0	45	100	0
Lamb, New Zealand, imported, loin chop, separable lean and fat, raw	15.4	26.19	0.22	298	0	63	69	0.22
Lamb, New Zealand, imported, frozen, loin, separable lean and fat, cooked, broiled	23.43	23.88	0	315	0	49	112	0
Lamb, New Zealand, imported, loin chop, separable lean only, raw	19.98	6.88	0	142	0	77	66	0
Lamb, New Zealand, imported, frozen, loin, separable lean only, cooked, broiled	29.31	8.24	0	199	0	55	114	0
Lamb, New Zealand, imported, rack - partly frenched, separable lean and fat, raw	18.12	18.52	0.13	240	0	61	66	0.13
Lamb, New Zealand, imported, rack - partly frenched, separable lean and fat, cooked, fast roasted	22.06	18.29	0.04	253	0	69	76	0.04
Lamb, New Zealand, imported, rack - partly frenched, separable lean only, raw	20.65	8.61	0	160	0	67	64	0
Lamb, New Zealand, imported, rack - partly frenched, separable lean only, cooked, fast roasted	24.43	10.63	0	193	0	72	76	0
Lamb, New Zealand, imported, square-cut shoulder, separable lean and fat, raw	16.16	22.89	0.24	272	0	64	60	0.24
Lamb, New Zealand, imported, frozen, shoulder, whole (arm and blade), separable lean and fat, cooked, braised	28.21	26.27	0	357	0	51	123	0
Lamb, New Zealand, imported, square-cut shoulder, separable lean only, raw	19.72	8.3	0	154	0	73	56	0
Lamb, New Zealand, imported, frozen, shoulder, whole (arm and blade), separable lean only, cooked, braised	34.06	15.5	0	285	0	56	127	0
Veal, composite of trimmed retail cuts, separable lean and fat, raw	19.35	6.77	0	144	0	82	82	0
Veal, composite of trimmed retail cuts, separable lean and fat, cooked	30.1	11.39	0	231	0	87	114	0
Veal, composite of trimmed retail cuts, separable lean only, raw	20.2	2.87	0	112	0	86	83	0
Veal, composite of trimmed retail cuts, separable lean only, cooked	31.9	6.58	0	196	0	89	118	0
Veal, composite of trimmed retail cuts, separable fat, raw	6.02	67.83	0	638	0	26	73	0
Veal, composite of trimmed retail cuts, separable fat, cooked	9.42	66.74	0	642	0	57	73	0
Veal, leg (top round), separable lean and fat, raw	20.98	3.08	0	117	0	63	78	0
Veal, leg (top round), separable lean and fat,	36.16	6.33	0	211	0	67	134	0

cooked, braised

Food Name ---> per 100 g	Protein (g)	Fat (g)	Carb (g)	Calories	Fiber (g)	Sodium (mg)	Cholesterol (mg)	Net Carb (g)
Veal, leg (top round), separable lean and fat, cooked, pan-fried, breaded	27.29	9.18	9.91	238	0.3	454	112	9.61
Veal, leg (top round), separable lean and fat, cooked, pan-fried, not breaded	31.75	8.35	0	211	0	76	105	0
Veal, leg (top round), separable lean and fat, cooked, roasted	27.7	4.65	0	160	0	68	103	0
Veal, leg (top round), separable lean only, raw	21.28	1.76	0	107	0	64	78	0
Veal, leg (top round), separable lean only, cooked, braised	36.71	5.09	0	203	0	67	135	0
Veal, leg (top round), separable lean only, cooked, pan-fried, breaded	28.41	6.27	9.84	216	0.2	455	113	9.64
Veal, leg (top round), separable lean only, cooked, pan-fried, not breaded	33.17	4.62	0	183	0	77	107	0
Veal, leg (top round), separable lean only, cooked, roasted	28.07	3.39	0	150	0	68	103	0
Veal, loin, separable lean and fat, raw	20.07	10.07	0.07	177	0	98	59	0.07
Veal, loin, separable lean and fat, cooked, braised	30.19	17.21	0	284	0	80	118	0
Veal, loin, separable lean and fat, cooked, roasted	24.8	12.32	0	217	0	93	103	0
Veal, loin, separable lean only, raw	21.85	2.9	0	114	0	99	55	0
Veal, loin, separable lean only, cooked, braised	33.57	9.15	0	226	0	84	125	0
Veal, loin, separable lean only, cooked, roasted	26.32	6.94	0	175	0	96	106	0
Veal, rib, separable lean and fat, raw	18.86	9.01	0	162	0	89	82	0
Veal, rib, separable lean and fat, cooked, braised	32.43	12.53	0	251	0	95	139	0
Veal, rib, separable lean and fat, cooked, roasted	23.96	13.96	0	228	0	92	110	0
Veal, rib, separable lean only, raw	19.97	3.89	0	120	0	95	83	0
Veal, rib, separable lean only, cooked, braised	34.44	7.81	0	218	0	99	144	0
Veal, rib, separable lean only, cooked, roasted	25.76	7.44	0	177	0	97	115	0
Veal, shoulder, whole (arm and blade), separable lean and fat, raw	19.27	5.28	0	130	0	91	87	0
Veal, shoulder, whole (arm and blade), separable lean and fat, cooked, braised	32.06	10.14	0	228	0	95	126	0
Veal, shoulder, whole (arm and blade), separable lean and fat, cooked, roasted	25.32	8.42	0	184	0	96	113	0
Veal, shoulder, whole (arm and blade), separable lean only, raw	19.79	3	0	112	0	92	86	0
Veal, shoulder, whole (arm and blade), separable lean only, cooked, braised	33.68	6.1	0	199	0	97	130	0
Veal, shoulder, whole (arm and blade), separable lean only, cooked, roasted	25.81	6.62	0	170	0	97	114	0
Veal, shoulder, arm, separable lean and fat, raw	19.34	5.44	0	132	0	83	82	0
Veal, shoulder, arm, separable lean and fat, cooked, braised	33.63	10.24	0	236	0	87	148	0
Veal, shoulder, arm, separable lean and fat, cooked, roasted	25.46	8.25	0	183	0	90	108	0
Veal, shoulder, arm, separable lean only, raw	20.04	2.16	0	105	0	86	83	0
Veal, shoulder, arm, separable lean only, cooked, braised	35.73	5.33	0	201	0	90	155	0
Veal, shoulder, arm, separable lean only, cooked, roasted	26.13	5.81	0	164	0	91	109	0
Veal, shoulder, blade chop, separable lean and fat, raw	18.72	7.61	0.03	148	0	91	62	0.03
Veal, shoulder, blade, separable lean and fat, cooked, braised	31.26	10.09	0	225	0	98	153	0
Veal, shoulder, blade, separable lean and fat,	25.15	8.67	0	186	0	100	117	0

Food Name ---> per 100 g	Protein (g)	Fat (g)	Carb (g)	Calories	Fiber (g)	Sodium (mg)	Cholesterol (mg)	Net Carb (g)
cooked, roasted								
Veal, shoulder, blade chop, separable lean only, raw	19.6	2.88	0	110	0	92	60	0
Veal, shoulder, blade, separable lean only, cooked, braised	32.66	6.48	0	198	0	101	158	0
Veal, shoulder, blade, separable lean only, cooked, roasted	25.64	6.88	0	171	0	102	119	0
Veal, sirloin, separable lean and fat, raw	19.07	7.81	0	152	0	76	78	0
Veal, sirloin, separable lean and fat, cooked, braised	31.26	13.14	0	252	0	79	108	0
Veal, sirloin, separable lean and fat, cooked, roasted	25.14	10.45	0	202	0	83	102	0
Veal, sirloin, separable lean only, raw	20.2	2.59	0	110	0	80	79	0
Veal, sirloin, separable lean only, cooked, braised	33.96	6.51	0	204	0	81	113	0
Veal, sirloin, separable lean only, cooked, roasted	26.32	6.22	0	168	0	85	104	0
Veal, cubed for stew (leg and shoulder), separable lean only, raw	20.27	2.5	0	109	0	83	84	0
Veal, cubed for stew (leg and shoulder), separable lean only, cooked, braised	34.94	4.31	0	188	0	93	145	0
Veal, ground, raw	18.58	13.06	0	197	0	103	49	0
Veal, ground, cooked, broiled	24.38	7.56	0	172	0	83	103	0
Game meat, antelope, raw	22.38	2.03	0	114	0	51	95	0
Game meat, antelope, cooked, roasted	29.45	2.67	0	150	0	54	126	0
Game meat, bear, raw	20.1	8.3	0	161	0	-	-	0
Game meat, bear, cooked, simmered	32.42	13.39	0	259	0	71	98	0
Bison, ground, grass-fed, cooked	25.45	8.62	0	179	0	76	71	0
Bison, ground, grass-fed, raw	20.23	7.21	0.05	146	0	70	55	0.05
Game meat, beaver, raw	24.05	4.8	0	146	0	51	-	0
Game meat, beaver, cooked, roasted	34.85	6.96	0	212	0	59	117	0
Game meat, beefalo, composite of cuts, raw	23.3	4.8	0	143	0	78	44	0
Game meat, beefalo, composite of cuts, cooked, roasted	30.66	6.32	0	188	0	82	58	0
Veal, Australian, separable fat, raw	9.91	52.17	0	509	0	44	66	0
Veal, Australian, rib, rib roast, separable lean and fat, raw	19.6	13.1	1.15	201	0	76	60	1.15
Game meat, bison, separable lean only, raw	21.62	1.84	0	109	0	54	62	0
Game meat, bison, separable lean only, cooked, roasted	28.44	2.42	0	143	0	57	82	0
Game meat, boar, wild, raw	21.51	3.33	0	122	0	-	-	0
Game meat, boar, wild, cooked, roasted	28.3	4.38	0	160	0	60	77	0
Game meat, buffalo, water, raw	20.39	1.37	0	99	0	53	46	0
Game meat, buffalo, water, cooked, roasted	26.83	1.8	0	131	0	56	61	0
Game meat, caribou, raw	22.63	3.36	0	127	0	57	83	0
Game meat, caribou, cooked, roasted	29.77	4.42	0	167	0	60	109	0
Game meat, deer, raw	22.96	2.42	0	120	0	51	85	0
Game meat, deer, cooked, roasted	30.21	3.19	0	158	0	54	112	0
Game meat, elk, raw	22.95	1.45	0	111	0	58	55	0
Game meat, elk, cooked, roasted	30.19	1.9	0	146	0	61	73	0
Goat, raw	20.6	2.31	0	109	0	82	57	0
Game meat, goat, cooked, roasted	27.1	3.03	0	143	0	86	75	0
Game meat, horse, raw	21.39	4.6	0	133	0	53	52	0
Game meat, horse, cooked, roasted	28.14	6.05	0	175	0	55	68	0
Game meat, moose, raw	22.24	0.74	0	102	0	65	59	0

Food Name ---> per 100 g	Protein (g)	Fat (g)	Carb (g)	Calories	Fiber (g)	Sodium (mg)	Cholesterol (mg)	Net Carb (g)
Game meat, moose, cooked, roasted	29.27	0.97	0	134	0	69	78	0
Game meat, muskrat, raw	20.76	8.1	0	162	0	82	-	0
Game meat, muskrat, cooked, roasted	30.09	11.74	0	234	0	95	121	0
Game meat, opossum, cooked, roasted	30.2	10.2	0	221	0	58	129	0
Game meat, rabbit, domesticated, composite of cuts, raw	20.05	5.55	0	136	0	41	57	0
Game meat, rabbit, domesticated, composite of cuts, cooked, roasted	29.06	8.05	0	197	0	47	82	0
Game meat, rabbit, domesticated, composite of cuts, cooked, stewed	30.38	8.41	0	206	0	37	86	0
Game meat, rabbit, wild, raw	21.79	2.32	0	114	0	50	81	0
Game meat, rabbit, wild, cooked, stewed	33.02	3.51	0	173	0	45	123	0
Game meat, raccoon, cooked, roasted	29.2	14.5	0	255	0	79	97	0
Game meat, squirrel, raw	21.23	3.21	0	120	0	103	83	0
Game meat, squirrel, cooked, roasted	30.77	4.69	0	173	0	119	121	0
Lamb, variety meats and by-products, brain, raw	10.4	8.58	0	122	0	112	1352	0
Lamb, variety meats and by-products, brain, cooked, braised	12.55	10.17	0	145	0	134	2043	0
Lamb, variety meats and by-products, brain, cooked, pan-fried	16.97	22.19	0	273	0	157	2504	0
Veal, variety meats and by-products, brain, raw	10.32	8.21	0	118	0	127	1590	0
Veal, variety meats and by-products, brain, cooked, braised	11.48	9.63	0	136	0	156	3100	0
Veal, variety meats and by-products, brain, cooked, pan-fried	14.48	16.75	0	213	0	176	2120	0
Lamb, variety meats and by-products, heart, raw	16.47	5.68	0.21	122	0	89	135	0.21
Lamb, variety meats and by-products, heart, cooked, braised	24.97	7.91	1.93	185	0	63	249	1.93
Veal, variety meats and by-products, heart, raw	17.18	3.98	0.08	110	0	77	104	0.08
Veal, variety meats and by-products, heart, cooked, braised	29.12	6.75	0.13	186	0	58	176	0.13
Lamb, variety meats and by-products, kidneys, raw	15.74	2.95	0.82	97	0	156	337	0.82
Lamb, variety meats and by-products, kidneys, cooked, braised	23.65	3.62	0.99	137	0	151	565	0.99
Veal, variety meats and by-products, kidneys, raw	15.76	3.12	0.85	99	0	178	364	0.85
Veal, variety meats and by-products, kidneys, cooked, braised	26.32	5.66	0	163	0	110	791	0
Lamb, variety meats and by-products, liver, raw	20.38	5.02	1.78	139	0	70	371	1.78
Lamb, variety meats and by-products, liver, cooked, braised	30.57	8.81	2.53	220	0	56	501	2.53
Lamb, variety meats and by-products, liver, cooked, pan-fried	25.53	12.65	3.78	238	0	124	493	3.78
Veal, variety meats and by-products, liver, raw	19.93	4.85	2.91	140	0	77	334	2.91
Veal, variety meats and by-products, liver, cooked, braised	28.42	6.26	3.77	192	0	78	511	3.77
Veal, variety meats and by-products, liver, cooked, pan-fried	27.37	6.51	4.47	193	0	85	485	4.47
Lamb, variety meats and by-products, lungs, raw	16.7	2.6	0	95	0	157	-	0
Lamb, variety meats and by-products, lungs, cooked, braised	19.88	3.1	0	113	0	84	284	0
Veal, variety meats and by-products, lungs, raw	16.3	2.3	0	90	0	108	229	0
Veal, variety meats and by-products, lungs, cooked, braised	18.74	2.64	0	104	0	56	263	0
Lamb, variety meats and by-products,	14.97	23.54	0	276	0	59	213	0

Food Name ---> per 100 g	Protein (g)	Fat (g)	Carb (g)	Calories	Fiber (g)	Sodium (mg)	Cholesterol (mg)	Net Carb (g)
mechanically separated, raw								
Lamb, variety meats and by-products, pancreas, raw	14.84	9.82	0	152	0	75	260	0
Lamb, variety meats and by-products, pancreas, cooked, braised	22.83	15.12	0	234	0	52	400	0
Veal, variety meats and by-products, pancreas, raw	15	13.1	0	182	0	67	173	0
Veal, variety meats and by-products, pancreas, cooked, braised	29.1	14.6	0	256	0	68	-	0
Lamb, variety meats and by-products, spleen, raw	17.2	3.1	0	101	0	84	250	0
Lamb, variety meats and by-products, spleen, cooked, braised	26.46	4.77	0	156	0	58	385	0
Veal, variety meats and by-products, spleen, raw	18.3	2.2	0	98	0	97	340	0
Veal, variety meats and by-products, spleen, cooked, braised	24.08	2.89	0	129	0	58	447	0
Veal, variety meats and by-products, thymus, raw	17.21	3.07	0	101	0	67	250	0
Veal, variety meats and by-products, thymus, cooked, braised	22.67	3.11	0	125	0	59	350	0
Lamb, variety meats and by-products, tongue, raw	15.7	17.17	0	222	0	78	156	0
Lamb, variety meats and by-products, tongue, cooked, braised	21.57	20.28	0	275	0	67	189	0
Veal, variety meats and by-products, tongue, raw	17.18	5.48	1.91	131	0	82	62	1.91
Veal, variety meats and by-products, tongue, cooked, braised	25.85	10.1	0	202	0	64	238	0
Lamb, ground, raw	16.56	23.41	0	282	0	59	73	0
Lamb, ground, cooked, broiled	24.75	19.65	0	283	0	81	97	0
Lamb, domestic, composite of trimmed retail cuts, separable lean and fat, trimmed to 1/8" fat, choice, raw	17.54	18.66	0	243	0	59	70	0
Lamb, domestic, composite of trimmed retail cuts, separable lean and fat, trimmed to 1/8" fat, choice, cooked	25.51	18.01	0	271	0	72	96	0
Lamb, domestic, foreshank, separable lean and fat, trimmed to 1/8" fat, choice, raw	18.91	13.38	0	201	0	72	72	0
Lamb, domestic, foreshank, separable lean and fat, trimmed to 1/8" fat, cooked, braised	28.37	13.46	0	243	0	72	106	0
Lamb, domestic, leg, whole (shank and sirloin), separable lean and fat, trimmed to 1/8" fat, choice, raw	18.47	14.42	0	209	0	57	68	0
Lamb, domestic, leg, whole (shank and sirloin), separable lean and fat, trimmed to 1/8" fat, choice, cooked, roasted	26.2	14.42	0	242	0	67	92	0
Lamb, domestic, leg, shank half, separable lean and fat, trimmed to 1/8" fat, choice, raw	18.99	11.5	0	185	0	58	67	0
Lamb, domestic, leg, shank half, separable lean and fat, trimmed to 1/8" fat, choice, cooked, roasted	26.73	11.4	0	217	0	65	90	0
Lamb, domestic, leg, sirloin half, separable lean and fat, trimmed to 1/8" fat, choice, raw	17.21	20.8	0	261	0	56	71	0
Lamb, domestic, leg, sirloin half, separable lean and fat, trimmed to 1/8" fat, choice, cooked, roasted	24.95	19.67	0	284	0	68	96	0
Lamb, domestic, loin, separable lean and fat, trimmed to 1/8" fat, choice, raw	17.18	22.75	0	279	0	59	72	0
Lamb, domestic, loin, separable lean and fat, trimmed to 1/8" fat, choice, cooked, broiled	26.06	20.61	0	297	0	78	99	0

Food Name ---> per 100 g	Protein (g)	Fat (g)	Carb (g)	Calories	Fiber (g)	Sodium (mg)	Cholesterol (mg)	Net Carb (g)
Lamb, domestic, loin, separable lean and fat, trimmed to 1/8" fat, choice, cooked, roasted	23.27	21.12	0	290	0	64	93	0
Lamb, domestic, rib, separable lean and fat, trimmed to 1/8" fat, choice, raw	15.32	30.71	0	342	0	58	74	0
Lamb, domestic, rib, separable lean and fat, trimmed to 1/8" fat, choice, cooked, broiled	23.06	26.82	0	340	0	77	98	0
Lamb, domestic, rib, separable lean and fat, trimmed to 1/8" fat, choice, cooked, roasted	21.82	27.53	0	341	0	74	96	0
Lamb, domestic, shoulder, whole (arm and blade), separable lean and fat, trimmed to 1/8" fat, choice, raw	17.07	18.96	0	244	0	63	71	0
Lamb, domestic, shoulder, whole (arm and blade), separable lean and fat, trimmed to 1/8" fat, choice, cooked, braised	29.46	23.57	0	338	0	74	117	0
Lamb, domestic, shoulder, whole (arm and blade), separable lean and fat, trimmed to 1/8" fat, choice, cooked, broiled	23.84	18.39	0	268	0	82	95	0
Lamb, domestic, shoulder, whole (arm and blade), separable lean and fat, trimmed to 1/8" fat, choice, cooked, roasted	22.7	19.08	0	269	0	66	91	0
Lamb, domestic, shoulder, arm, separable lean and fat, trimmed to 1/8" fat, choice, raw	17.19	18.94	0	244	0	61	70	0
Lamb, domestic, shoulder, arm, separable lean and fat, trimmed to 1/8" fat, choice, cooked, braised	31.1	22.65	0	337	0	72	120	0
Lamb, domestic, shoulder, arm, separable lean and fat, trimmed to 1/8" fat, cooked, broiled	24.91	18.05	0	269	0	78	96	0
Lamb, domestic, shoulder, arm, separable lean and fat, trimmed to 1/8" fat, choice, roasted	22.93	18.75	0	267	0	65	91	0
Lamb, domestic, shoulder, blade, separable lean and fat, trimmed to 1/8" fat, choice, raw	17.01	18.97	0	244	0	63	71	0
Lamb, domestic, shoulder, blade, separable lean and fat, trimmed to 1/8" fat, choice, cooked, braised	28.92	23.88	0	339	0	75	116	0
Lamb, domestic, shoulder, blade, separable lean and fat, trimmed to 1/8" fat, choice, cooked, broiled	23.48	18.5	0	267	0	83	95	0
Lamb, domestic, shoulder, blade, separable lean and fat, trimmed to 1/8" fat, choice, cooked, roasted	22.62	19.19	0	270	0	67	92	0
Lamb, New Zealand, imported, frozen, composite of trimmed retail cuts, separable lean and fat, trimmed to 1/8" fat, raw	17.95	17.2	0	232	0	41	77	0
Lamb, New Zealand, imported, frozen, composite of trimmed retail cuts, separable lean and fat, trimmed to 1/8" fat, cooked	25.26	17.98	0	270	0	46	106	0
Lamb, New Zealand, imported, frozen, foreshank, separable lean and fat, trimmed to 1/8" fat, raw	18.04	16.15	0	223	0	45	71	0
Lamb, New Zealand, imported, frozen, foreshank, separable lean and fat, trimmed to 1/8" fat, cooked, braised	26.97	15.83	0	258	0	47	102	0
Lamb, New Zealand, imported, frozen, leg, whole (shank and sirloin), separable lean and fat, trimmed to 1/8" fat, raw	18.76	13.37	0	201	0	41	75	0
Lamb, New Zealand, imported, frozen, leg, whole (shank and sirloin), separable lean and fat, trimmed to 1/8" fat, cooked, roasted	25.34	13.95	0	234	0	44	101	0

Food Name ---> per 100 g	Protein (g)	Fat (g)	Carb (g)	Calories	Fiber (g)	Sodium (mg)	Cholesterol (mg)	Net Carb (g)
Lamb, New Zealand, imported, frozen, loin, separable lean and fat, trimmed to 1/8" fat, raw	17.18	22.1	0	273	0	39	82	0
Lamb, New Zealand, imported, frozen, loin, separable lean and fat, trimmed to 1/8" fat, cooked, broiled	24.41	21.28	0	296	0	50	113	0
Lamb, new zealand, imported, frozen, rib, separable lean and fat, trimmed to 1/8" fat, raw	15.87	27	0	311	0	42	80	0
Lamb, New Zealand, imported, frozen, rib, separable lean and fat, trimmed to 1/8" fat, cooked, roasted	19.86	25.74	0	317	0	44	99	0
Lamb, New Zealand, imported, frozen, shoulder, whole (arm and blade), separable lean and fat, trimmed to 1/8" fat, raw	17.19	19.74	0	251	0	42	74	0
Lamb, New Zealand, imported, frozen, shoulder, whole (arm and blade), separable lean and fat, trimmed to 1/8" fat, cooked, braised	29.43	24.03	0	342	0	52	123	0
Game meat, bison, top sirloin, separable lean only, trimmed to 0" fat, raw	21.4	2.4	0	113	-	51	71	0
Game meat, bison, ribeye, separable lean only, trimmed to 0" fat, raw	22.1	2.4	0	116	-	48	62	0
Game meat, bison, shoulder clod, separable lean only, trimmed to 0" fat, raw	21.1	2.1	0	109	-	59	66	0
Veal, breast, separable fat, cooked	9.4	53.35	0	521	0	49	95	0
Veal, breast, whole, boneless, separable lean and fat, raw	17.47	14.75	0	208	-	71	71	0
Veal, breast, whole, boneless, separable lean and fat, cooked, braised	26.97	16.77	0	266	-	65	113	0
Veal, breast, plate half, boneless, separable lean and fat, cooked, braised	25.93	18.95	0	282	-	64	112	0
Veal, breast, point half, boneless, separable lean and fat, cooked, braised	28.23	14.16	0	248	-	66	114	0
Veal, breast, whole, boneless, separable lean only, cooked, braised	30.32	9.8	0	218	-	68	116	0
Veal, shank (fore and hind), separable lean and fat, raw	19.15	3.48	0	113	-	84	75	0
Veal, shank (fore and hind), separable lean and fat, cooked, braised	31.54	6.2	0	191	-	93	124	0
Veal, shank (fore and hind), separable lean only, raw	19.28	2.83	0	108	-	85	75	0
Veal, shank (fore and hind), separable lean only, cooked, braised	32.22	4.33	0	177	0	94	126	0
Lamb, Australian, imported, fresh, composite of trimmed retail cuts, separable lean and fat, trimmed to 1/8" fat, raw	17.84	16.97	0	229	-	74	66	0
Lamb, Australian, imported, fresh, composite of trimmed retail cuts, separable lean and fat, trimmed to 1/8" fat, cooked	24.52	16.82	0	256	-	76	87	0
Lamb, Australian, imported, fresh, composite of trimmed retail cuts, separable lean only, trimmed to 1/8" fat, raw	20.25	6.18	0	142	-	83	64	0
Lamb, Australian, imported, fresh, composite of trimmed retail cuts, separable lean only, trimmed to 1/8" fat, cooked	26.71	9.63	0	201	-	80	87	0
Lamb, Australian, imported, fresh, separable fat, raw	6.27	68.87	0	648	-	33	77	0
Lamb, Australian, imported, fresh, separable fat, cooked	9.42	66.4	0	639	-	51	83	0

Food Name ---> per 100 g	Protein (g)	Fat (g)	Carb (g)	Calories	Fiber (g)	Sodium (mg)	Cholesterol (mg)	Net Carb (g)
Lamb, Australian, imported, fresh, foreshank, separable lean and fat, trimmed to 1/8" fat, raw	18.85	12.68	0	195	-	96	67	0
Lamb, Australian, imported, fresh, foreshank, separable lean and fat, trimmed to 1/8" fat, cooked, braised	24.78	14.44	0	236	-	93	91	0
Lamb, Australian, imported, fresh, foreshank, separable lean only, trimmed to 1/8" fat, raw	20.83	3.81	0	123	-	106	66	0
Lamb, Australian, imported, fresh, foreshank, separable lean only, trimmed to 1/8" fat, cooked, braised	27.5	5.22	0	165	-	100	92	0
Lamb, Australian, imported, fresh, leg, whole (shank and sirloin), separable lean and fat, trimmed to 1/8" fat, raw	18.24	15.19	0	215	-	73	66	0
Lamb, Australian, imported, fresh, leg, whole (shank and sirloin), separable lean and fat, trimmed to 1/8" fat, cooked, roasted	25.16	15.13	0	244	-	70	88	0
Lamb, Australian, imported, fresh, leg, whole (shank and sirloin), separable lean only, trimmed to 1/8" fat, raw	20.46	5.23	0	135	-	81	64	0
Lamb, Australian, imported, fresh, leg, whole (shank and sirloin), separable lean only, trimmed to 1/8" fat, cooked, roasted	27.31	8.1	0	190	-	72	89	0
Lamb, Australian, imported, fresh, leg, shank half, separable lean and fat, trimmed to 1/8" fat, raw	18.59	13.48	0	201	-	75	66	0
Lamb, Australian, imported, fresh, leg, shank half, separable lean and fat, trimmed to 1/8" fat, cooked, roasted	25.25	13.69	0	231	-	67	83	0
Lamb, Australian, imported, fresh, leg, shank half, separable lean only, trimmed to 1/8" fat, raw	20.45	5.1	0	133	-	81	64	0
Lamb, Australian, imported, fresh, leg, shank half, separable lean only, trimmed to 1/8" fat, cooked, roasted	27.18	7.27	0	182	-	69	83	0
Lamb, Australian, imported, fresh, leg, sirloin half, boneless, separable lean and fat, trimmed to 1/8" fat, raw	17.25	20	0	254	-	70	66	0
Lamb, Australian, imported, fresh, leg, sirloin half, boneless, separable lean and fat, trimmed to 1/8" fat, cooked, roasted	24.88	19.38	0	281	-	78	102	0
Lamb, Australian, imported, fresh, leg, sirloin half, boneless, separable lean only, trimmed to 1/8" fat, raw	20.48	5.64	0	138	-	80	63	0
Lamb, Australian, imported, fresh, leg, sirloin half, boneless, separable lean only, trimmed to 1/8" fat, cooked, roasted	27.75	10.65	0	215	-	83	105	0
Lamb, Australian, imported, fresh, leg, sirloin chops, boneless, separable lean and fat, trimmed to 1/8" fat, raw	18.33	14.38	0	208	-	59	66	0
Lamb, Australian, imported, fresh, leg, sirloin chops, boneless, separable lean and fat, trimmed to 1/8" fat, cooked, broiled	25.75	13.83	0	235	-	64	85	0
Lamb, Australian, imported, fresh, leg, sirloin chops, boneless, separable lean only, trimmed to 1/8" fat, raw	20.43	4.91	0	132	-	64	64	0
Lamb, Australian, imported, fresh, leg, sirloin chops, boneless, separable lean only, trimmed to 1/8" fat, cooked, broiled	27.63	7.8	0	188	-	66	85	0
Lamb, Australian, imported, fresh, leg, center	19.17	12.56	0	195	-	61	65	0

Food Name ---> per 100 g	Protein (g)	Fat (g)	Carb (g)	Calories	Fiber (g)	Sodium (mg)	Cholesterol (mg)	Net Carb (g)
slice, bone-in, separable lean and fat, trimmed to 1/8" fat, raw								
Lamb, Australian, imported, fresh, leg, center slice, bone-in, separable lean and fat, trimmed to 1/8" fat, cooked, broiled	25.54	11.78	0	215	-	65	85	0
Lamb, Australian, imported, fresh, leg, center slice, bone-in, separable lean only, trimmed to 1/8" fat, raw	20.65	6.08	0	143	-	64	64	0
Lamb, Australian, imported, fresh, leg, center slice, bone-in, separable lean only, trimmed to 1/8" fat, cooked, broiled	26.75	7.68	0	183	-	66	85	0
Lamb, Australian, imported, fresh, loin, separable lean and fat, trimmed to 1/8" fat, raw	19.32	13.38	0	203	-	70	66	0
Lamb, Australian, imported, fresh, loin, separable lean and fat, trimmed to 1/8" fat, cooked, broiled	25.49	12.25	0	219	-	78	82	0
Lamb, Australian, imported, fresh, loin, separable lean only, trimmed to 1/8" fat, raw	21	6.24	0	146	-	75	64	0
Lamb, Australian, imported, fresh, loin, separable lean only, trimmed to 1/8" fat, cooked, broiled	26.53	8.75	0	192	-	80	81	0
Lamb, Australian, imported, fresh, rib chop/rack roast, frenched, bone-in, separable lean and fat, trimmed to 1/8" fat, raw	21.26	16.89	0	237	0	69	69	0
Lamb, Australian, imported, fresh, rib chop, frenched, bone-in, separable lean and fat, trimmed to 1/8" fat, cooked, grilled	28.48	21.2	0	305	0	79	91	0
Lamb, Australian, imported, fresh, rib chop/rack roast, frenched, bone-in, separable lean only, trimmed to 1/8" fat, raw	24.07	5.59	0	147	0	71	66	0
Lamb, Australian, imported, fresh, rib chop, frenched, bone-in, separable lean only, trimmed to 1/8" fat, cooked, grilled	32.16	11.68	0	234	0	85	92	0
Lamb, Australian, imported, fresh, shoulder, whole (arm and blade), separable lean and fat, trimmed to 1/8" fat, raw	16.68	20.47	0	256	-	76	66	0
Lamb, Australian, imported, fresh, shoulder, whole (arm and blade), separable lean and fat, trimmed to 1/8" fat, cooked	23.58	21.65	0	296	-	85	89	0
Lamb, Australian, imported, fresh, shoulder, whole (arm and blade), separable lean only, trimmed to 1/8" fat, raw	19.36	8.01	0	155	-	88	64	0
Lamb, Australian, imported, fresh, shoulder, whole (arm and blade), separable lean only, trimmed to 1/8" fat, cooked	26.18	13.44	0	233	-	91	91	0
Lamb, Australian, imported, fresh, shoulder, arm, separable lean and fat, trimmed to 1/8" fat, raw	17.06	18.89	0	243	-	72	65	0
Lamb, Australian, imported, fresh, shoulder, arm, separable lean and fat, trimmed to 1/8" fat, cooked, braised	29.7	20.38	0	311	-	73	106	0
Lamb, Australian, imported, fresh, shoulder, arm, separable lean only, trimmed to 1/8" fat, raw	19.88	5.81	0	137	-	83	62	0
Lamb, Australian, imported, fresh, shoulder, arm, separable lean only, trimmed to 1/8" fat, cooked, braised	34.17	10.23	0	238	-	78	111	0
Lamb, Australian, imported, fresh, shoulder, blade, separable lean and fat, trimmed to 1/8" fat, raw	16.48	21.28	0	262	-	78	67	0
Lamb, Australian, imported, fresh, shoulder,	21.71	22.03	0	291	-	88	84	0

Food Name ---> per 100 g	Protein (g)	Fat (g)	Carb (g)	Calories	Fiber (g)	Sodium (mg)	Cholesterol (mg)	Net Carb (g)
blade, separable lean and fat, trimmed to 1/8" fat, cooked, broiled								
Lamb, Australian, imported, fresh, shoulder, blade, separable lean only, trimmed to 1/8" fat, raw	19.1	9.09	0	164	-	90	64	0
Lamb, Australian, imported, fresh, shoulder ,blade, separable lean only, trimmed to 1/8" fat, cooked, broiled	23.83	14.38	0	231	-	94	85	0
Game meat , bison, ground, raw	18.67	15.93	0	223	0	66	70	0
Game meat, bison, ground, cooked, pan-broiled	23.77	15.13	0	238	0	73	83	0
Game meat , bison, top sirloin, separable lean only, 1" steak, cooked, broiled	28.05	5.65	0	171	0	53	86	0
Game meat, bison, chuck, shoulder clod, separable lean only, cooked, braised	33.78	5.43	0	193	0	57	111	0
Game meat, bison, chuck, shoulder clod, separable lean only, raw	21.12	3.15	0	119	0	62	64	0
Game meat, bison, ribeye, separable lean only, 1" steak, cooked, broiled	29.45	5.67	0	177	0	52	79	0
Game meat, bison, top round, separable lean only, 1" steak, cooked, broiled	30.18	4.96	0	174	0	41	85	0
Game meat, bison, top round, separable lean only, 1" steak, raw	23.32	2.43	0	122	0	47	65	0
Game meat, elk, ground, raw	21.76	8.82	0	172	0	79	66	0
Game meat, elk, ground, cooked, pan-broiled	26.64	8.74	0	193	0	85	78	0
Game meat, elk, loin, separable lean only, cooked, broiled	31	3.84	0	167	0	54	75	0
Game meat, elk, round, separable lean only, cooked, broiled	30.94	2.64	0	156	0	51	78	0
Game meat, elk, tenderloin, separable lean only, cooked, broiled	30.76	3.41	0	162	0	50	72	0
Game meat, deer, ground, raw	21.78	7.13	0	157	0	75	80	0
Game meat, deer, ground, cooked, pan-broiled	26.45	8.22	0	187	0	78	98	0
Game meat, deer, loin, separable lean only, 1" steak, cooked, broiled	30.2	2.38	0	150	0	57	79	0
Game meat, deer, shoulder clod, separable lean only, cooked, braised	36.28	3.95	0	191	0	52	113	0
Game meat, deer, tenderloin, separable lean only, cooked, broiled	29.9	2.35	0	149	0	57	88	0
Game meat, deer, top round, separable lean only, 1" steak, cooked, broiled	31.47	1.92	0	152	0	45	85	0
Veal, Australian, shank, fore, bone-in, separable lean only, raw	20.18	4.65	0	123	0	112	65	0
Veal, Australian, shank, fore, bone-in, separable lean and fat, raw	19.58	7.42	0	145	0	108	65	0
Veal, Australian, shank, hind, bone-in, separable lean only, raw	20.37	4.47	0	122	0	98	59	0
Veal, Australian, shank, hind, bone-in, separable lean and fat	19.78	7.2	0	144	0	95	60	0
Lamb, Australian, ground, 85% lean / 15% fat, raw	17.14	20.71	0	255	-	77	73	0
Lamb, New Zealand, imported, Intermuscular fat, cooked	8.53	62.44	0	596	0	52	82	0
Lamb, New Zealand, imported, Intermuscular fat, raw	4.63	68.53	1.26	640	0	34	75	1.26
Lamb, New Zealand, imported, subcutaneous fat, raw	3.87	76.16	0.55	703	0	28	78	0.55

Food Name ---> per 100 g	Protein (g)	Fat (g)	Carb (g)	Calories	Fiber (g)	Sodium (mg)	Cholesterol (mg)	Net Carb (g)
Lamb, New Zealand, imported, brains, cooked, soaked and fried	14.03	10.92	0	154	0	101	2559	0
Lamb, New Zealand, imported, brains, raw	11.33	8.03	0	118	0	117	2100	0
Lamb, New Zealand, imported, breast, separable lean only, cooked, braised	28.16	17.53	0	270	0	86	102	0
Lamb, New Zealand, imported, breast, separable lean only, raw	18.31	7.98	1.02	149	0	107	65	1.02
Lamb, New Zealand, imported, chump, boneless, separable lean only, cooked, fast roasted	23.69	5.27	0	142	0	61	74	0
Lamb, New Zealand, imported, subcutaneous fat, cooked	5.24	72.28	0.62	674	0	43	66	0.62
Lamb, New Zealand, imported, chump, boneless, separable lean only, raw	21.68	3.83	0	121	0	62	65	0
Lamb, New Zealand, imported, kidney, cooked, soaked and fried	19.78	3.56	0.18	112	0	199	508	0.18
Lamb, New Zealand, imported, flap, boneless, separable lean only, cooked, braised	27.88	13.6	0	234	0	54	78	0
Lamb, New Zealand, imported, flap, boneless, separable lean only, raw	21.72	10.31	0	180	0	87	58	0
Lamb, New Zealand, imported, kidney, raw	15.21	2.54	0.03	84	0	168	369	0.03
Lamb, New Zealand, imported, liver, cooked, soaked and fried	25.8	6.56	1.48	168	0	59	566	1.48
Lamb, New Zealand, imported, liver, raw	20.7	4.92	2.22	136	0	59	386	2.22
Lamb, New Zealand, imported, ground lamb, cooked, braised	22.6	11.34	0	192	0	34	71	0
Lamb, New Zealand, imported, ground lamb, raw	20.33	12.41	0	193	0	57	63	0
Lamb, New Zealand, imported, heart, cooked, soaked and simmered	26.26	6.21	0	161	0	67	186	0
Lamb, New Zealand, imported, heart, raw	18.09	3.68	0	105	0	94	119	0
Lamb, New Zealand, imported, sweetbread, cooked, soaked and simmered	21.13	6.61	0	144	0	52	462	0
Lamb, New Zealand, imported, sweetbread, raw	11	3.16	0	72	0	39	160	0
Lamb, New Zealand, imported, testes, cooked, soaked and fried	21.01	4.56	0	125	0	118	523	0
Lamb, New Zealand, imported, testes, raw	11.4	2.38	0.14	68	0	119	393	0.14
Lamb, New Zealand, imported, tongue - swiss cut, cooked, soaked and simmered	17.51	22.04	0.86	272	0	52	126	0.86
Lamb, New Zealand, imported, tongue - swiss cut, raw	14.27	18.61	0	225	0	77	88	0
Lamb, New Zealand, imported, tunnel-boned leg, chump off, shank, separable lean only, cooked, slow roasted	25.29	6.44	0	159	0	62	79	0
Lamb, New Zealand, imported, tunnel-boned leg, chump off, shank off, separable lean only, raw	20.93	4.09	0	121	0	60	64	0
Lamb, New Zealand, imported, square-cut shoulder chops, separable lean only, cooked, braised	31.06	14.56	0	255	0	59	99	0
Lamb, New Zealand, imported, square-cut shoulder chops, separable lean only, raw	20.62	9.08	0	164	0	82	59	0
Lamb, New Zealand, imported, tenderloin, separable lean only, cooked, fast fried	27.94	4.81	0	155	0	59	94	0
Lamb, New Zealand, imported, tenderloin, separable lean only, raw	20.53	3.81	0	116	0	49	69	0
Lamb, New Zealand, imported, loin saddle, separable lean only, cooked, fast roasted	25.53	6.7	0	162	0	76	78	0
Lamb, New Zealand, imported, loin saddle,	20.86	5.32	0	131	0	75	66	0

Food Name ---> per 100 g	Protein (g)	Fat (g)	Carb (g)	Calories	Fiber (g)	Sodium (mg)	Cholesterol (mg)	Net Carb (g)
separable lean only, raw								
Lamb, New Zealand, imported, loin, boneless, separable lean only, cooked, fast roasted	28.99	4.49	0	156	0	57	86	0
Lamb, New Zealand, imported, loin, boneless, separable lean only, raw	21.5	3.77	0	120	0	60	66	0
Lamb, New Zealand, imported, hind-shank, separable lean only, cooked, braised	32.5	7.37	0	196	0	72	115	0
Lamb, New Zealand, imported, hind-shank, separable lean only, raw	20.4	3.35	0.73	115	0	82	62	0.73
Lamb, New Zealand, imported, neck chops, separable lean only, raw	19.84	7.97	0	151	0	81	71	0
Lamb, New Zealand, imported, neck chops, separable lean only, cooked, braised	31.4	15.36	0	264	0	97	121	0
Lamb, New Zealand, imported, netted shoulder, rolled, boneless, separable lean only, cooked, slow roasted	25.14	10.91	0	199	0	65	79	0
Lamb, New Zealand, imported, netted shoulder, rolled, boneless, separable lean only, raw	20.2	6.88	0	143	0	65	58	0
Lamb, New Zealand, imported, rack - fully frenched, separable lean only, cooked, fast roasted	24.39	8.38	0	173	0	67	72	0
Lamb, New Zealand, imported, rack - fully frenched, separable lean only, raw	20.61	7.12	0	147	0	63	62	0
Lamb, New Zealand, imported, loin chop, separable lean only, cooked, fast fried	27.43	10.7	0.41	208	0	84	85	0.41
Lamb, New Zealand, imported, square-cut shoulder, separable lean only, cooked, slow roasted	25.08	10.13	0	192	0	80	71	0
Lamb, New Zealand, imported, leg chop/steak, bone-in, separable lean only, cooked	26.31	6.35	0	162	0	67	78	0
Lamb, New Zealand, imported, flap, boneless, separable lean and fat, cooked, braised	20.48	32.63	0.14	376	0	51	76	0.14
Lamb, New Zealand, imported, flap, boneless, separable lean and fat, raw	16.17	30.14	0.27	337	0	69	64	0.27
Lamb, New Zealand, imported, hind-shank, separable lean and fat, cooked, braised	29.59	14.22	0.04	247	0	69	111	0.04
Lamb, New Zealand, imported, hind-shank, separable lean and fat, raw	18.39	12.12	0.73	186	0	76	64	0.73
Lamb, New Zealand, imported, leg chop/steak, bone-in, separable lean and fat, cooked, fast fried	24.26	12.76	0.04	212	0	65	78	0.04
Lamb, New Zealand, imported, loin chop, separable lean and fat, cooked, fast fried	21.5	27.11	0.41	332	0	73	81	0.41
Lamb, New Zealand, imported, loin saddle, separable lean and fat, cooked, fast roasted	21.13	20.98	0.1	274	0	69	76	0.1
Lamb, New Zealand, imported, loin saddle, separable lean and fat, raw	16.56	22.9	0.2	273	0	63	69	0.2
Lamb, New Zealand, imported, loin, boneless, separable lean and fat, cooked, fast roasted	28.96	4.57	0	157	0	57	86	0
Lamb, New Zealand, imported, loin, boneless, separable lean and fat, raw	21.44	3.99	0	122	0	60	66	0
Lamb, New Zealand, imported, neck chops, separable lean and fat, cooked, braised	28.53	21.43	0.03	307	0	91	116	0.03
Lamb, New Zealand, imported, neck chops, separable lean and fat, raw	17.43	17.9	0.14	231	0	73	72	0.14
Lamb, New Zealand, imported, netted shoulder, rolled, boneless, separable lean and fat, cooked, slow roasted	21.45	22.33	0.05	287	0	61	78	0.05

Food Name ---> per 100 g	Protein (g)	Fat (g)	Carb (g)	Calories	Fiber (g)	Sodium (mg)	Cholesterol (mg)	Net Carb (g)
Lamb, New Zealand, imported, netted shoulder, rolled, boneless, separable lean and fat, raw	16.9	20.36	0.2	252	0	58	61	0.2
Lamb, New Zealand, imported, square-cut shoulder chops, separable lean and fat, cooked, braised	26.79	23.86	0.05	322	0	57	95	0.05
Lamb, New Zealand, imported, square-cut shoulder chops, separable lean and fat, raw	17.02	22.84	0.23	275	0	71	63	0.23
Lamb, New Zealand, imported, square-cut shoulder, separable lean and fat, cooked, slow roasted	20.88	23.39	0.03	294	0	72	72	0.03
Lamb, New Zealand, imported, tenderloin, separable lean and fat, cooked, fast fried	27.87	5	0	157	0	59	94	0
Lamb, New Zealand, imported, rack - fully frenched, separable lean and fat, cooked, fast roasted	23.56	11.2	0.01	195	0	67	72	0.01
Lamb, New Zealand, imported, rack - fully frenched, separable lean and fat, raw	19.88	9.96	0.05	169	0	62	62	0.05
Lamb, New Zealand, imported, tunnel-boned leg, chump off, shank off, separable lean and fat, cooked, slow roasted	23.41	12.68	0.03	208	0	61	79	0.03
Lamb, New Zealand, imported, tunnel-boned leg, chump off, shank off, separable lean and fat, raw	20.93	4.09	0	121	-	60	64	0
Lamb, New Zealand, imported, tenderloin, separable lean and fat, raw	20.43	4.22	0.01	120	0	49	69	0.01
Veal, ground, cooked, pan-fried	25.83	11.78	1.51	215	0	146	77	1.51
Veal, leg, top round, cap off, cutlet, boneless, cooked, grilled	31.89	2.63	0	151	0	88	72	0
Veal, leg, top round, cap off, cutlet, boneless, raw	22.07	2.07	0	107	0	86	56	0
Veal, loin, chop, separable lean only, cooked, grilled	29.75	4.44	0.07	159	0	85	78	0.07
Veal, shank, separable lean only, raw	19.77	1.64	0	94	0	109	62	0
Veal, foreshank, osso buco, separable lean only, cooked, braised	29.12	4.51	0	157	0	90	92	0
Veal, shoulder, blade chop, separable lean only, cooked, grilled	27.33	5.53	0	159	0	113	77	0
Veal, external fat only, raw	8.85	51.6	0.89	503	0	89	86	0.89
Veal, external fat only, cooked	15.28	53.23	0	540	0	103	85	0
Veal, seam fat only, raw	12.53	43.75	0	444	0	89	83	0
Veal, seam fat only, cooked	11.16	50.17	2.11	505	0	87	82	2.11
Veal, shank, separable lean and fat, raw	19.28	3.3	0	107	0	107	63	0
Veal, foreshank, osso buco, separable lean and fat, cooked, braised	27.94	7.77	0.11	182	0	90	92	0.11
Veal, loin, chop, separable lean and fat, cooked, grilled	28.04	9.48	0.16	198	0	86	79	0.16
Veal, shoulder, blade chop, separable lean and fat, cooked, grilled	25.72	10.57	0.15	199	0	111	78	0.15
Lamb, Australian, imported, fresh, leg, bottom, boneless, separable lean only, trimmed to 1/8" fat, cooked, roasted	28.6	8.35	0	190	0	70	107	0
Lamb, Australian, imported, fresh, leg, hindshank, heel on, bone-in, separable lean only, trimmed to 1/8" fat, cooked, braised	30.73	5.63	0	174	0	86	111	0
Lamb, Australian, imported, fresh, leg, hindshank, heel on, bone-in, separable lean only, trimmed to 1/8" fat, raw	22.49	3.53	0	122	0	93	54	0
Lamb, Australian, imported, fresh, tenderloin,	30.97	6.71	0	184	0	61	111	0

Food Name ---> per 100 g	Protein (g)	Fat (g)	Carb (g)	Calories	Fiber (g)	Sodium (mg)	Cholesterol (mg)	Net Carb (g)
boneless, separable lean only, trimmed to 1/8" fat, cooked, roasted								
Lamb, Australian, imported, fresh, tenderloin, boneless, separable lean only, trimmed to 1/8" fat, raw	23.42	4.73	0	136	0	73	76	0
Lamb, Australian, imported, fresh, leg, bottom, boneless, separable lean only, trimmed to 1/8" fat, raw	22.28	5.24	0	136	0	83	61	0
Lamb, Australian, imported, fresh, leg, trotter off, bone-in, separable lean only, trimmed to 1/8" fat, cooked, roasted	32.08	9.59	0	215	0	80	117	0
Lamb, Australian, imported, fresh, leg, trotter off, bone-in, separable lean only, trimmed to 1/8" fat, raw	23.11	4.33	0	131	0	77	76	0
Lamb, Australian, imported, fresh, rack, roast, frenched, denuded, bone-in, separable lean only, trimmed to 0" fat, cooked, roasted	26.52	7.63	0	175	0	72	97	0
Lamb, Australian, imported, fresh, rack, roast, frenched, bone-in, separable lean only, trimmed to 1/8" fat, cooked, roasted	28.01	14.64	0	244	0	67	96	0
Lamb, Australian, imported, fresh, external fat, cooked	16.9	52.3	0	538	0	58	81	0
Lamb, Australian, imported, fresh, external fat, raw	12.59	48.5	0	487	0	69	71	0
Lamb, Australian, imported, fresh, seam fat, cooked	13.81	54.72	1.55	554	0	53	110	1.55
Lamb, Australian, imported, fresh, seam fat, raw	15.65	44.01	0	459	0	55	90	0
Lamb, Australian, imported, fresh, leg, bottom, boneless, separable lean and fat, trimmed to 1/8" fat, cooked, roasted	27.54	12.04	0	219	0	69	106	0
Lamb, Australian, imported, fresh, leg, bottom, boneless, separable lean and fat, trimmed to 1/8" fat, raw	20.97	11.43	0	187	0	80	63	0
Lamb, Australian, imported, fresh, leg, hindshank, heel on, bone-in, separable lean and fat, trimmed to 1/8" fat, cooked, braised	29.52	9.5	0	204	0	84	110	0
Lamb, Australian, imported, fresh, leg, hindshank, heel on, bone-in, separable lean and fat, trimmed to 1/8" fat, raw	20.58	12.68	0	196	0	87	59	0
Lamb, Australian, imported, fresh, leg, trotter off, bone-in, separable lean and fat, trimmed to 1/8" fat, cooked, roasted	30.15	11.64	0.08	226	0	77	113	0.08
Lamb, Australian, imported, fresh, leg, trotter off, bone-in, separable lean and fat, trimmed to 1/8" fat, raw	21.95	9.73	0	175	0	75	76	0
Lamb, Australian, imported, fresh, tenderloin, boneless, separable lean and fat, trimmed to 1/8" fat, cooked, roasted	30.87	7.02	0	187	0	61	110	0
Lamb, Australian, imported, fresh, tenderloin, boneless, separable lean and fat, trimmed to 1/8" fat, raw	23.23	5.52	0	143	0	73	76	0
Lamb, Australian, imported, fresh, rib chop, frenched, denuded, bone-in, separable lean only, trimmed to 0" fat, cooked, grilled	33.17	11.5	0	236	0	85	103	0
Lamb, Australian, imported, fresh, rack, roast, frenched, denuded, bone-in, separable lean and fat, trimmed to 0" fat, cooked, roasted	25.95	9.91	0	193	0	71	97	0

Food Name ---> per 100 g	Protein (g)	Fat (g)	Carb (g)	Calories	Fiber (g)	Sodium (mg)	Cholesterol (mg)	Net Carb (g)
Lamb, Australian, imported, fresh, rack, roast, frenched, bone-in, separable lean and fat, trimmed to 1/8" fat, cooked, roasted	25.96	20.77	0	291	0	65	97	0
Lamb, Australian, imported, fresh, rib chop, frenched, denuded, bone-in, separable lean and fat, trimmed to 0" fat, cooked, grilled	30.9	16.96	0	276	0	82	101	0

Legumes and Legume Products

Food Name ---> per 100 g	Protein (g)	Fat (g)	Carb (g)	Calories	Fiber (g)	Sodium (mg)	Cholesterol (mg)	Net Carb (g)
Beans, adzuki, mature seeds, raw	19.87	0.53	62.9	329	12.7	5	0	50.2
Beans, adzuki, mature seeds, cooked, boiled, without salt	7.52	0.1	24.77	128	7.3	8	0	17.47
Beans, adzuki, mature seeds, canned, sweetened	3.8	0.03	55.01	237	-	218	0	55.01
Yokan, prepared from adzuki beans and sugar	3.29	0.12	60.72	260	-	83	0	60.72
Beans, baked, home prepared	5.54	5.15	21.63	155	5.5	422	5	16.13
Beans, baked, canned, plain or vegetarian	4.75	0.37	21.14	94	4.1	343	0	17.04
Beans, baked, canned, with beef	6.38	3.45	16.91	121	-	475	22	16.91
Beans, baked, canned, with franks	6.75	6.57	15.39	142	6.9	430	6	8.49
Beans, baked, canned, with pork	5.19	1.55	19.99	106	5.5	414	7	14.49
Beans, baked, canned, with pork and sweet sauce	4.52	0.89	21.57	105	4.4	391	7	17.17
Beans, baked, canned, with pork and tomato sauce	5.15	0.93	18.69	94	4	437	7	14.69
Beans, black, mature seeds, raw	21.6	1.42	62.36	341	15.5	5	0	46.86
Beans, black, mature seeds, cooked, boiled, without salt	8.86	0.54	23.71	132	8.7	1	0	15.01
Beans, black turtle, mature seeds, raw	21.25	0.9	63.25	339	15.5	9	0	47.75
Beans, black turtle, mature seeds, cooked, boiled, without salt	8.18	0.35	24.35	130	8.3	3	0	16.05
Beans, black turtle, mature seeds, canned	6.03	0.29	16.55	91	6.9	384	0	9.65
Beans, cranberry (roman), mature seeds, raw	23.03	1.23	60.05	335	24.7	6	0	35.35
Beans, cranberry (roman), mature seeds, cooked, boiled, without salt	9.34	0.46	24.46	136	8.6	1	0	15.86
Beans, cranberry (roman), mature seeds, canned	5.54	0.28	15.12	83	6.3	332	0	8.82
Beans, french, mature seeds, raw	18.81	2.02	64.11	343	25.2	18	0	38.91
Beans, french, mature seeds, cooked, boiled, without salt	7.05	0.76	24.02	129	9.4	6	0	14.62
Beans, great northern, mature seeds, raw	21.86	1.14	62.37	339	20.2	14	0	42.17
Beans, great northern, mature seeds, cooked, boiled, without salt	8.33	0.45	21.09	118	7	2	0	14.09
Beans, great northern, mature seeds, canned	7.37	0.39	21.02	114	4.9	370	0	16.12
Beans, kidney, all types, mature seeds, raw	23.58	0.83	60.01	333	24.9	24	0	35.11
Beans, kidney, all types, mature seeds, cooked, boiled, without salt	8.67	0.5	22.8	127	6.4	1	0	16.4
Beans, kidney, all types, mature seeds, canned	5.22	0.6	14.5	84	4.3	296	0	10.2
Beans, kidney, california red, mature seeds, raw	24.37	0.25	59.8	330	24.9	11	0	34.9
Beans, kidney, california red, mature seeds, cooked, boiled, without salt	9.13	0.09	22.41	124	9.3	4	0	13.11
Beans, kidney, red, mature seeds, raw	22.53	1.06	61.29	337	15.2	12	0	46.09
Beans, kidney, red, mature seeds, cooked, boiled, without salt	8.67	0.5	22.8	127	7.4	2	0	15.4
Beans, kidney, red, mature seeds, canned, solids and liquids	5.22	0.36	14.83	81	4.3	256	0	10.53
Beans, kidney, royal red, mature seeds, raw	25.33	0.45	58.33	329	24.9	13	0	33.43
Beans, kidney, royal red, mature seeds, cooked, boiled, without salt	9.49	0.17	21.85	123	9.3	5	0	12.55
Beans, navy, mature seeds, raw	22.33	1.5	60.75	337	15.3	5	-	45.45
Beans, navy, mature seeds, cooked, boiled, without salt	8.23	0.62	26.05	140	10.5	0	-	15.55

Food Name ---> per 100 g	Protein (g)	Fat (g)	Carb (g)	Calories	Fiber (g)	Sodium (mg)	Cholesterol (mg)	Net Carb (g)
Beans, navy, mature seeds, canned	7.53	0.43	20.45	113	5.1	336	0	15.35
Beans, pink, mature seeds, raw	20.96	1.13	64.19	343	12.7	8	0	51.49
Beans, pink, mature seeds, cooked, boiled, without salt	9.06	0.49	27.91	149	5.3	2	0	22.61
Beans, pinto, mature seeds, raw	21.42	1.23	62.55	347	15.5	12	0	47.05
Beans, pinto, mature seeds, cooked, boiled, without salt	9.01	0.65	26.22	143	9	1	0	17.22
Beans, pinto, mature seeds, canned, solids and liquids	4.6	0.56	15.18	82	4.6	268	0	10.58
Beans, small white, mature seeds, raw	21.11	1.18	62.25	336	24.9	12	0	37.35
Beans, small white, mature seeds, cooked, boiled, without salt	8.97	0.64	25.81	142	10.4	2	0	15.41
Beans, yellow, mature seeds, raw	22	2.6	60.7	345	25.1	12	0	35.6
Beans, yellow, mature seeds, cooked, boiled, without salt	9.16	1.08	25.28	144	10.4	5	0	14.88
Beans, white, mature seeds, raw	23.36	0.85	60.27	333	15.2	16	0	45.07
Beans, white, mature seeds, cooked, boiled, without salt	9.73	0.35	25.09	139	6.3	6	0	18.79
Beans, white, mature seeds, canned	7.26	0.29	21.2	114	4.8	340	0	16.4
Broadbeans (fava beans), mature seeds, raw	26.12	1.53	58.29	341	25	13	0	33.29
Broadbeans (fava beans), mature seeds, cooked, boiled, without salt	7.6	0.4	19.65	110	5.4	5	0	14.25
Broadbeans (fava beans), mature seeds, canned	5.47	0.22	12.41	71	3.7	453	0	8.71
Carob flour	4.62	0.65	88.88	222	39.8	35	0	49.08
Chickpeas (garbanzo beans, bengal gram), mature seeds, raw	20.47	6.04	62.95	378	12.2	24	0	50.75
Chickpeas (garbanzo beans, bengal gram), mature seeds, cooked, boiled, without salt	8.86	2.59	27.42	164	7.6	7	0	19.82
Chickpeas (garbanzo beans, bengal gram), mature seeds, canned, solids and liquids	4.92	1.95	13.49	88	4.4	278	0	9.09
Chili with beans, canned	6.12	3.76	13.24	103	3.3	423	17	9.94
Cowpeas, catjang, mature seeds, raw	23.85	2.07	59.64	343	10.7	58	0	48.94
Cowpeas, catjang, mature seeds, cooked, boiled, without salt	8.13	0.71	20.32	117	3.6	19	0	16.72
Cowpeas, common (blackeyes, crowder, southern), mature seeds, raw	23.52	1.26	60.03	336	10.6	16	0	49.43
Cowpeas, common (blackeyes, crowder, southern), mature seeds, cooked, boiled, without salt	7.73	0.53	20.76	116	6.5	4	0	14.26
Cowpeas, common (blackeyes, crowder, southern), mature seeds, canned, plain	4.74	0.55	13.63	77	3.3	293	0	10.33
Cowpeas, common (blackeyes, crowder, southern), mature seeds, canned with pork	2.74	1.6	16.53	83	3.3	350	7	13.23
Hyacinth beans, mature seeds, raw	23.9	1.69	60.74	344	25.6	21	0	35.14
Hyacinth beans, mature seeds, cooked, boiled, without salt	8.14	0.58	20.69	117	-	7	0	20.69
Lentils, raw	24.63	1.06	63.35	352	10.7	6	0	52.65
Lentils, mature seeds, cooked, boiled, without salt	9.02	0.38	20.13	116	7.9	2	0	12.23
Lima beans, large, mature seeds, raw	21.46	0.69	63.38	338	19	18	0	44.38
Lima beans, large, mature seeds, cooked, boiled, without salt	7.8	0.38	20.88	115	7	2	0	13.88
Lima beans, large, mature seeds, canned	4.93	0.17	14.91	79	4.8	336	0	10.11
Lima beans, thin seeded (baby), mature seeds, raw	20.62	0.93	62.83	335	20.6	13	0	42.23
Lima beans, thin seeded (baby), mature seeds,	8.04	0.38	23.31	126	7.7	3	0	15.61

Food Name ---> per 100 g	Protein (g)	Fat (g)	Carb (g)	Calories	Fiber (g)	Sodium (mg)	Cholesterol (mg)	Net Carb (g)
cooked, boiled, without salt								
Lupins, mature seeds, raw	36.17	9.74	40.37	371	18.9	15	0	21.47
Lupins, mature seeds, cooked, boiled, without salt	15.57	2.92	9.88	119	2.8	4	0	7.08
Mothbeans, mature seeds, raw	22.94	1.61	61.52	343	-	30	0	61.52
Mothbeans, mature seeds, cooked, boiled, without salt	7.81	0.55	20.96	117	-	10	0	20.96
Mung beans, mature seeds, raw	23.86	1.15	62.62	347	16.3	15	0	46.32
Mung beans, mature seeds, cooked, boiled, without salt	7.02	0.38	19.15	105	7.6	2	0	11.55
Noodles, chinese, cellophane or long rice (mung beans), dehydrated	0.16	0.06	86.09	351	0.5	10	0	85.59
Mungo beans, mature seeds, raw	25.21	1.64	58.99	341	18.3	38	0	40.69
Mungo beans, mature seeds, cooked, boiled, without salt	7.54	0.55	18.34	105	6.4	7	0	11.94
Peas, green, split, mature seeds, raw	23.82	1.16	63.74	352	25.5	15	0	38.24
Peas, split, mature seeds, cooked, boiled, without salt	8.34	0.39	21.1	118	8.3	2	0	12.8
Peanuts, all types, raw	25.8	49.24	16.13	567	8.5	18	0	7.63
Peanuts, all types, cooked, boiled, with salt	13.5	22.01	21.26	318	8.8	751	0	12.46
Peanuts, all types, oil-roasted, with salt	28.03	52.5	15.26	599	9.4	320	0	5.86
Peanuts, all types, dry-roasted, with salt	24.35	49.66	21.26	587	8.4	410	0	12.86
Peanuts, spanish, raw	26.15	49.6	15.83	570	9.5	22	0	6.33
Peanuts, spanish, oil-roasted, with salt	28.01	49.04	17.45	579	8.9	433	0	8.55
Peanuts, valencia, raw	25.09	47.58	20.91	570	8.7	1	0	12.21
Peanuts, valencia, oil-roasted, with salt	27.04	51.24	16.3	589	8.9	772	0	7.4
Peanuts, virginia, raw	25.19	48.75	16.54	563	8.5	10	0	8.04
Peanuts, virginia, oil-roasted, with salt	25.87	48.62	19.86	578	8.9	433	0	10.96
Peanut butter, chunk style, with salt	24.06	49.94	21.57	589	8	486	0	13.57
Peanut butter, smooth style, with salt	22.21	51.36	22.31	598	5	426	0	17.31
Peanut flour, defatted	52.2	0.55	34.7	327	15.8	180	0	18.9
Peanut flour, low fat	33.8	21.9	31.27	428	15.8	1	0	15.47
Pigeon peas (red gram), mature seeds, raw	21.7	1.49	62.78	343	15	17	0	47.78
Pigeon peas (red gram), mature seeds, cooked, boiled, without salt	6.76	0.38	23.25	121	6.7	5	0	16.55
Refried beans, canned, traditional style (includes USDA commodity)	4.98	2.01	13.55	90	3.7	370	0	9.85
Bacon, meatless	11.69	29.52	5.31	309	2.6	1465	0	2.71
Meat extender	41.71	2.97	34.71	311	17.5	10	0	17.21
Sausage, meatless	20.28	18.16	8.09	255	2.8	888	0	5.29
Soybeans, mature seeds, raw	36.49	19.94	30.16	446	9.3	2	0	20.86
Soybeans, mature cooked, boiled, without salt	18.21	8.97	8.36	172	6	1	0	2.36
Soybeans, mature seeds, roasted, salted	38.55	25.4	30.22	469	17.7	163	0	12.52
Soybeans, mature seeds, dry roasted	43.32	21.62	28.98	449	8.1	2	0	20.88
Miso	12.79	6.01	25.37	198	5.4	3728	0	19.97
Natto	19.4	11	12.68	211	5.4	7	0	7.28
Tempeh	20.29	10.8	7.64	192	-	9	0	7.64
Soy flour, full-fat, raw	37.81	20.65	31.92	434	9.6	13	0	22.32
Soy flour, full-fat, roasted	38.09	21.86	30.38	439	9.7	12	0	20.68
Soy flour, defatted	51.46	1.22	33.92	327	17.5	20	0	16.42
Soy flour, low-fat	49.81	8.9	30.63	372	16	9	0	14.63
Soy meal, defatted, raw	49.2	2.39	35.89	337	-	3	0	35.89
Soymilk, original and vanilla, unfortified	3.27	1.75	6.28	54	0.6	51	0	5.68
Soy protein concentrate, produced by alcohol	63.63	0.46	25.41	328	5.5	3	0	19.91

Food Name ---> per 100 g	Protein (g)	Fat (g)	Carb (g)	Calories	Fiber (g)	Sodium (mg)	Cholesterol (mg)	Net Carb (g)
extraction								
Soy protein isolate	88.32	3.39	0	335	0	1005	0	0
Soy sauce made from soy and wheat (shoyu)	8.14	0.57	4.93	53	0.8	5493	0	4.13
Soy sauce made from soy (tamari)	10.51	0.1	5.57	60	0.8	5586	0	4.77
Soy sauce made from hydrolyzed vegetable protein	7	0.51	7.84	60	0.5	6820	0	7.34
Tofu, firm, prepared with calcium sulfate and magnesium chloride (nigari)	9.04	4.17	2.85	78	0.9	12	0	1.95
Tofu, soft, prepared with calcium sulfate and magnesium chloride (nigari)	7.17	3.69	1.18	61	0.2	8	0	0.98
Tofu, dried-frozen (koyadofu)	52.47	30.34	10.03	477	7.2	6	0	2.83
Tofu, fried	18.82	20.18	8.86	270	3.9	16	0	4.96
Okara	3.52	1.73	12.23	76	-	9	0	12.23
Tofu, salted and fermented (fuyu)	8.92	8	4.38	116	-	2873	0	4.38
Yardlong beans, mature seeds, raw	24.33	1.31	61.91	347	11	17	0	50.91
Yardlong beans, mature seeds, cooked, boiled, without salt	8.29	0.45	21.09	118	3.8	5	0	17.29
Winged beans, mature seeds, raw	29.65	16.32	41.71	409	25.9	38	0	15.81
Winged beans, mature seeds, cooked, boiled, without salt	10.62	5.84	14.94	147	-	13	0	14.94
Hummus, home prepared	4.86	8.59	20.12	177	4	242	0	16.12
Falafel, home-prepared	13.31	17.8	31.84	333	-	294	0	31.84
Soymilk, original and vanilla, with added calcium, vitamins A and D	2.6	1.47	4.92	43	0.2	47	0	4.72
Lentils, pink or red, raw	23.91	2.17	63.1	358	10.8	7	0	52.3
Beans, kidney, red, mature seeds, canned, drained solids	7.98	1.05	21.49	124	5.5	231	0	15.99
Beans, pinto, canned, drained solids	6.99	0.9	20.22	114	5.5	239	0	14.72
Veggie burgers or soyburgers, unprepared	15.7	6.3	14.27	177	4.9	569	5	9.37
Peanut spread, reduced sugar	24.8	54.89	14.23	650	7.8	292	0	6.43
Peanut butter, smooth, reduced fat	25.9	34	35.65	520	5.2	540	0	30.45
Peanut butter, smooth, vitamin and mineral fortified	25.72	50.81	18.75	591	5.6	420	0	13.15
Peanut butter, chunky, vitamin and mineral fortified	26.06	51.47	17.69	593	5.7	366	0	11.99
Chickpea flour (besan)	22.39	6.69	57.82	387	10.8	64	0	47.02
Hummus, commercial	7.9	9.6	14.29	166	6	379	0	8.29
Tofu, extra firm, prepared with nigari	9.98	5.26	1.18	83	1	4	0	0.18
Tofu, hard, prepared with nigari	12.68	9.99	4.39	145	0.6	2	0	3.79
MORI-NU, Tofu, silken, soft	4.8	2.7	2.9	55	0.1	5	0	2.8
MORI-NU, Tofu, silken, firm	6.9	2.7	2.4	62	0.1	36	0	2.3
MORI-NU, Tofu, silken, extra firm	7.4	1.9	2	55	0.1	63	0	1.9
MORI-NU, Tofu, silken, lite firm	6.3	0.8	1.1	37	0	85	0	1.1
MORI-NU, Tofu, silken, lite extra firm	7	0.7	1	38	0	98	0	1
Soymilk, chocolate, unfortified	2.26	1.53	9.95	63	0.4	53	0	9.55
USDA Commodity, Peanut Butter, smooth	21.93	49.54	23.98	588	5.7	476	0	18.28
Soymilk, chocolate, with added calcium, vitamins A and D	2.26	1.53	9.95	63	0.4	53	0	9.55
Refried beans, canned, vegetarian	5.28	0.87	13.5	83	4.7	430	-	8.8
Refried beans, canned, fat-free	5.34	0.45	13.5	79	4.7	438	0	8.8
Frijoles rojos volteados (Refried beans, red, canned)	5	6.93	15.47	144	4.7	375	-	10.77
Tempeh, cooked	19.91	11.38	7.62	195	-	14	-	7.62

Food Name ---> per 100 g	Protein (g)	Fat (g)	Carb (g)	Calories	Fiber (g)	Sodium (mg)	Cholesterol (mg)	Net Carb (g)
Campbell's Brown Sugar And Bacon Flavored Baked Beans	3.85	1.92	23.08	123	6.2	362	4	16.88
Campbell's Pork and Beans	4.62	1.15	19.23	108	5.4	338	4	13.83
PACE, Traditional Refried Beans	4.17	0	10.83	67	4.2	575	0	6.63
PACE, Salsa Refried Beans	3.33	0	11.67	60	3.3	492	0	8.37
PACE, Spicy Jalapeno Refried Beans	4.17	0	11.67	63	4.2	492	0	7.47
Vitasoy USA, Nasoya Lite Firm Tofu	8.3	1.7	1.3	54	0.6	34	0	0.7
Vitasoy USA, Organic Nasoya Super Firm Cubed Tofu	12.4	6.3	2.8	118	2	6	0	0.8
Vitasoy USA, Organic Nasoya Extra Firm Tofu	10.1	5.2	2.6	98	1.3	4	0	1.3
Vitasoy USA, Organic Nasoya Firm Tofu	8.9	4.4	2.3	84	0.8	4	0	1.5
Vitasoy USA, Organic Nasoya Silken Tofu	4.8	2.5	1.4	47	0.3	2	0	1.1
Vitasoy USA, Vitasoy Organic Creamy Original Soymilk	2.9	1.6	4.5	44	0.4	66	0	4.1
Vitasoy USA, Vitasoy Organic Classic Original Soymilk	3.2	1.8	4.5	47	0.4	66	0	4.1
Vitasoy USA, Vitasoy Light Vanilla Soymilk	1.6	0.82	4.1	30	0.1	49	0	4
Soymilk (all flavors), unsweetened, with added calcium, vitamins A and D	2.86	1.61	1.74	33	0.5	37	0	1.24
Soymilk (All flavors), enhanced	2.94	1.99	3.45	45	0.4	50	0	3.05
Soymilk, original and vanilla, light, with added calcium, vitamins A and D	2.38	0.77	3.51	30	0.3	48	0	3.21
Soymilk, chocolate and other flavors, light, with added calcium, vitamins A and D	2.1	0.64	8.24	47	0.7	46	0	7.54
Soymilk, original and vanilla, light, unsweetened, with added calcium, vitamins A and D	2.62	0.85	3.85	34	0.6	63	0	3.25
Soymilk (All flavors), lowfat, with added calcium, vitamins A and D	1.65	0.62	7.2	43	0.8	37	0	6.4
Soymilk (all flavors), nonfat, with added calcium, vitamins A and D	2.47	0.04	4.14	28	0.2	57	0	3.94
Soymilk, chocolate, nonfat, with added calcium, vitamins A and D	2.47	0.04	8.51	44	0.2	57	0	8.31
SILK Plain, soymilk	2.88	1.65	3.29	41	0.4	49	0	2.89
SILK Vanilla, soymilk	2.47	1.44	4.12	41	0.4	39	0	3.72
SILK Chocolate, soymilk	2.06	1.44	9.47	58	0.8	41	0	8.67
SILK Light Plain, soymilk	2.47	0.82	3.29	29	0.4	49	0	2.89
SILK Light Vanilla, soymilk	2.47	0.82	4.12	33	0.4	39	0	3.72
SILK Light Chocolate, soymilk	2.06	0.62	9.05	49	0.8	41	0	8.25
SILK Plus Omega-3 DHA, soymilk	2.88	2.06	3.29	45	0.4	49	0	2.89
SILK Plus for Bone Health, soymilk	2.47	1.44	4.53	41	0.8	39	0	3.73
SILK Plus Fiber, soymilk	2.47	1.44	5.76	41	2.1	39	0	3.66
SILK Unsweetened, soymilk	2.88	1.65	1.65	33	0.4	35	0	1.25
SILK Very Vanilla, soymilk	2.47	1.65	7.82	53	0.4	58	0	7.42
SILK Nog, soymilk	2.46	1.64	12.3	74	0	61	0	12.3
SILK Chai, soymilk	2.47	1.44	7.82	53	0	41	0	7.82
SILK Mocha, soymilk	2.06	1.44	9.05	58	0	41	0	9.05
SILK Coffee, soymilk	2.06	1.44	10.29	62	0	41	0	10.29
SILK Vanilla soy yogurt (family size)	2.64	1.76	13.66	79	0.4	13	0	13.26
SILK Vanilla soy yogurt (single serving size)	2.94	1.76	14.71	88	0.6	12	0	14.11
SILK Plain soy yogurt	2.64	1.76	9.69	66	0.4	13	0	9.29
SILK Strawberry soy yogurt	2.35	1.18	18.24	94	0.6	15	0	17.64
SILK Raspberry soy yogurt	2.35	1.18	17.65	88	0.6	15	0	17.05
SILK Peach soy yogurt	2.35	1.18	18.82	94	0.6	15	0	18.22

Food Name ---> per 100 g	Protein (g)	Fat (g)	Carb (g)	Calories	Fiber (g)	Sodium (mg)	Cholesterol (mg)	Net Carb (g)
SILK Black Cherry soy yogurt	2.35	1.18	17.06	88	0.6	12	0	16.46
SILK Blueberry soy yogurt	2.35	1.18	17.06	88	0.6	15	0	16.46
SILK Key Lime soy yogurt	2.35	1.18	17.65	88	0.6	15	0	17.05
SILK Banana-Strawberry soy yogurt	2.35	1.18	17.06	88	0.6	15	0	16.46
SILK Original Creamer	0	6.67	6.67	100	0	67	0	6.67
SILK French Vanilla Creamer	0	6.67	20	133	0	67	0	20
SILK Hazelnut Creamer	0	6.67	20	133	0	67	0	20
Vitasoy USA Organic Nasoya, Soft Tofu	8.76	3.5	0.74	70	0.6	4	0	0.14
Vitasoy USA Nasoya, Lite Silken Tofu	8.21	1.1	0	43	-	79	0	0
Vitasoy USA Organic Nasoya, Tofu Plus Extra Firm	10.18	4.9	1.82	92	1	7	0	0.82
Vitasoy USA Organic Nasoya, Tofu Plus Firm	9.19	3.4	1.71	74	0.8	4	0	0.91
Vitasoy USA Organic Nasoya Sprouted, Tofu Plus Super Firm	13.24	5.9	2.16	115	1.2	28	0	0.96
Vitasoy USA Azumaya, Extra Firm Tofu	10.07	4.6	1.53	88	0.9	26	0	0.63
Vitasoy USA Azumaya, Firm Tofu	9.08	4.2	1.52	80	0.6	23	0	0.92
Vitasoy USA Azumaya, Silken Tofu	4.82	2.4	0.58	43	0.2	2	0	0.38
HOUSE FOODS Premium Soft Tofu	6.38	2.71	2.19	59	0.8	34	0	1.39
HOUSE FOODS Premium Firm Tofu	10.92	4.19	0.97	85	0.9	33	0	0.07
Beans, adzuki, mature seed, cooked, boiled, with salt	7.52	0.1	24.77	128	7.3	244	0	17.47
Beans, black, mature seeds, cooked, boiled, with salt	8.86	0.54	23.71	132	8.7	237	0	15.01
Beans, black, mature seeds, canned, low sodium	6.03	0.29	16.55	91	6.9	138	0	9.65
Beans, black turtle, mature seeds, cooked, boiled, with salt	8.18	0.35	24.35	130	8.3	239	0	16.05
Beans, cranberry (roman), mature seeds, cooked, boiled, with salt	9.34	0.46	24.46	136	8.6	237	0	15.86
Beans, french, mature seeds, cooked, boiled, with salt	7.05	0.76	24.02	129	9.4	242	0	14.62
Beans, great northern, mature seeds, cooked, boiled, with salt	8.33	0.45	21.09	118	7	238	0	14.09
Beans, great northern, mature seeds, canned, low sodium	7.37	0.39	21.02	114	4.9	177	0	16.12
Beans, kidney, all types, mature seeds, cooked, boiled, with salt	8.67	0.5	22.8	127	6.4	238	0	16.4
Beans, kidney, california red, mature seeds, cooked, boiled, with salt	9.13	0.09	22.41	124	9.3	240	0	13.11
Beans, kidney, red, mature seeds, cooked, boiled, with salt	8.67	0.5	22.8	127	7.4	238	0	15.4
Beans, kidney, red, mature seeds, canned, drained solids, rinsed in tap water	8.12	0.93	20.8	121	6	208	0	14.8
Beans, kidney, royal red, mature seeds, cooked, boiled with salt	9.49	0.17	21.85	123	9.3	241	0	12.55
Beans, kidney, red, mature seeds, canned, solids and liquid, low sodium	5.22	0.36	14.83	81	5.3	117	0	9.53
Beans, navy, mature seeds, cooked, boiled, with salt	8.23	0.62	26.05	140	10.5	237	0	15.55
Beans, pink, mature seeds, cooked, boiled, with salt	9.06	0.49	27.91	149	5.3	238	0	22.61
Beans, pinto, mature seeds, cooked, boiled, with salt	9.01	0.65	26.22	143	9	238	0	17.22
Beans, pinto, mature seeds, canned, drained solids, rinsed in tap water	7.04	0.97	20.77	117	-	212	0	20.77
Beans, small white, mature seeds, cooked, boiled,	8.97	0.64	25.81	142	10.4	238	0	15.41

Food Name ---> per 100 g	Protein (g)	Fat (g)	Carb (g)	Calories	Fiber (g)	Sodium (mg)	Cholesterol (mg)	Net Carb (g)
with salt								
Beans, pinto, mature seeds, canned, solids and liquids, low sodium	4.6	0.56	15.18	82	4.6	146	0	10.58
Beans, yellow, mature seeds, cooked, boiled, with salt	9.16	1.08	25.28	144	10.4	241	0	14.88
Beans, white, mature seeds, cooked, boiled, with salt	9.73	0.35	25.09	139	6.3	242	0	18.79
Broadbeans (fava beans), mature seeds, cooked, boiled, with salt	7.6	0.4	19.65	110	5.4	241	0	14.25
Chickpeas (garbanzo beans, bengal gram), mature seeds, cooked, boiled, with salt	8.86	2.59	27.42	164	7.6	243	0	19.82
Chickpeas (garbanzo beans, bengal gram), mature seeds, canned, drained solids	7.05	2.77	22.53	139	6.4	246	0	16.13
Chickpeas (garbanzo beans, bengal gram), mature seeds, canned, drained, rinsed in tap water	7.04	2.47	22.87	138	6.3	212	0	16.57
Chickpeas (garbanzo beans, bengal gram), mature seeds, canned, solids and liquids, low sodium	4.92	1.95	13.49	88	4.4	132	0	9.09
Cowpeas, catjang, mature seeds, cooked, boiled, with salt	8.13	0.71	20.32	117	3.6	255	0	16.72
Cowpeas, common (blackeyes, crowder, southern), mature seeds, cooked, boiled, with salt	7.73	0.53	20.76	116	6.5	240	0	14.26
Hyacinth beans, mature seeds, cooked, boiled, with salt	8.14	0.58	20.7	117	-	243	0	20.7
Lentils, mature seeds, cooked, boiled, with salt	9.02	0.38	19.54	114	7.9	238	0	11.64
Lima beans, large, mature seeds, cooked, boiled, with salt	7.8	0.38	20.88	115	7	238	0	13.88
Lima beans, thin seeded (baby), mature seeds, cooked, boiled, with salt	8.04	0.38	23.31	126	7.7	239	0	15.61
Lupins, mature seeds, cooked, boiled, with salt	15.57	2.92	9.29	116	2.8	240	0	6.49
Mothbeans, mature seeds, cooked, boiled, with salt	7.81	0.55	20.96	117	-	246	0	20.96
Mung beans, mature seeds, cooked, boiled, with salt	7.02	0.38	19.15	105	7.6	238	0	11.55
Mungo beans, mature seeds, cooked, boiled, with salt	7.54	0.55	18.34	105	6.4	243	0	11.94
Peas, split, mature seeds, cooked, boiled, with salt	8.34	0.39	20.51	116	8.3	238	0	12.21
Peanuts, all types, oil-roasted, without salt	28.03	52.5	15.26	599	9.4	6	0	5.86
Peanuts, all types, dry-roasted, without salt	24.35	49.66	21.26	587	8.4	6	0	12.86
Peanuts, spanish, oil-roasted, without salt	28.01	49.04	17.45	579	8.9	6	0	8.55
Peanuts, valencia, oil-roasted, without salt	27.04	51.24	16.3	589	8.9	6	0	7.4
Peanuts, virginia, oil-roasted, without salt	25.87	48.62	19.86	578	8.9	6	0	10.96
Peanut butter, chunk style, without salt	24.06	49.94	21.57	589	8	17	0	13.57
Peanut butter, smooth style, without salt	22.21	51.36	22.31	598	5	17	0	17.31
Peanut butter with omega-3, creamy	24.47	54.17	17	608	6.1	356	-	10.9
Pigeon peas (red gram), mature seeds, cooked, boiled, with salt	6.76	0.38	23.25	121	6.7	241	0	16.55
Refried beans, canned, traditional, reduced sodium	4.98	2.01	13.55	89	3.7	138	0	9.85
Soybeans, mature seeds, cooked, boiled, with salt	18.21	8.97	8.36	172	6	237	0	2.36
Soybeans, mature seeds, roasted, no salt added	38.55	25.4	30.22	469	17.7	4	0	12.52
Soy protein concentrate, produced by acid wash	63.63	0.46	25.41	328	5.5	900	0	19.91
Soy protein isolate, potassium type	88.32	0.53	2.59	321	0	50	0	2.59
Soy sauce made from soy and wheat (shoyu), low sodium	9.05	0.3	5.59	57	0.7	3598	0	4.89
Soy sauce, reduced sodium, made from	8.19	0.31	14.44	90	0.3	2890	0	14.14

hydrolyzed vegetable protein

Food Name ---> per 100 g	Protein (g)	Fat (g)	Carb (g)	Calories	Fiber (g)	Sodium (mg)	Cholesterol (mg)	Net Carb (g)
Tofu, raw, firm, prepared with calcium sulfate	17.27	8.72	2.78	144	2.3	14	0	0.48
Tofu, raw, regular, prepared with calcium sulfate	8.08	4.78	1.87	76	0.3	7	0	1.57
Tofu, dried-frozen (koyadofu), prepared with calcium sulfate	52.43	30.34	8.3	470	1.2	6	0	7.1
Tofu, fried, prepared with calcium sulfate	18.82	20.18	8.86	270	3.9	16	0	4.96
Tofu, salted and fermented (fuyu), prepared with calcium sulfate	8.15	8	5.15	116	-	2873	0	5.15
Yardlong beans, mature seeds, cooked, boiled, with salt	8.29	0.45	21.09	118	3.8	241	0	17.29
Winged beans, mature seeds, cooked, boiled, with salt	10.62	5.84	14.94	147	-	249	0	14.94
LOMA LINDA Little Links, canned, unprepared	19.4	13.5	5.5	221	4.2	472	0	1.3
LOMA LINDA Low Fat Big Franks, canned, unprepared	23.1	4.7	4.9	154	4.1	481	0	0.8
LOMA LINDA Tender Rounds with Gravy, canned, unprepared	16.3	5.6	7.4	145	3.5	443	1	3.9
LOMA LINDA Swiss Stake with Gravy, canned, unprepared	10.2	6.2	10.4	138	3.2	471	1	7.2
LOMA LINDA Vege-Burger, canned, unprepared	22.2	1.2	3.7	114	2.6	222	0	1.1
LOMA LINDA Redi-Burger, canned, unprepared	21.9	2.8	8.2	146	4.3	508	0	3.9
LOMA LINDA Tender Bits, canned, unprepared	15.1	4.6	8.3	135	4.3	613	0	4
LOMA LINDA Linketts, canned, unprepared	21.3	11.8	4.4	209	3	401	0	1.4
WORTHINGTON Chili, canned, unprepared	10.4	4.5	10.9	126	3.4	453	0	7.5
WORTHINGTON Choplets, canned, unprepared	19.4	1	4.1	103	2.8	456	0	1.3
WORTHINGTON Diced Chik, canned, unprepared	14.7	0.7	3.7	80	1.4	344	1	2.3
WORTHINGTON FriChik Original, canned, unprepared	13.4	10.3	3.4	160	1.5	401	1	1.9
WORTHINGTON Low Fat Fri Chik, canned, unprepared	14.3	2.7	4.9	102	1	416	1	3.9
WORTHINGTON Low Fat Veja-Links, canned, unprepared	15.8	4.8	4.3	123	1.2	612	2	3.1
WORTHINGTON Multigrain Cutlets, canned, unprepared	23.29	1.5	7.3	117	4.5	371	0	2.8
WORTHINGTON Prime Stakes, canned, unprepared	10.2	7.2	7.5	135	1.4	480	1	6.1
WORTHINGTON Saucettes, canned, unprepared	15	15.2	5.6	219	2.8	532	2	2.8
WORTHINGTON Super Links, canned, unprepared	14.5	15.5	5.5	219	1.8	708	1	3.7
WORTHINGTON Vegetable Skallops, canned, unprepared	19.9	1.2	4.6	109	3.4	460	0	1.2
WORTHINGTON Vegetable Steaks, canned, unprepared	20.7	1.2	5.1	113	2.2	417	0	2.9
WORTHINGTON Vegetarian Burger, canned, unprepared	18.6	2.9	6.2	124	2.7	451	0	3.5
WORTHINGTON Veja-Links, canned, unprepared	14.6	8.9	4.1	155	3.3	530	3	0.8
WORTHINGTON Chic-Ketts, frozen, unprepared	23.6	9.7	5.1	200	1.2	642	0	3.9
WORTHINGTON Meatless Chicken Roll, frozen, unprepared	16.1	8	4.3	154	2.4	452	1	1.9
WORTHINGTON Meatless Corned Beef Roll, frozen, unprepared	18.6	14.5	9.9	245	0	758	1	9.9
WORTHINGTON Dinner Roast, frozen, unprepared	16	13.5	6.9	213	3.1	671	1	3.8

Food Name ---> per 100 g	Protein (g)	Fat (g)	Carb (g)	Calories	Fiber (g)	Sodium (mg)	Cholesterol (mg)	Net Carb (g)
WORTHINGTON FriPats, frozen, unprepared	23.7	9.1	8	209	2.8	517	2	5.2
WORTHINGTON Prosage Links, frozen, unprepared	20.2	4.7	5	143	2.8	819	2	2.2
WORTHINGTON Prosage Roll, frozen, unprepared	19.6	17.6	6	261	3.5	667	2	2.5
WORTHINGTON Smoked Turkey Roll, frozen, unprepared	18.5	16.1	7.9	251	1.1	859	0	6.8
WORTHINGTON Stakelets, frozen, unprepared	19.7	10.4	9.6	211	2.8	651	1	6.8
WORTHINGTON Stripples, frozen, unprepared	12.4	26.6	14.3	346	5.1	1463	2	9.2
WORTHINGTON Wham (roll), frozen, unprepared	17.8	11.3	5.7	196	0	717	0	5.7
MORNINGSTAR FARMS Breakfast Pattie with Organic Soy, frozen, unprepared	23.7	8.3	12.6	220	7.6	690	0	5
MORNINGSTAR FARMS Breakfast Bacon Strips, frozen, unprepared	12.4	26.6	14.3	346	5.1	1463	2	9.2
MORNINGSTAR FARMS Breakfast Sausage Links, frozen, unprepared	19.2	6.1	6.8	159	4	670	2	2.8
MORNINGSTAR FARMS Grillers Original, frozen, unprepared	23.9	9.3	8.5	213	4.4	422	3	4.1
MORNINGSTAR FARMS Grillers Prime, frozen, unprepared	24	13.2	5.9	238	2.6	501	1	3.3
MORNINGSTAR FARMS Asian Veggie Patties, frozen, unprepared	11.4	6.2	18.2	158	5.1	741	0	13.1
MORNINGSTAR FARMS Mushroom Lover's Burger, frozen, unprepared	14.3	8.2	9.2	168	5.1	445	0	4.1
MORNINGSTAR FARMS Tomato & Basil Pizza Burger, frozen, unprepared	15.5	8.6	14	161	9.1	414	10	4.9
MORNINGSTAR FARMS Buffalo Wings, frozen, unprepared	14.1	11	22.6	232	4.8	642	0	17.8
MORNINGSTAR FARMS Chik'n Nuggets, frozen, unprepared	14.4	10	21.8	221	4.9	702	0	16.9
MORNINGSTAR FARMS Chik Patties, frozen, unprepared	11.8	7	22.9	197	3	835	0	19.9
MORNINGSTAR FARMS Italian Herb Chik'n Pattie, frozen, unprepared	13.6	7	31.1	236	3.4	682	0	27.7
MORNINGSTAR FARMS Corn Dog, frozen, unprepared	11.2	3.5	36	208	3.8	666	0	32.2
MORNINGSTAR FARMS Corn Dog Mini, frozen, unprepared	13.2	4.7	32.6	219	2.6	678	0	30
MORNINGSTAR FARMS Sausage Style Recipe Crumbles, frozen, unprepared	20.2	4.6	9.9	159	4.6	758	0	5.3
GARDENBURGER Black Bean Chipotle Burger, frozen, unprepared	6.5	3.9	22	133	6.1	545	0	15.9
GARDENBURGER Original, frozen, unprepared	7.2	4.6	22.1	155	5	684	9	17.1
GARDENBURGER Flame Grilled Burger, frozen, unprepared	15.2	4.4	6.8	122	3.7	445	0	3.1
GARDENBURGER Savory Portabella Veggie Burger, frozen, unprepared	5.9	3.3	22.1	138	7.1	633	4	15
GARDENBURGER Sun-Dried Tomato Basil Burger, frozen, unprepared	5.5	3.6	23.7	137	5.2	387	4	18.5
GARDENBURGER Veggie Medley Burger, frozen, unprepared	4.1	3.6	24	121	7.1	559	0	16.9
MORNINGSTAR FARMS Breakfast Sausage Patties Maple Flavored, frozen, unprepared	26.3	7.2	13.6	222	2	656	1	11.6
MORNINGSTAR FARMS Chik'n Grill Veggie Patties, frozen, unprepared	12.8	4.8	10.2	118	5.7	519	0	4.5

Food Name ---> per 100 g	Protein (g)	Fat (g)	Carb (g)	Calories	Fiber (g)	Sodium (mg)	Cholesterol (mg)	Net Carb (g)
MORNINGSTAR FARMS BBQ Riblets, frozen, unprepared	11.4	2.3	24.6	150	4.7	438	0	19.9
WORTHINGTON Leanies, frozen, unprepared	19.5	16.5	6.1	251	3.8	1078	3	2.3
MORNINGSTAR FARMS California Turk'y Burger, frozen, unprepared	14.9	7.7	12.6	155	7.6	690	1	5
MORNINGSTAR FARMS Hot and Spicy Veggie Sausage Patties, frozen, unprepared	21.8	7.4	8.5	185	2.3	551	1	6.2
MORNINGSTAR FARMS Lasagna with Veggie Sausage, frozen, unprepared	7.1	2.3	14.4	96	2.3	208	4	12.1
MORNINGSTAR FARMS Grillers Quarter Pound Veggie Burger, frozen, unprepared	22.8	10.5	8.9	219	2.5	429	1	6.4
MORNINGSTAR FARMS Sesame Chik'n Entree, frozen, unprepared	5.3	3.5	17.3	116	1.3	196	0	16
MORNINGSTAR FARMS Grillers Chik'n Veggie Patties, frozen, unprepared	12.8	4.8	10.2	118	5.7	519	0	4.5
MORNINGSTAR FARMS Meal Starters Veggie Meatballs, frozen, unprepared	17.7	5.8	9.9	158	3.6	487	0	6.3
MORNINGSTAR FARMS Breakfast Biscuit Sausage, Egg & Cheese, frozen, unprepared	9.3	8.1	37.5	257	1.5	568	22	36
MORNINGSTAR FARMS Mediterranean Chickpea, frozen, unprepared	15.5	6.5	19.8	200	10.1	357	1	9.7
MORNINGSTAR FARMS Buffalo Chik Patties, frozen, unprepared	12.1	12.8	25.2	255	5.1	757	1	20.1
MORNINGSTAR FARMS Chik Patties Original, frozen, unprepared	11.2	9.1	20.5	197	3.7	676	0	16.8
MORNINGSTAR FARMS Breakfast Pattie, frozen, unprepared	23.7	8.3	12.6	195	7.6	690	0	5
MORNINGSTAR FARMS Roasted Garlic & Quinoa Burger, frozen, unprepared	10.7	12.1	17.8	192	10.1	522	1	7.7
MORNINGSTAR FARMS Parmesan Garlic Wings, frozen, unprepared	14.2	8.6	24.1	227	3.1	616	1	21
MORNINGSTAR FARMS Breakfast Sandwich Veggie Sausage Egg & Cheese English Muffin, frozen, unprepared	14.3	9.4	18.7	205	3.8	639	67	14.9
MORNINGSTAR FARMS Breakfast Sandwich Veggie Scramble & Cheese English Muffin, frozen, unprepared	10.4	4.8	18.9	149	2.9	562	10	16
MORNINGSTAR FARMS Chipotle Black Bean Crumbles, frozen, unprepared	14.4	4.1	10.2	122	4.3	491	0	5.9
MORNINGSTAR FARMS Garden Veggie Nuggets, frozen, unprepared	9.6	12.2	16.9	197	6.9	420	1	10
MORNINGSTAR FARMS Spicy Black Bean Enchilada Entree, frozen, unprepared	5.8	5.2	15.9	123	2.6	277	7	13.3
MORNINGSTAR FARMS Spicy Indian Veggie Burger, frozen, unprepared	9.2	11.6	17	189	7.8	555	0	9.2
MORNINGSTAR FARMS Tuscan Greens & Beans, frozen, unprepared	5.9	6.3	11.7	112	3.8	161	12	7.9
Papad	25.56	3.25	59.87	371	18.6	1745	4	41.27
Peanut butter, reduced sodium	24	49.9	21.83	590	6.6	203	0	15.23
Beans, chili, barbecue, ranch style, cooked	5	1	16.9	97	4.2	725	0	12.7
Vermicelli, made from soy	0.1	0.1	82.32	331	3.9	4	0	78.42
Beans, liquid from stewed kidney beans	1.8	3.2	2.8	47	0.1	2	4	2.7
Chicken, meatless	23.64	12.73	3.64	224	3.6	709	0	0.04
Frankfurter, meatless	19.61	13.73	7.7	233	3.9	471	0	3.8
Luncheon slices, meatless	17.78	11.11	4.44	189	1.1	711	0	3.34
Meatballs, meatless	21	9	8	197	4.6	550	0	3.4

Food Name ---> per 100 g	Protein (g)	Fat (g)	Carb (g)	Calories	Fiber (g)	Sodium (mg)	Cholesterol (mg)	Net Carb (g)
Vegetarian fillets	23	18	9	290	6.1	490	0	2.9
Sandwich spread, meatless	8	9	9	149	3.3	630	0	5.7
Vegetarian meatloaf or patties	21	9	8	197	4.6	550	0	3.4
Bacon bits, meatless	32	25.9	28.6	476	10.2	1770	0	18.4
Soybean, curd cheese	12.5	8.1	6.9	151	0	20	0	6.9
Chicken, meatless, breaded, fried	21.28	12.77	8.51	234	4.3	400	0	4.21
Beans, baked, canned, no salt added	4.8	0.4	20.49	105	5.5	1	0	14.99
Tofu yogurt	3.5	1.8	15.96	94	0.2	35	0	15.76

Nut and Seed Products

Food Name ---> per 100 g	Protein (g)	Fat (g)	Carb (g)	Calories	Fiber (g)	Sodium (mg)	Cholesterol (mg)	Net Carb (g)
Seeds, breadfruit seeds, raw	7.4	5.59	29.24	191	5.2	25	0	24.04
Seeds, breadfruit seeds, boiled	5.3	2.3	32	168	4.8	23	0	27.2
Seeds, breadnut tree seeds, raw	5.97	0.99	46.28	217	-	31	0	46.28
Seeds, breadnut tree seeds, dried	8.62	1.68	79.39	367	14.9	53	0	64.49
Seeds, chia seeds, dried	16.54	30.74	42.12	486	34.4	16	0	7.72
Seeds, cottonseed flour, partially defatted (glandless)	40.96	6.2	40.54	359	3	35	0	37.54
Seeds, cottonseed flour, low fat (glandless)	49.83	1.41	36.1	332	-	35	0	36.1
Seeds, cottonseed meal, partially defatted (glandless)	49.1	4.77	38.43	367	-	37	0	38.43
Seeds, hemp seed, hulled	31.56	48.75	8.67	553	4	5	0	4.67
Seeds, lotus seeds, dried	15.41	1.97	64.47	332	-	5	0	64.47
Seeds, pumpkin and squash seed kernels, dried	30.23	49.05	10.71	559	6	7	0	4.71
Seeds, pumpkin and squash seed kernels, roasted, without salt	29.84	49.05	14.71	574	6.5	18	0	8.21
Seeds, safflower seed kernels, dried	16.18	38.45	34.29	517	-	3	0	34.29
Seeds, safflower seed meal, partially defatted	35.62	2.39	48.73	342	-	3	0	48.73
Seeds, sesame seeds, whole, dried	17.73	49.67	23.45	573	11.8	11	0	11.65
Seeds, sesame seeds, whole, roasted and toasted	16.96	48	25.74	565	14	11	0	11.74
Seeds, sesame seed kernels, toasted, without salt added (decorticated)	16.96	48	26.04	567	16.9	39	0	9.14
Seeds, sesame flour, partially defatted	40.32	11.89	35.14	382	-	41	0	35.14
Seeds, sesame flour, low-fat	50.14	1.75	35.51	333	-	39	0	35.51
Seeds, sesame meal, partially defatted	16.96	48	26.04	567	-	39	0	26.04
Seeds, sunflower seed kernels, dried	20.78	51.46	20	584	8.6	9	0	11.4
Seeds, sunflower seed kernels, dry roasted, without salt	19.33	49.8	24.07	582	11.1	3	0	12.97
Seeds, sunflower seed kernels, oil roasted, without salt	20.06	51.3	22.89	592	10.6	3	0	12.29
Seeds, sunflower seed kernels, toasted, without salt	17.21	56.8	20.59	619	11.5	3	0	9.09
Seeds, sunflower seed butter, without salt	17.28	55.2	23.32	617	5.7	3	0	17.62
Seeds, sunflower seed flour, partially defatted	48.06	1.61	35.83	326	5.2	3	0	30.63
Nuts, acorns, raw	6.15	23.86	40.75	387	-	0	0	40.75
Nuts, acorns, dried	8.1	31.41	53.66	509	-	0	0	53.66
Nuts, acorn flour, full fat	7.49	30.17	54.65	501	-	0	0	54.65
Nuts, almonds	21.15	49.93	21.55	579	12.5	1	0	9.05
Nuts, almonds, blanched	21.4	52.52	18.67	590	9.9	19	0	8.77
Nuts, almonds, dry roasted, without salt added	20.96	52.54	21.01	598	10.9	3	0	10.11
Nuts, almonds, oil roasted, without salt added	21.23	55.17	17.68	607	10.5	1	0	7.18
Nuts, almond paste	9	27.74	47.81	458	4.8	9	0	43.01
Nuts, beechnuts, dried	6.2	50	33.5	576	-	38	0	33.5
Nuts, brazilnuts, dried, unblanched	14.32	67.1	11.74	659	7.5	3	0	4.24
Nuts, butternuts, dried	24.9	56.98	12.05	612	4.7	1	0	7.35
Nuts, cashew nuts, dry roasted, without salt added	15.31	46.35	32.69	574	3	16	0	29.69
Nuts, cashew nuts, oil roasted, without salt added	16.84	47.77	29.87	580	3.3	13	0	26.57
Nuts, cashew nuts, raw	18.22	43.85	30.19	553	3.3	12	0	26.89
Nuts, cashew butter, plain, without salt added	17.56	49.41	27.57	587	2	15	0	25.57
Nuts, chestnuts, chinese, raw	4.2	1.11	49.07	224	-	3	0	49.07

Food Name ---> per 100 g	Protein (g)	Fat (g)	Carb (g)	Calories	Fiber (g)	Sodium (mg)	Cholesterol (mg)	Net Carb (g)
Nuts, chestnuts, chinese, dried	6.82	1.81	79.76	363	-	5	0	79.76
Nuts, chestnuts, chinese, boiled and steamed	2.88	0.76	33.64	153	-	2	0	33.64
Nuts, chestnuts, chinese, roasted	4.48	1.19	52.36	239	-	4	0	52.36
Nuts, chestnuts, european, raw, unpeeled	2.42	2.26	45.54	213	8.1	3	0	37.44
Nuts, chestnuts, european, raw, peeled	1.63	1.25	44.17	196	-	2	0	44.17
Nuts, chestnuts, european, dried, unpeeled	6.39	4.45	77.31	374	11.7	37	0	65.61
Nuts, chestnuts, european, dried, peeled	5.01	3.91	78.43	369	-	37	0	78.43
Nuts, chestnuts, european, boiled and steamed	2	1.38	27.76	131	-	27	0	27.76
Nuts, coconut meat, raw	3.33	33.49	15.23	354	9	20	0	6.23
Nuts, coconut meat, dried (desiccated), not sweetened	6.88	64.53	23.65	660	16.3	37	0	7.35
Nuts, coconut meat, dried (desiccated), sweetened, flaked, packaged	3.13	27.99	51.85	456	9.9	285	0	41.95
Nuts, coconut meat, dried (desiccated), sweetened, flaked, canned	3.35	31.69	40.91	443	4.5	20	0	36.41
Nuts, coconut meat, dried (desiccated), toasted	5.3	47	44.4	592	-	37	0	44.4
Nuts, coconut cream, raw (liquid expressed from grated meat)	3.63	34.68	6.65	330	2.2	4	0	4.45
Nuts, coconut cream, canned, sweetened	1.17	16.31	53.21	357	0.2	36	0	53.01
Nuts, coconut milk, raw (liquid expressed from grated meat and water)	2.29	23.84	5.54	230	2.2	15	0	3.34
Nuts, coconut milk, canned (liquid expressed from grated meat and water)	2.02	21.33	2.81	197	-	13	0	2.81
Nuts, coconut water (liquid from coconuts)	0.72	0.2	3.71	19	1.1	105	0	2.61
Nuts, hazelnuts or filberts	14.95	60.75	16.7	628	9.7	0	0	7
Nuts, hazelnuts or filberts, blanched	13.7	61.15	17	629	11	0	0	6
Nuts, hazelnuts or filberts, dry roasted, without salt added	15.03	62.4	17.6	646	9.4	0	0	8.2
Nuts, ginkgo nuts, raw	4.32	1.68	37.6	182	-	7	0	37.6
Nuts, ginkgo nuts, dried	10.35	2	72.45	348	-	13	0	72.45
Nuts, ginkgo nuts, canned	2.29	1.62	22.1	111	9.3	307	0	12.8
Nuts, hickorynuts, dried	12.72	64.37	18.25	657	6.4	1	0	11.85
Nuts, macadamia nuts, raw	7.91	75.77	13.82	718	8.6	5	0	5.22
Nuts, macadamia nuts, dry roasted, without salt added	7.79	76.08	13.38	718	8	4	0	5.38
Nuts, mixed nuts, dry roasted, with peanuts, without salt added	19.5	53.5	22.42	607	6.4	4	0	16.02
Nuts, mixed nuts, dry roasted, with peanuts, salt added, PLANTERS pistachio blend	21.95	49.3	22.51	580	8.1	232	-	14.41
Nuts, mixed nuts, oil roasted, with peanuts, without salt added	20.04	53.95	21.05	607	7	5	0	14.05
Nuts, mixed nuts, oil roasted, without peanuts, without salt added	15.52	56.17	22.27	615	5.5	11	0	16.77
Nuts, formulated, wheat-based, unflavored, with salt added	13.82	57.7	23.68	622	5.2	505	0	18.48
Nuts, mixed nuts, dry roasted, with peanuts, salt added, CHOSEN ROASTER	18	58.8	19.02	632	7.1	113	-	11.92
Nuts, pecans	9.17	71.97	13.86	691	9.6	0	0	4.26
Nuts, pecans, dry roasted, without salt added	9.5	74.27	13.55	710	9.4	1	0	4.15
Nuts, pecans, oil roasted, without salt added	9.2	75.23	13.01	715	9.5	1	0	3.51
Nuts, pilinuts, dried	10.8	79.55	3.98	719	-	3	0	3.98
Nuts, pine nuts, dried	13.69	68.37	13.08	673	3.7	2	0	9.38
Nuts, pine nuts, pinyon, dried	11.57	60.98	19.3	629	10.7	72	0	8.6
Nuts, pistachio nuts, raw	20.16	45.32	27.17	560	10.6	1	0	16.57

Food Name ---> per 100 g	Protein (g)	Fat (g)	Carb (g)	Calories	Fiber (g)	Sodium (mg)	Cholesterol (mg)	Net Carb (g)
Nuts, pistachio nuts, dry roasted, without salt added	21.05	45.82	28.28	572	10.3	6	0	17.98
Nuts, walnuts, black, dried	24.06	59.33	9.58	619	6.8	2	0	2.78
Nuts, walnuts, english	15.23	65.21	13.71	654	6.7	2	0	7.01
Nuts, walnuts, glazed	8.28	35.71	47.59	500	3.6	446	0	43.99
Nuts, walnuts, dry roasted, with salt added	14.29	60.71	17.86	643	7.1	643	0	10.76
Seeds, breadfruit seeds, roasted	6.2	2.7	40.1	207	6	28	0	34.1
Seeds, cottonseed kernels, roasted (glandless)	32.59	36.29	21.9	506	5.5	25	0	16.4
Seeds, pumpkin and squash seeds, whole, roasted, without salt	18.55	19.4	53.75	446	18.4	18	0	35.35
Seeds, sesame butter, tahini, from roasted and toasted kernels (most common type)	17	53.76	21.19	595	9.3	115	0	11.89
Nuts, chestnuts, european, roasted	3.17	2.2	52.96	245	5.1	2	0	47.86
Seeds, sesame butter, paste	18.08	50.87	24.05	586	5.5	12	0	18.55
Seeds, sesame flour, high-fat	30.78	37.1	26.62	526	-	41	0	26.62
Seeds, sesame butter, tahini, from unroasted kernels (non-chemically removed seed coat)	17.95	56.44	17.89	607	9.3	1	0	8.59
Seeds, watermelon seed kernels, dried	28.33	47.37	15.31	557	-	99	0	15.31
Nuts, chestnuts, japanese, dried	5.25	1.24	81.43	360	-	34	0	81.43
Nuts, coconut milk, frozen (liquid expressed from grated meat and water)	1.61	20.8	5.58	202	-	12	0	5.58
Nuts, coconut meat, dried (desiccated), creamed	5.3	69.08	21.52	684	-	37	0	21.52
Nuts, coconut meat, dried (desiccated), sweetened, shredded	2.88	35.49	47.67	501	4.5	262	0	43.17
Seeds, sisymbrium sp. seeds, whole, dried	12.14	4.6	58.26	318	-	92	0	58.26
Nuts, almond butter, plain, without salt added	20.96	55.5	18.82	614	10.3	7	0	8.52
Seeds, sesame butter, tahini, from raw and stone ground kernels	17.81	48	26.19	570	9.3	74	0	16.89
Nuts, formulated, wheat-based, all flavors except macadamia, without salt	13.11	62.3	20.79	647	5.2	91	0	15.59
Seeds, sesame seed kernels, dried (decorticated)	20.45	61.21	11.73	631	11.6	47	0	0.13
Nuts, chestnuts, japanese, raw	2.25	0.53	34.91	154	-	14	0	34.91
Nuts, chestnuts, japanese, boiled and steamed	0.82	0.19	12.64	56	-	5	0	12.64
Nuts, chestnuts, japanese, roasted	2.97	0.8	45.13	201	-	19	0	45.13
Seeds, lotus seeds, raw	4.13	0.53	17.28	89	-	1	0	17.28
Nuts, almonds, honey roasted, unblanched	18.17	49.9	27.9	594	13.7	130	0	14.2
Seeds, flaxseed	18.29	42.16	28.88	534	27.3	30	0	1.58
Seeds, pumpkin and squash seed kernels, roasted, with salt added	29.84	49.05	14.71	574	6.5	256	0	8.21
Seeds, sesame seed kernels, toasted, with salt added (decorticated)	16.96	48	26.04	567	16.9	588	0	9.14
Seeds, sunflower seed kernels from shell, dry roasted, with salt added	19.33	49.8	15.31	546	9	6008	0	6.31
Seeds, sunflower seed kernels, dry roasted, with salt added	19.33	49.8	24.07	582	9	655	0	15.07
Seeds, sunflower seed kernels, oil roasted, with salt added	20.06	51.3	22.89	592	10.6	733	0	12.29
Seeds, sunflower seed kernels, toasted, with salt added	17.21	56.8	20.59	619	11.5	613	0	9.09
Seeds, sunflower seed butter, with salt added	17.28	55.2	23.32	617	5.7	331	0	17.62
Nuts, almonds, dry roasted, with salt added	20.96	52.54	21.01	598	10.9	498	0	10.11
Nuts, almonds, oil roasted, with salt added	21.23	55.17	17.68	607	10.5	339	0	7.18
Nuts, almonds, oil roasted, with salt added, smoke flavor	21.43	55.89	17.86	607	10.7	548	0	7.16

Food Name ---> per 100 g	Protein (g)	Fat (g)	Carb (g)	Calories	Fiber (g)	Sodium (mg)	Cholesterol (mg)	Net Carb (g)
Nuts, cashew nuts, dry roasted, with salt added	15.31	46.35	32.69	574	3	640	0	29.69
Nuts, cashew nuts, oil roasted, with salt added	16.84	47.77	30.16	581	3.3	308	0	26.86
Nuts, cashew butter, plain, with salt added	12.12	53.03	30.3	609	3	295	0	27.3
Nuts, macadamia nuts, dry roasted, with salt added	7.79	76.08	12.83	716	8	353	0	4.83
Nuts, mixed nuts, dry roasted, with peanuts, with salt added	17.3	51.45	25.35	594	9	345	0	16.35
Nuts, mixed nuts, oil roasted, with peanuts, with salt added	20.04	53.95	21.05	607	7	273	0	14.05
Nuts, mixed nuts, oil roasted, without peanuts, with salt added	15.52	56.17	22.27	615	5.5	306	0	16.77
Nuts, pecans, dry roasted, with salt added	9.5	74.27	13.55	710	9.4	383	0	4.15
Nuts, pecans, oil roasted, with salt added	9.2	75.23	13.01	715	9.5	393	0	3.51
Nuts, pistachio nuts, dry roasted, with salt added	21.05	45.82	27.55	569	10.3	428	0	17.25
Seeds, pumpkin and squash seeds, whole, roasted, with salt added	18.55	19.4	53.75	446	18.4	2541	0	35.35
Nuts, almonds, oil roasted, lightly salted	21.23	55.17	17.68	607	10.5	143	0	7.18
Nuts, almond butter, plain, with salt added	20.96	55.5	18.82	614	10.3	227	0	8.52
Seeds, sesame butter, tahini, type of kernels unspecified	17.4	53.01	21.5	592	4.7	35	0	16.8
Nuts, mixed nuts, oil roasted, with peanuts, lightly salted	20.04	53.95	21.05	607	7	161	0	14.05
Nuts, mixed nuts, oil roasted, without peanuts, lightly salted	17.86	50	25	607	7.1	143	0	17.9

Pork Products

Food Name ---> per 100 g	Protein (g)	Fat (g)	Carb (g)	Calories	Fiber (g)	Sodium (mg)	Cholesterol (mg)	Net Carb (g)
Pork, fresh, composite of separable fat, with added solution, cooked	10.06	60.42	0.32	585	0	125	81	0.32
Pork, fresh, carcass, separable lean and fat, raw	13.91	35.07	0	376	0	42	74	0
Pork, fresh, composite of trimmed retail cuts (leg, loin, shoulder), separable lean only, raw	21.2	4.86	0	134	0	59	64	0
Pork, fresh, composite of trimmed leg, loin, shoulder, and spareribs, (includes cuts to be cured), separable lean and fat, raw	18.22	14.79	0	211	0	57	69	0
Pork, fresh, backfat, raw	2.92	88.69	0	812	0	11	57	0
Pork, fresh, belly, raw	9.34	53.01	0	518	0	32	72	0
Pork, fresh, separable fat, raw	9.25	65.7	0	632	0	47	72	0
Pork, fresh, separable fat, cooked	7.06	66.1	0	626	0	56	79	0
Pork, fresh, leg (ham), whole, separable lean and fat, raw	17.43	18.87	0	245	0	47	73	0
Pork, fresh, leg (ham), whole, separable lean and fat, cooked, roasted	26.83	17.61	0	273	0	60	94	0
Pork, fresh, leg (ham), whole, separable lean only, raw	20.48	5.41	0	136	0	55	68	0
Pork, fresh, leg (ham), whole, separable lean only, cooked, roasted	29.41	9.44	0	211	0	64	94	0
Pork, fresh, leg (ham), rump half, separable lean and fat, raw	20.27	10.63	0	182	0	73	63	0
Pork, fresh, leg (ham), rump half, separable lean and fat, cooked, roasted	27.03	10.32	0	209	0	77	85	0
Pork, fresh, leg (ham), rump half, separable lean only, raw	21.81	2.93	0	120	0	76	62	0
Pork, fresh, leg (ham), rump half, separable lean only, cooked, roasted	28.86	4.62	0	165	0	80	86	0
Pork, fresh, leg (ham), shank half, separable lean and fat, raw	19.87	11.96	0	193	0	84	67	0
Pork, fresh, leg (ham), shank half, separable lean and fat, cooked, roasted	25.96	13.42	0	232	0	81	91	0
Pork, fresh, leg (ham), shank half, separable lean only, raw	21.66	2.95	0	119	0	90	66	0
Pork, fresh, leg (ham), shank half, separable lean only, cooked, roasted	28.69	5.83	0	175	0	84	93	0
Pork, fresh, loin, whole, separable lean and fat, raw	19.74	12.58	0	198	0	50	63	0
Pork, fresh, loin, whole, separable lean and fat, cooked, braised	27.23	13.62	0	239	0	48	80	0
Pork, fresh, loin, whole, separable lean and fat, cooked, broiled	27.32	13.92	0	242	0	62	80	0
Pork, fresh, loin, whole, separable lean and fat, cooked, roasted	27.09	14.65	0	248	0	59	82	0
Pork, fresh, loin, whole, separable lean only, raw	21.43	5.66	0	143	0	52	59	0
Pork, fresh, loin, whole, separable lean only, cooked, braised	28.57	9.12	0	204	0	50	79	0
Pork, fresh, loin, whole, separable lean only, cooked, broiled	28.57	9.8	0	210	0	64	79	0
Pork, fresh, loin, whole, separable lean only, cooked, roasted	28.62	9.63	0	209	0	58	81	0

Food Name ---> per 100 g	Protein (g)	Fat (g)	Carb (g)	Calories	Fiber (g)	Sodium (mg)	Cholesterol (mg)	Net Carb (g)
Pork, fresh, loin, blade (chops or roasts), bone-in and fat, raw	19.56	12.27	0	194	0	69	63	0
Pork, fresh, loin, blade (chops), bone-in, separable lean and fat, cooked, braised	26.54	15.71	0	255	0	69	86	0
Pork, fresh, loin, blade (chops), bone-in, separable lean and fat, cooked, broiled	23.72	14.35	0	231	0	74	78	0
Pork, fresh, loin, blade (roasts), bone-in, separable lean and fat, cooked, roasted	24.29	16.71	0	254	0	76	83	0
Pork, fresh, loin, blade (chops or roasts), bone-in, separable lean only, raw	21.22	5.84	0	143	0	73	59	0
Pork, fresh, loin, blade (chops), bone-in, separable lean only, cooked, braised	28.02	11.29	0	222	0	70	87	0
Pork, fresh, loin, blade (chops), bone-in, separable lean only, cooked, broiled	24.99	9.56	0	193	0	76	78	0
Pork, fresh, loin, blade (roasts), bone-in, separable lean only, cooked, roasted	25.7	11.89	0	217	0	78	83	0
Pork, fresh, loin, center loin (chops), bone-in, separable lean and fat, raw	20.71	9.03	0	170	0	55	69	0
Pork, fresh, loin, center loin (chops), bone-in, separable lean and fat, cooked, braised	28.21	13.51	0	242	0	73	81	0
Pork, fresh, loin, center loin (chops), bone-in, separable lean and fat, cooked, broiled	25.61	11.06	0	209	0	55	84	0
Pork, fresh, loin, center loin (roasts), bone-in, separable lean and fat, cooked, roasted	27.01	12.8	0	231	0	83	76	0
Pork, fresh, loin, center loin (chops), bone-in, separable lean only, raw	21.99	3.71	0	127	0	58	69	0
Pork, fresh, loin, center loin (chops), bone-in, separable lean only, cooked, braised	30.2	7.86	0	200	0	75	81	0
Pork, fresh, loin, center loin (chops), bone-in, separable lean only, cooked, broiled	26.76	7.29	0	180	0	56	84	0
Pork, fresh, loin, center loin (roasts), bone-in, separable lean only, cooked, roasted	28.58	7.95	0	194	0	86	75	0
Pork, fresh, loin, center rib (chops or roasts), bone-in, separable lean and fat, raw	20.28	11.04	0	186	0	56	58	0
Pork, fresh, loin, center rib (chops), bone-in, separable lean and fat, cooked, braised	26.66	16.28	0	261	0	70	79	0
Pork, fresh, loin, center rib (chops), bone-in, separable lean and fat, cooked, broiled	24.42	13.04	0	222	0	55	67	0
Pork, fresh, loin, center rib (roasts), bone-in, separable lean and fat, cooked, roasted	26.99	14.68	0	248	0	91	78	0
Pork, fresh, loin, center rib (chops or roasts), bone-in, separable lean only, raw	21.79	4.8	0	136	0	60	56	0
Pork, fresh, loin, center rib (chops), bone-in, separable lean only, cooked, braised	29.03	9.32	0	208	0	72	79	0
Pork, fresh, loin, center rib (chops), bone-in, separable lean only, cooked, broiled	25.79	8.36	0	186	0	57	66	0
Pork, fresh, loin, center rib (roasts), bone-in, separable lean only, cooked, roasted	28.82	9.21	0	206	0	95	78	0
Pork, fresh, loin, sirloin (chops or roasts), bone-in, separable lean and fat, raw	20.48	8.96	0	168	0	57	70	0
Pork, fresh, loin, sirloin (chops), bone-in, separable lean and fat, cooked, braised	28.81	12.31	0	234	0	58	87	0
Pork, fresh, loin, sirloin (chops), bone-in, separable lean and fat, cooked, broiled	26.96	11.82	0	222	0	86	87	0
Pork, fresh, loin, sirloin (roasts), bone-in, separable lean and fat, cooked, roasted	26.64	12.87	0	230	0	57	89	0

Food Name ---> per 100 g	Protein (g)	Fat (g)	Carb (g)	Calories	Fiber (g)	Sodium (mg)	Cholesterol (mg)	Net Carb (g)
Pork, fresh, loin, sirloin (chops or roasts), bone-in, separable lean only, raw	21.65	4.02	0	129	0	59	69	0
Pork, fresh, loin, sirloin (chops), bone-in, separable lean only, cooked, braised	31	6.9	0	195	0	58	88	0
Pork, fresh, loin, sirloin (chops), bone-in, separable lean only, cooked, broiled	29.29	5.45	0	174	0	89	88	0
Pork, fresh, loin, sirloin (roasts), bone-in, separable lean only, cooked, roasted	27.78	9.44	0	204	0	59	89	0
Pork, fresh, loin, tenderloin, separable lean only, raw	20.95	2.17	0	109	0	53	65	0
Pork, fresh, loin, tenderloin, separable lean only, cooked, roasted	26.17	3.51	0	143	0	57	73	0
Pork, fresh, loin, top loin (chops), boneless, separable lean and fat, raw	21.55	6.94	0	155	0	48	67	0
Pork, fresh, loin, top loin (chops), boneless, separable lean and fat, cooked, braised	29.2	8.31	0	200	0	66	72	0
Pork, fresh, loin, top loin (chops), boneless, separable lean and fat, cooked, broiled	26.62	9.14	0	196	0	44	73	0
Pork, fresh, loin, top loin (roasts), boneless, separable lean and fat, cooked, roasted	26.45	8.82	0	192	0	46	80	0
Pork, fresh, loin, top loin (chops), boneless, separable lean only, raw	22.41	3.42	0	127	0	49	66	0
Pork, fresh, loin, top loin (chops), boneless, separable lean only, cooked, braised	30.54	4.34	0	170	0	67	71	0
Pork, fresh, loin, top loin (chops), boneless, separable lean only, cooked, broiled	27.58	6.08	0	173	0	45	72	0
Pork, fresh, loin, top loin (roasts), boneless, separable lean only, cooked, roasted	27.23	6.28	0	173	0	47	79	0
Pork, fresh, spareribs, separable lean and fat, raw	15.47	23.4	0	277	0	81	80	0
Pork, fresh, spareribs, separable lean and fat, cooked, braised	29.06	30.3	0	397	0	93	121	0
Pork, fresh, composite of trimmed retail cuts (leg, loin, and shoulder), separable lean only, cooked	27.51	9.21	0	201	0	55	84	0
Pork, fresh, loin, center loin (chops), boneless, separable lean only, raw	23.75	3.09	0	123	0	87	56	0
Pork, fresh, variety meats and by-products, brain, raw	10.28	9.21	0	127	0	120	2195	0
Pork, fresh, variety meats and by-products, brain, cooked, braised	12.14	9.51	0	138	0	91	2552	0
Pork, fresh, variety meats and by-products, chitterlings, raw	7.64	16.61	0	182	0	24	154	0
Pork, fresh, variety meats and by-products, chitterlings, cooked, simmered	12.49	20.32	0	233	0	18	277	0
Pork, fresh, variety meats and by-products, ears, frozen, raw	22.45	15.1	0.6	234	0	191	82	0.6
Pork, fresh, variety meats and by-products, ears, frozen, cooked, simmered	15.95	10.8	0.2	166	0	167	90	0.2
Pork, fresh, variety meats and by-products, feet, raw	23.16	12.59	0	212	0	132	88	0
Pork, fresh, variety meats and by-products, heart, raw	17.27	4.36	1.33	118	0	56	131	1.33
Pork, fresh, variety meats and by-products, heart, cooked, braised	23.6	5.05	0.4	148	0	35	221	0.4
Pork, fresh, variety meats and by-products, jowl, raw	6.38	69.61	0	655	0	25	90	0

Food Name ---> per 100 g	Protein (g)	Fat (g)	Carb (g)	Calories	Fiber (g)	Sodium (mg)	Cholesterol (mg)	Net Carb (g)
Pork, fresh, variety meats and by-products, kidneys, raw	16.46	3.25	0	100	0	121	319	0
Pork, fresh, variety meats and by-products, kidneys, cooked, braised	25.4	4.7	0	151	0	80	480	0
Pork, fresh, variety meats and by-products, leaf fat, raw	1.76	94.16	0	857	0	5	110	0
Pork, fresh, variety meats and by-products, liver, raw	21.39	3.65	2.47	134	0	87	301	2.47
Pork, fresh, variety meats and by-products, liver, cooked, braised	26.02	4.4	3.76	165	0	49	355	3.76
Pork, fresh, variety meats and by-products, lungs, raw	14.08	2.72	0	85	0	153	320	0
Pork, fresh, variety meats and by-products, lungs, cooked, braised	16.6	3.1	0	99	0	81	387	0
Pork, fresh, variety meats and by-products, mechanically separated, raw	15.03	26.54	0	304	0	50	77	0
Pork, fresh, variety meats and by-products, pancreas, raw	18.56	13.24	0	199	0	44	193	0
Pork, fresh, variety meats and by-products, pancreas, cooked, braised	28.5	10.8	0	219	0	42	315	0
Pork, fresh, variety meats and by-products, spleen, raw	17.86	2.59	0	100	0	98	363	0
Pork, fresh, variety meats and by-products, spleen, cooked, braised	28.2	3.2	0	149	0	107	504	0
Pork, fresh, variety meats and by-products, stomach, raw	16.85	10.14	0	159	0	75	223	0
Pork, fresh, loin, blade (chops), bone-in, separable lean only, cooked, pan-fried	26.38	12.14	0	222	0	88	82	0
Pork, fresh, variety meats and by-products, tongue, raw	16.3	17.2	0	225	0	110	101	0
Pork, fresh, variety meats and by-products, tongue, cooked, braised	24.1	18.6	0	271	0	109	146	0
Pork, cured, bacon, unprepared	12.62	39.69	1.28	417	0	662	66	1.28
Pork, cured, breakfast strips, raw or unheated	11.74	37.16	0.7	388	0	987	69	0.7
Canadian bacon, unprepared	20.31	2.62	1.34	110	0	751	48	1.34
Pork, cured, feet, pickled	11.63	10.02	0.01	140	0	946	83	0.01
Pork, cured, ham, boneless, extra lean (approximately 5% fat), roasted	20.93	5.53	1.5	145	0	1203	53	1.5
Pork, cured, ham, boneless, regular (approximately 11% fat), roasted	22.62	9.02	0	178	0	1500	59	0
Pork, cured, ham, extra lean (approximately 4% fat), canned, unheated	18.49	4.56	0	120	0	1255	38	0
Pork, cured, ham, extra lean (approximately 4% fat), canned, roasted	21.16	4.88	0.52	136	0	1135	30	0.52
Pork, cured, ham, regular (approximately 13% fat), canned, roasted	20.53	15.2	0.42	226	0	941	62	0.42
Pork, cured, ham, center slice, country-style, separable lean only, raw	27.8	8.32	0.3	195	0	2695	70	0.3
Pork, cured, ham, center slice, separable lean and fat, unheated	20.17	12.9	0.05	203	0	1386	54	0.05
Pork, cured, ham, patties, unheated	12.78	28.19	1.69	315	0	1088	70	1.69
Pork, cured, ham, steak, boneless, extra lean, unheated	19.56	4.25	0	122	0	1269	45	0
Pork, cured, ham, whole, separable lean and fat, unheated	18.49	18.52	0.06	246	0	1284	56	0.06
Pork, cured, ham, whole, separable lean only,	22.32	5.71	0.05	147	0	1516	52	0.05

unheated

Food Name ---> per 100 g	Protein (g)	Fat (g)	Carb (g)	Calories	Fiber (g)	Sodium (mg)	Cholesterol (mg)	Net Carb (g)
Pork, cured, ham, whole, separable lean only, roasted	25.05	5.5	0	157	0	1327	55	0
USDA Commodity, pork, canned	19.4	12.95	0.59	196	0	213	75	0.59
Pork, fresh, loin, center loin (chops), boneless, separable lean only, cooked, pan-broiled	30.02	4.65	0	162	0	91	74	0
Pork, fresh, loin, center loin (chops), boneless, separable lean and fat, raw	21.14	12.96	0	201	0	82	59	0
Pork, cured, salt pork, raw	5.05	80.5	0	748	0	2684	86	0
Pork, cured, separable fat (from ham and arm picnic), unheated	5.68	61.41	0.09	579	0	505	68	0.09
Pork, cured, separable fat (from ham and arm picnic), roasted	7.64	61.86	0	591	0	624	86	0
Pork, cured, shoulder, arm picnic, separable lean and fat, roasted	20.43	21.35	0	280	0	1072	58	0
Pork, cured, shoulder, arm picnic, separable lean only, roasted	24.94	7.04	0	170	0	1231	48	0
Pork, cured, shoulder, blade roll, separable lean and fat, unheated	16.47	21.98	0	269	0	1250	53	0
Pork, cured, shoulder, blade roll, separable lean and fat, roasted	17.28	23.48	0.37	287	0	973	67	0.37
Pork, fresh, variety meats and by-products, feet, cooked, simmered	21.94	16.05	0	238	0	73	107	0
Pork, fresh, variety meats and by-products, tail, raw	17.75	33.5	0	378	0	63	97	0
Pork, fresh, variety meats and by-products, tail, cooked, simmered	17	35.8	0	396	0	25	129	0
Pork, fresh, loin, center loin (chops), bone-in, separable lean only, cooked, pan-fried	29.56	7.66	0	195	0	99	78	0
Pork, fresh, loin, center rib (chops), bone-in, separable lean only, cooked, pan-fried	28.84	9.73	0	211	0	88	77	0
Pork, fresh, loin, blade (chops), bone-in, separable lean and fat, cooked, pan-fried	25.02	16.56	0	256	0	85	82	0
Pork, fresh, loin, center loin (chops), bone-in, separable lean and fat, cooked, pan-fried	27.63	13.32	0	238	0	94	79	0
Pork, fresh, loin, center rib (chops), bone-in, separable lean and fat, cooked, pan-fried	26.81	15.71	0	256	0	84	78	0
Pork, fresh, loin, top loin (chops), boneless, separable lean only, cooked, pan-fried	30.46	4.62	0	172	0	87	69	0
Pork, cured, ham, boneless, extra lean and regular, unheated	18.26	8.39	2.28	162	0	1278	53	2.28
Pork, cured, ham, boneless, extra lean and regular, roasted	21.97	7.66	0.5	165	0	1385	57	0.5
Pork, cured, ham, extra lean and regular, canned, unheated	17.97	7.46	0	144	0	1276	38	0
Pork, cured, ham, extra lean and regular, canned, roasted	20.94	8.43	0.49	167	0	1068	41	0.49
Pork, fresh, loin, top loin (chops), boneless, separable lean and fat, cooked, pan-fried	29.36	7.86	0	196	0	86	70	0
Pork, fresh, composite of trimmed retail cuts (leg, loin, shoulder, and spareribs), separable lean and fat, raw	18.95	14.95	0	216	0	55	67	0
Pork, fresh, composite of trimmed retail cuts (leg, loin, shoulder, and spareribs), separable lean and fat, cooked	26.36	13.89	0	238	0	57	88	0
Pork, fresh, loin, center loin (chops), boneless,	26.68	13.6	0	229	0	86	75	0

Food Name ---> per 100 g	Protein (g)	Fat (g)	Carb (g)	Calories	Fiber (g)	Sodium (mg)	Cholesterol (mg)	Net Carb (g)
separable lean and fat, cooked, pan-broiled								
Pork, fresh, backribs, separable lean and fat, raw	19.07	16.33	0	224	0	87	69	0
Pork, fresh, backribs, separable lean and fat, cooked, roasted	23.01	21.51	0	292	0	94	84	0
Pork, fresh, loin, center rib (chops or roasts), boneless, separable lean and fat, raw	19.9	14.01	0	211	0	42	60	0
Pork, fresh, loin, center rib (chops), boneless, separable lean and fat, cooked, braised	26.29	15.79	0	255	0	40	73	0
Pork, fresh, loin, center rib (chops), boneless, separable lean and fat, cooked, broiled	27.63	15.76	0	260	0	62	82	0
Pork, fresh, loin, center rib (chops), boneless, separable lean and fat, cooked, pan-fried	25.82	18.05	0	273	0	50	73	0
Pork, fresh, loin, center rib (roasts), boneless, separable lean and fat, cooked, roasted	26.99	15.15	0	252	0	48	81	0
Pork, fresh, loin, center rib (chops or roasts), boneless, separable lean only, raw	21.8	6.48	0	152	0	45	55	0
Pork, fresh, loin, center rib (chops), boneless, separable lean only, cooked, braised	27.95	10.14	0	211	0	41	71	0
Pork, fresh, loin, center rib (chops), boneless, separable lean only, cooked, broiled	29.46	10.05	0	216	0	65	81	0
Pork, fresh, loin, center rib (chops), boneless, separable lean only, cooked, pan-fried	27.68	11.8	0	224	0	52	70	0
Pork, fresh, loin, center rib (roasts), boneless, separable lean only, cooked, roasted	28.81	10.13	0	214	0	50	83	0
Pork, fresh, loin, country-style ribs, separable lean and fat, raw	19.34	11.82	0	189	0	63	74	0
Pork, fresh, loin, country-style ribs, separable lean and fat, cooked, braised	26.49	17.71	0	273	0	58	103	0
Pork, fresh, loin, country-style ribs, separable lean and fat, bone-in, cooked, roasted	21.75	29.46	0	359	0	52	91	0
Pork, fresh, loin, country-style ribs, separable lean only, raw	20.76	5.64	0	140	0	67	74	0
Pork, fresh, loin, country-style ribs, separable lean only, cooked, braised	27.74	14.26	0	247	0	60	105	0
Pork, fresh, loin, country-style ribs, separable lean only, bone-in, cooked, roasted	29.2	11.38	0	227	0	91	99	0
Pork, fresh, loin, sirloin (chops or roasts), boneless, separable lean and fat, raw	22.49	4.05	0	133	0	63	63	0
Pork, fresh, loin, sirloin (chops), boneless, separable lean and fat, cooked, braised	28.41	5.47	0	171	0	56	80	0
Pork, fresh, loin, sirloin (chops), boneless, separable lean and fat, cooked, broiled	28.19	5.53	0	170	0	65	76	0
Pork, fresh, loin, sirloin (roasts), boneless, separable lean and fat, cooked, roasted	29.62	7.32	0	192	0	66	84	0
Pork, fresh, loin, sirloin (chops or roasts), boneless, separable lean only, raw	22.81	2.59	0	121	0	63	63	0
Pork, fresh, loin, sirloin (chops), boneless, separable lean only, cooked, braised	28.75	4.5	0	163	0	56	80	0
Pork, fresh, loin, sirloin (chops), boneless, separable lean only, cooked, broiled	28.6	4.36	0	161	0	66	76	0
Pork, fresh, loin, sirloin (roasts), boneless, separable lean only, cooked, roasted	30.39	5.31	0	178	0	66	84	0
Pork, fresh, loin, tenderloin, separable lean and fat, raw	20.65	3.53	0	120	0	52	65	0
Pork, fresh, ground, raw	16.88	21.19	0	263	0	56	72	0
Pork, fresh, ground, cooked	25.69	20.77	0	297	0	73	94	0

Food Name ---> per 100 g	Protein (g)	Fat (g)	Carb (g)	Calories	Fiber (g)	Sodium (mg)	Cholesterol (mg)	Net Carb (g)
Pork, fresh, loin, tenderloin, separable lean and fat, cooked, broiled	29.86	8.11	0	201	0	64	94	0
Pork, fresh, loin, tenderloin, separable lean and fat, cooked, roasted	26.04	3.96	0	147	0	57	73	0
Pork, fresh, loin, tenderloin, separable lean only, cooked, broiled	30.42	6.33	0	187	0	65	94	0
Pork, fresh, loin, top loin (roasts), boneless, separable lean and fat, raw	21.34	8.33	0	166	0	47	64	0
Pork, fresh, loin, top loin (roasts), boneless, separable lean only, raw	22.39	4.06	0	132	0	49	63	0
Pork, fresh, composite of trimmed retail cuts (loin and shoulder blade), separable lean and fat, raw	20.08	10.14	0	177	0	54	65	0
Pork, fresh, composite of trimmed retail cuts (loin and shoulder blade), separable lean and fat, cooked	26.07	13.66	0	235	0	55	83	0
Pork, fresh, composite of trimmed retail cuts (loin and shoulder blade), separable lean only, raw	21.23	5.88	0	144	0	54	60	0
Pork, fresh, composite of trimmed retail cuts (loin and shoulder blade), separable lean only, cooked	29.47	9.44	0	211	0	57	85	0
USDA Commodity, pork, cured, ham, boneless, cooked, heated	18.84	7.62	0	149	0	1155	73	0
USDA Commodity, pork, ground, fine/coarse, frozen, cooked	23.55	18.19	0	265	0	76	105	0
USDA Commodity, pork, cured, ham, boneless, cooked, unheated	17.44	6.16	0.69	133	0	1210	71	0.69
USDA Commodity, pork, ground, fine/coarse, frozen, raw	15.41	17.18	0	221	0	58	58	0
HORMEL, Cure 81 Ham	18.43	3.59	0.21	106	-	1038	51	0.21
HORMEL ALWAYS TENDER, Pork Tenderloin, Teriyaki-Flavored	18.2	3.07	4.63	119	-	413	46	4.63
HORMEL ALWAYS TENDER, Pork Tenderloin, Peppercorn-Flavored	17.21	3.8	1.82	110	-	594	47	1.82
HORMEL ALWAYS TENDER, Pork Loin Filets, Lemon Garlic-Flavored	17.83	4.16	1.79	118	-	590	42	1.79
HORMEL ALWAYS TENDER, Center Cut Chops, Fresh Pork	18.74	9.62	0.84	167	-	378	52	0.84
HORMEL ALWAYS TENDER, Boneless Pork Loin, Fresh Pork	19.02	7.18	0.76	145	-	358	49	0.76
HORMEL Canadian Style Bacon	16.88	4.94	1.87	122	-	1016	49	1.87
Pork, fresh, loin, top loin (chops), boneless, separable lean only, with added solution, cooked, pan-broiled	28.95	5	0	169	0	209	75	0
Pork, fresh, loin, top loin (chops), boneless, separable lean and fat, with added solution, cooked, pan-broiled	28.35	7.66	0	190	0	205	75	0
Pork, cured, bacon, cooked, baked	35.73	43.27	1.35	548	0	2193	107	1.35
Pork, cured, bacon, cooked, microwaved	39.01	34.12	0.48	476	0	1783	111	0.48
Pork, cured, bacon, pre-sliced, cooked, pan-fried	33.92	35.09	1.7	468	0	1684	99	1.7
Pork, fresh, variety meats and by-products, stomach, cooked, simmered	21.4	7.26	0.09	157	0	40	316	0.09
Pork, bacon, rendered fat, cooked	0.07	99.5	0	898	0	27	97	0
Pork, cured, ham -- water added, rump, bone-in, separable lean only, heated, roasted	21.41	3.56	0.87	121	0	1150	62	0.87

Food Name ---> per 100 g	Protein (g)	Fat (g)	Carb (g)	Calories	Fiber (g)	Sodium (mg)	Cholesterol (mg)	Net Carb (g)
Pork, cured, ham -- water added, rump, bone-in, separable lean only, unheated	15.43	3.48	0.67	95	0	1170	53	0.67
Pork, cured, ham -- water added, shank, bone-in, separable lean only, heated, roasted	20.92	4.43	1.2	128	0	1060	65	1.2
Pork, cured, ham -- water added, slice, bone-in, separable lean only, heated, pan-broil	22.04	4.3	1.48	131	0	1374	65	1.48
Pork, cured, ham and water product, slice, bone-in, separable lean only, heated, pan-broil	20.9	3.63	1.35	122	0	1237	64	1.35
Pork, cured, ham and water product, slice, boneless, separable lean only, heated, pan-broil	15.09	5.06	4.69	123	0	1390	45	4.69
Pork, cured, ham and water product, whole, boneless, separable lean only, heated, roasted	13.88	5.46	4.61	123	0	1335	43	4.61
Pork, cured, ham and water product, whole, boneless, separable lean only, unheated	14.07	4.86	4.22	116	0	1310	43	4.22
Pork, cured, ham with natural juices, rump, bone-in, separable lean only, heated, roasted	24.14	4.25	0.48	137	0	861	72	0.48
Pork, cured, ham with natural juices, shank, bone-in, separable lean only, heated, roasted	24.95	4.97	0.34	145	0	820	74	0.34
Pork, cured, ham with natural juices, slice, bone-in, separable lean only, heated, pan-broil	27.75	4.38	0	150	0	835	80	0
Pork, cured, ham with natural juices, spiral slice, meat only, boneless, separable lean only, heated, roasted	22.56	3.78	1.08	126	0	986	63	1.08
Pork, cured, ham and water product, rump, bone-in, separable lean only, heated, roasted	21.28	4.7	1.15	131	0	1267	66	1.15
Pork, cured, ham -- water added, slice, boneless, separable lean only, heated, pan-broil	18.82	4.09	1.75	119	0	1223	54	1.75
Pork, cured, ham -- water added, whole, boneless, separable lean only, heated, roasted	17.99	4.39	1.57	117	0	1193	53	1.57
Pork, cured, ham -- water added, whole, boneless, separable lean only, unheated	17.34	3.97	1.45	110	0	1141	50	1.45
Pork, cured, ham and water product, shank, bone-in, separable lean only, heated, roasted	21.69	4.45	1.26	132	0	1045	72	1.26
Pork, cured, ham with natural juices, slice, boneless, separable lean only, heated, pan-broil	20.95	3.16	1.05	116	0	1163	57	1.05
Pork, cured, ham with natural juices, whole, boneless, separable lean only, heated, roasted	20.57	3.01	0.84	113	0	1180	56	0.84
Pork, cured, ham with natural juices, whole, boneless, separable lean only, unheated	19.44	3.21	1.03	111	0	1098	53	1.03
Pork, cured, ham -- water added, shank, bone-in, separable lean only, unheated	18.65	1.87	0.71	91	0	1040	50	0.71
Pork, cured, ham -- water added, slice, bone-in, separable lean only, unheated	17.38	2.29	1.23	95	0	1090	54	1.23
Pork, cured, ham and water product, rump, bone-in, separable lean only, unheated	17.93	3.38	1.24	107	0	1070	58	1.24
Pork, cured, ham and water product, slice, bone-in, separable lean only, unheated	14.47	3.78	2.82	103	0	1160	49	2.82
Pork, cured, ham and water product, shank, bone-in, unheated, separable lean only	17.53	4.18	1.2	113	0	1090	52	1.2
Pork, cured, ham with natural juices, rump, bone-in, separable lean only, unheated	22.71	3.47	0.43	122	0	893	68	0.43
Pork, cured, ham with natural juices, shank, bone-in, separable lean only, unheated	25.11	3.33	0.3	130	0	809	63	0.3
Pork, cured, ham with natural juices, slice, bone-in, separable lean only, unheated	24.34	2.87	0	123	0	861	63	0
Pork, cured, ham with natural juices, spiral slice,	19.25	3.26	1.22	109	0	895	57	1.22

Food Name ---> per 100 g	Protein (g)	Fat (g)	Carb (g)	Calories	Fiber (g)	Sodium (mg)	Cholesterol (mg)	Net Carb (g)
boneless, separable lean only, unheated								
Pork, cured, ham, separable fat, boneless, heated	8.77	51.57	2	507	0	677	72	2
Pork, cured, ham, separable fat, boneless, unheated	7.5	53	1.87	515	0	616	61	1.87
Pork, pickled pork hocks	19.11	10.54	0	171	0	1050	89	0
Pork, cured, ham, slice, bone-in, separable lean only, heated, pan-broil	27.18	4.09	0.74	148	0	870	73	0.74
Pork, cured, ham with natural juices, whole, boneless, separable lean and fat, unheated	19.38	3.43	1.02	112	0	1096	53	1.02
Pork, cured, ham with natural juices, spiral slice, boneless, separable lean and fat, unheated	18.66	5.75	1.18	129	0	881	57	1.18
Pork, cured, ham with natural juices, slice, bone-in, separable lean and fat, unheated	22.82	7.4	0.17	159	0	839	63	0.17
Pork, cured, ham with natural juices, shank, bone-in, separable lean and fat, unheated	22.35	11.11	0.32	191	0	779	62	0.32
Pork, cured, ham with natural juices, rump, bone-in, separable lean and fat, unheated	19.7	13.26	0.43	200	0	838	67	0.43
Pork, cured, ham and water product, whole, boneless, separable lean and fat, unheated	14.05	4.99	4.21	117	0	1308	43	4.21
Pork, cured, ham and water product, slice, bone-in, separable lean and fat, unheated	13.69	9.29	2.72	149	0	1099	50	2.72
Pork, cured, ham and water product, shank, bone-in, separable lean and fat, unheated	14.28	20	1.42	243	0	936	55	1.42
Pork, cured, ham and water product, rump, bone-in, separable lean and fat, unheated	16.09	12.13	1.35	179	0	990	58	1.35
Pork, cured, ham -- water added, whole, boneless, separable lean and fat, unheated	17.06	5.38	1.42	121	0	1126	50	1.42
Pork, cured, ham -- water added, slice, bone-in, separable lean and fat, unheated	15.73	10.77	1.1	164	0	1011	55	1.1
Pork, cured, ham -- water added, shank, bone-in, separable lean and fat, unheated	16.65	11.02	0.66	167	0	964	52	0.66
Pork, cured, ham -- water added, rump, bone-in, separable lean and fat, unheated	13.99	12.5	0.8	172	0	1069	54	0.8
Pork, cured, ham -- water added, rump, bone-in, separable lean and fat, heated, roasted	20.1	8.56	0.99	161	0	1101	63	0.99
Pork, cured, ham -- water added, shank, bone-in, separable lean and fat, heated, roasted	18.62	13.37	1.35	200	0	988	66	1.35
Pork, cured, ham -- water added, slice, bone-in, separable lean and fat, heated, pan-broil	20.8	8.73	1.54	166	0	1309	66	1.54
Pork, cured, ham -- water added, slice, boneless, separable lean and fat, heated, pan-broil	18.62	5.05	1.72	125	0	1212	54	1.72
Pork, cured, ham -- water added, whole, boneless, separable lean and fat, heated, roasted	17.77	5.48	1.54	126	0	1181	54	1.54
Pork, cured, ham and water product, rump, bone-in, separable lean and fat, heated, roasted	19.46	11.48	1.15	186	0	1181	67	1.15
Pork, cured, ham and water product, shank, bone-in, separable lean and fat, heated, roasted	18.17	17.29	1.42	234	0	945	72	1.42
Pork, cured, ham and water product, slice, bone-in, separable lean and fat, heated, pan-broil	19.85	7.78	1.41	155	0	1188	64	1.41
Pork, cured, ham and water product, slice, boneless, separable lean and fat, heated, pan-broil	15.08	5.13	4.69	124	0	1389	45	4.69
Pork, cured, ham and water product, whole, boneless, separable lean and fat, heated, roasted	13.88	5.46	4.61	123	0	1335	43	4.61
Pork, cured, ham with natural juices, rump, bone-in, separable lean and fat, heated, roasted	22.47	9.39	0.6	177	0	841	72	0.6

Food Name ---> per 100 g	Protein (g)	Fat (g)	Carb (g)	Calories	Fiber (g)	Sodium (mg)	Cholesterol (mg)	Net Carb (g)
Pork, cured, ham with natural juices, shank, bone-in, separable lean and fat, heated, roasted	22.88	10.93	0.33	191	0	801	74	0.33
Pork, cured, ham with natural juices, slice, bone-in, separable lean and fat, heated, pan-broil	26.18	8.28	0.17	180	0	821	80	0.17
Pork, cured, ham with natural juices, slice, boneless, separable lean and fat, heated, pan-broil	20.89	3.4	1.04	118	0	1160	58	1.04
Pork, cured, ham with natural juices, spiral slice, boneless, separable lean and fat, heated, roasted	22.18	5.1	1.06	139	0	977	64	1.06
Pork, cured, ham with natural juices, whole, boneless, separable lean and fat, heated, roasted	20.54	3.13	0.84	114	0	1179	56	0.84
Pork, cured, ham, rump, bone-in, separable lean and fat, heated, roasted	23.95	8.88	0.64	177	0	826	71	0.64
Pork, cured, ham, rump, bone-in, separable lean only, heated, roasted	26.02	3.07	0.68	132	0	846	71	0.68
Pork, cured, ham, rump, bone-in, separable lean only, unheated	24.46	2.92	0.32	125	0	737	63	0.32
Pork, cured, ham, shank, bone-in, separable lean only, heated, roasted	26.49	3.68	0.68	139	0	828	70	0.68
Pork, cured, ham, shank, bone-in, separable lean only, unheated	23.79	3.19	0.18	125	0	846	61	0.18
Pork, cured, ham, shank, bone-in, separable lean and fat, heated, roasted	24.39	9.35	0.64	191	0	810	70	0.64
Pork, cured, ham, shank, bone-in, separable lean and fat, unheated	21.61	9.85	0.41	177	0	816	61	0.41
Pork, cured, ham, slice, bone-in, separable lean and fat, heated, pan-broil	25.48	8.48	0.7	181	0	852	73	0.7
Pork, cured, ham, slice, bone-in, separable lean only, unheated	24.36	3.59	0	130	0	760	65	0
Pork, cured, ham, slice, bone-in, separable lean and fat, unheated	22.45	9.17	0.21	173	0	744	65	0.21
Pork, fresh, spareribs, separable lean and fat, cooked, roasted	20.89	30.86	0	361	0	91	105	0
Pork, fresh, composite of separable fat, with added solution, raw	9.27	52.33	0	508	0	81	83	0
Pork, fresh, loin, tenderloin, separable lean only, with added solution, cooked, roasted	21.61	3.15	0.31	116	0	231	57	0.31
Pork, fresh, enhanced, loin, tenderloin, separable lean only, raw	20.39	2.09	0	106	0	243	48	0
Pork, fresh, shoulder, (Boston butt), blade (steaks), separable lean only, with added solution cooked, braised	27.58	12.14	0	227	0	154	98	0
Pork, fresh, shoulder, (Boston butt), blade (steaks), separable lean only, with added solution, raw	18.29	5.36	0.18	122	0	165	59	0.18
Pork, fresh, loin, top loin (chops), boneless, separable lean only, with added solution, cooked, broiled	29.65	5.73	0	170	0	315	70	0
Pork, fresh, loin, top loin (chops), boneless, separable lean only, with added solution, raw	21.09	3.48	0.22	117	0	278	51	0.22
Pork, fresh, loin, top loin (chops), boneless, separable lean and fat, with added solution, raw	19.45	10.26	0	171	0	251	56	0
Pork, fresh, loin, top loin (chops), boneless, separable lean and fat, with added solution, cooked, broiled	28.33	9.42	0.02	198	0	302	71	0.02
Pork, fresh, loin, tenderloin, separable lean and fat, with added solution, raw	20.16	3.14	0	114	0	239	49	0

Food Name ---> per 100 g	Protein (g)	Fat (g)	Carb (g)	Calories	Fiber (g)	Sodium (mg)	Cholesterol (mg)	Net Carb (g)
Pork, fresh, loin, tenderloin, separable lean and fat, with added solution, cooked, roasted	21.5	3.7	0.31	121	0	230	57	0.31
Pork, fresh, shoulder, (Boston butt), blade (steaks), separable lean and fat,with added solution, raw	17.19	11.12	0.16	169	0	155	62	0.16
Pork, fresh, shoulder, (Boston butt), blade (steaks), separable lean and fat, with added solution, cooked, braised	25.84	16.94	0.03	263	0	151	97	0.03
Pork, cured, ham, rump, bone-in, separable lean and fat, unheated	22.27	9.38	0.52	176	0	722	62	0.52
Pork, loin, leg cap steak, boneless, separable lean and fat, cooked, broiled	27.57	4.41	0	158	0	76	81	0
Pork, Leg Cap Steak, boneless, separable lean and fat, raw	21.64	3.39	0	123	0	73	63	0
Pork, Shoulder breast, boneless, separable lean and fat, raw	22.54	3.4	0	127	0	54	60	0
Pork, Shoulder breast, boneless, separable lean and fat, cooked, broiled	28.47	4.49	0	162	0	54	78	0
Pork, shoulder, petite tender, boneless, separable lean and fat, cooked, broiled	27.47	4.23	0	155	0	53	82	0
Pork, Shoulder petite tender, boneless, separable lean and fat, raw	21.65	3.91	0	128	0	50	66	0
Pork, Leg sirloin tip roast, boneless, separable lean and fat, cooked, braised	31.11	2.56	0	156	0	43	84	0
Pork, Leg sirloin tip roast, boneless, separable lean and fat, raw	22.88	1.71	0	113	0	50	62	0
Pork, ground, 84% lean / 16% fat, raw	17.99	16	0.44	218	0	68	68	0.44
Pork, ground, 96% lean / 4% fat, raw	21.1	4	0.21	121	0	67	59	0.21
Pork, ground, 72% lean / 28% fat, cooked, crumbles	22.83	32.93	1.39	393	0	94	100	1.39
Pork, ground, 84% lean / 16% fat, cooked, crumbles	26.69	20.04	0.58	289	0	89	89	0.58
Pork, ground, 96% lean / 4% fat, cooked, crumbles	30.55	7.15	0	187	0	84	78	0
Pork, ground, 72% lean / 28% fat, cooked, pan-broiled	22.59	31.42	1.08	377	0	91	99	1.08
Pork, ground, 84% lean / 16% fat, cooked, pan-broiled	27.14	21.39	0	301	0	89	97	0
Pork, ground, 96% lean / 4% fat, cooked, pan-broiled	31.69	6.2	0.57	185	0	88	85	0.57
Pork loin, fresh, backribs, bone-in, raw, lean only	20.85	9.84	0	172	0	95	66	0
Pork loin, fresh, backribs, bone-in, cooked-roasted, lean only	24.15	17.65	0	255	0	98	84	0
Pork, fresh, loin, blade (chops or roasts), boneless, separable lean only, raw	21.35	3.78	0.82	123	0	65	58	0.82
Pork, fresh, loin, blade (roasts), boneless, separable lean only, cooked, roasted	27.58	7.14	0	175	0	68	76	0
Pork, fresh, loin, blade (chops), boneless, separable lean only, boneless, cooked, broiled	26.14	6.74	0.89	169	0	58	76	0.89
Pork, fresh, loin, country-style ribs, separable lean only, boneless, cooked, broiled	27.83	11.65	0	216	0	58	89	0
Pork, fresh, loin, country-style ribs, separable lean only, bone-in, cooked, broiled	27.83	11.65	0	216	0	84	89	0
Pork, fresh, loin, country-style ribs, separable lean only, boneless, cooked, roasted	29.2	11.38	0	219	0	72	99	0

185

Food Name ---> per 100 g	Protein (g)	Fat (g)	Carb (g)	Calories	Fiber (g)	Sodium (mg)	Cholesterol (mg)	Net Carb (g)
Pork, fresh, blade, (chops), boneless, separable lean and fat, cooked, broiled	24.73	11.13	0.83	202	0	58	77	0.83
Pork, fresh, loin, blade (chops or roasts), boneless, separable lean and fat only, raw	20.54	7.94	0.76	157	0	64	59	0.76
Pork, fresh, loin, blade (roasts), boneless, separable lean and fat, cooked, roasted	26.48	10.32	0	199	0	67	76	0
Pork, fresh, loin, country-style ribs, separable lean and fat, boneless, cooked, broiled	26.28	15.73	0	247	0	58	88	0
Pork, fresh, loin, country-style ribs, separable lean and fat, bone-in, cooked, broiled	25.58	17.56	0	260	0	81	87	0
Pork, fresh, loin, country-style ribs, separable lean and fat, boneless, cooked, roasted	26.4	18.31	0	270	0	70	96	0
Bacon, pre-sliced, reduced/low sodium, unprepared	12.53	39.27	0.83	407	0	470	-	0.83
Canadian bacon, cooked, pan-fried	28.31	2.78	1.8	146	0	993	67	1.8
Pork, oriental style, dehydrated	11.8	62.4	1.4	615	0	685	67	1.4
Pork, cured, ham, boneless, low sodium, extra lean and regular, roasted	22	7.7	0.5	165	0	969	57	0.5
Pork, cured, ham, low sodium, lean and fat, cooked	22.3	8.3	0.3	172	0	969	58	0.3
Pork, cured, ham, boneless, low sodium, extra lean (approximately 5% fat), roasted	20.9	5.5	1.5	145	0	969	53	1.5
Pork, cured, bacon, cooked, broiled, pan-fried or roasted, reduced sodium	37.04	41.78	1.43	541	0	1030	110	1.43

Poultry Products

Food Name ---> per 100 g	Protein (g)	Fat (g)	Carb (g)	Calories	Fiber (g)	Sodium (mg)	Cholesterol (mg)	Net Carb (g)
Chicken, broiler, rotisserie, BBQ, breast meat only	28.04	3.57	0	144	0	328	86	0
Chicken, broilers or fryers, meat and skin and giblets and neck, raw	18.33	14.83	0.13	213	0	70	90	0.13
Chicken, broilers or fryers, meat and skin and giblets and neck, cooked, fried, batter	22.84	17.53	9.03	291	-	284	103	9.03
Chicken, broilers or fryers, meat and skin and giblets and neck, cooked, fried, flour	28.57	15.27	3.27	272	-	86	112	3.27
Chicken, broilers or fryers, meat and skin and giblets and neck, roasted	26.78	13.27	0.06	234	0	79	107	0.06
Chicken, broilers or fryers, meat and skin and giblets and neck, stewed	24.49	12.37	0.06	216	0	66	97	0.06
Chicken, broilers or fryers, meat and skin, raw	18.6	15.06	0	215	0	70	75	0
Chicken, broilers or fryers, meat and skin, cooked, fried, batter	22.54	17.35	9.42	289	0.3	292	87	9.12
Chicken, broilers or fryers, meat and skin, cooked, fried, flour	28.56	14.92	3.15	269	0.1	84	90	3.05
Chicken, broilers or fryers, meat and skin, cooked, roasted	27.3	13.6	0	239	0	82	88	0
Chicken, broilers or fryers, meat and skin, cooked, stewed	24.68	12.56	0	219	0	67	78	0
Chicken, broilers or fryers, meat only, raw	21.39	3.08	0	119	0	77	70	0
Chicken, broilers or fryers, meat only, cooked, fried	30.57	9.12	1.69	219	0.1	91	94	1.59
Chicken, broilers or fryers, meat only, roasted	28.93	7.41	0	190	0	86	89	0
Chicken, broilers or fryers, meat only, stewed	27.29	6.71	0	177	0	70	83	0
Chicken, broilers or fryers, skin only, raw	13.33	32.35	0	349	0	63	109	0
Chicken, broilers or fryers, skin only, cooked, fried, batter	10.32	28.83	23.15	394	-	581	74	23.15
Chicken, broilers or fryers, skin only, cooked, fried, flour	19.09	42.58	9.34	502	-	53	73	9.34
Chicken, broilers or fryers, skin only, cooked, roasted	20.36	40.68	0	454	0	65	83	0
Chicken, broilers or fryers, skin only, cooked, stewed	15.22	33.04	0	363	0	56	63	0
Chicken, broilers or fryers, giblets, raw	17.88	4.47	1.8	124	0	77	262	1.8
Chicken, broilers or fryers, giblets, cooked, fried	32.54	13.46	4.35	277	0	113	446	4.35
Chicken, broilers or fryers, giblets, cooked, simmered	27.15	4.5	0	157	0	67	442	0
Chicken, gizzard, all classes, raw	17.66	2.06	0	94	0	69	240	0
Chicken, gizzard, all classes, cooked, simmered	30.39	2.68	0	154	0	56	370	0
Chicken, heart, all classes, raw	15.55	9.33	0.71	153	0	74	136	0.71
Chicken, heart, all classes, cooked, simmered	26.41	7.92	0.1	185	0	48	242	0.1
Chicken, liver, all classes, raw	16.92	4.83	0.73	119	0	71	345	0.73
Chicken, liver, all classes, cooked, simmered	24.46	6.51	0.87	167	0	76	563	0.87
Chicken, broilers or fryers, light meat, meat and skin, raw	20.27	11.07	0	186	0	65	67	0
Chicken, broilers or fryers, light meat, meat and skin, cooked, fried, batter	23.55	15.44	9.5	277	-	287	84	9.5
Chicken, broilers or fryers, light meat, meat and skin, cooked, fried, flour	30.45	12.09	1.82	246	0.1	77	87	1.72
Chicken, broilers or fryers, light meat, meat and	29.02	10.85	0	222	0	75	84	0

Food Name ---> per 100 g	Protein (g)	Fat (g)	Carb (g)	Calories	Fiber (g)	Sodium (mg)	Cholesterol (mg)	Net Carb (g)
skin, cooked, roasted								
Chicken, broilers or fryers, light meat, meat and skin, cooked, stewed	26.14	9.97	0	201	0	63	74	0
Chicken, broilers or fryers, dark meat, meat and skin, raw	16.69	18.34	0	237	0	73	81	0
Chicken, broilers or fryers, dark meat, meat and skin, cooked, fried, batter	21.85	18.64	9.38	298	-	295	89	9.38
Chicken, broilers or fryers, dark meat, meat and skin, cooked, fried, flour	27.22	16.91	4.08	285	0	89	92	4.08
Chicken, broilers or fryers, dark meat, meat and skin, cooked, roasted	25.97	15.78	0	253	0	87	91	0
Chicken, broilers or fryers, dark meat, meat and skin, cooked, stewed	23.5	14.66	0	233	0	70	82	0
Chicken, broilers or fryers, light meat, meat only, raw	23.2	1.65	0	114	0	68	58	0
Chicken, broilers or fryers, light meat, meat only, cooked, fried	32.82	5.54	0.42	192	0	81	90	0.42
Chicken, broilers or fryers, light meat, meat only, cooked, roasted	30.91	4.51	0	173	0	77	85	0
Chicken, broilers or fryers, light meat, meat only, cooked, stewed	28.88	3.99	0	159	0	65	77	0
Chicken, broilers or fryers, dark meat, meat only, raw	20.08	4.31	0	125	0	85	80	0
Chicken, broilers or fryers, dark meat, meat only, cooked, fried	28.99	11.62	2.59	239	0	97	96	2.59
Chicken, broilers or fryers, dark meat, meat only, cooked, roasted	27.37	9.73	0	205	0	93	93	0
Chicken, broilers or fryers, dark meat, meat only, cooked, stewed	25.97	8.98	0	192	0	74	88	0
Chicken, broilers or fryers, separable fat, raw	3.73	67.95	0	629	0	32	58	0
Chicken, broilers or fryers, back, meat and skin, raw	14.05	28.74	0	319	0	64	79	0
Chicken, broilers or fryers, back, meat and skin, cooked, fried, batter	21.97	21.91	10.25	331	-	317	88	10.25
Chicken, broilers or fryers, back, meat and skin, cooked, fried, flour	27.79	20.74	6.5	331	-	90	89	6.5
Chicken, broilers or fryers, back, meat and skin, cooked, roasted	25.95	20.97	0	300	0	87	88	0
Chicken, broilers or fryers, back, meat and skin, cooked, stewed	22.18	18.14	0	258	0	64	78	0
Chicken, broilers or fryers, back, meat only, raw	19.56	5.92	0	137	0	82	81	0
Chicken, broilers or fryers, back, meat only, cooked, fried	29.99	15.32	5.68	288	0	99	93	5.68
Chicken, broilers or fryers, back, meat only, cooked, roasted	28.19	13.16	0	239	0	96	90	0
Chicken, broilers or fryers, back, meat only, cooked, stewed	25.31	11.19	0	209	0	67	85	0
Chicken, broilers or fryers, breast, meat and skin, raw	20.85	9.25	0	172	0	63	64	0
Chicken, broilers or fryers, breast, meat and skin, cooked, fried, batter	24.84	13.2	8.99	260	0.3	275	85	8.69
Chicken, broilers or fryers, breast, meat and skin, cooked, fried, flour	31.84	8.87	1.64	222	0.1	76	89	1.54
Chicken, broilers or fryers, breast, meat and skin, cooked, roasted	29.8	7.78	0	197	0	71	84	0
Chicken, broilers or fryers, breast, meat and skin, cooked, stewed	27.39	7.42	0	184	0	62	75	0
Chicken, broiler or fryers, breast, skinless, boneless, meat only, raw	22.5	2.62	0	120	0	45	73	0

Food Name ---> per 100 g	Protein (g)	Fat (g)	Carb (g)	Calories	Fiber (g)	Sodium (mg)	Cholesterol (mg)	Net Carb (g)
Chicken, broilers or fryers, breast, meat only, cooked, fried	33.44	4.71	0.51	187	0	79	91	0.51
Chicken, broilers or fryers, breast, meat only, cooked, roasted	31.02	3.57	0	165	0	74	85	0
Chicken, broilers or fryers, breast, meat only, cooked, stewed	28.98	3.03	0	151	0	63	77	0
Chicken, broilers or fryers, drumstick, meat and skin, raw	18.08	9.2	0.11	161	0	106	92	0.11
Chicken, broilers or fryers, drumstick, meat and skin, cooked, fried, batter	21.95	15.75	8.28	268	0.3	269	86	7.98
Chicken, broilers or fryers, drumstick, meat and skin, cooked, fried, flour	26.96	13.72	1.63	245	0.1	89	90	1.53
Chicken, broilers or fryers, drumstick, meat and skin, cooked, roasted	23.35	10.15	0	191	0	123	130	0
Chicken, broilers or fryers, drumstick, meat and skin, cooked, stewed	25.32	10.64	0	204	0	76	83	0
Chicken, broilers or fryers, dark meat, drumstick, meat only, raw	19.41	3.71	0	116	0	114	89	0
Chicken, broilers or fryers, drumstick, meat only, cooked, fried	28.62	8.08	0	195	0	96	94	0
Chicken, broilers or fryers, dark meat, drumstick, meat only, cooked, roasted	24.24	5.7	0	155	0	128	130	0
Chicken, broilers or fryers, drumstick, meat only, cooked, stewed	27.5	5.71	0	169	0	80	88	0
Chicken, broilers or fryers, leg, meat and skin, raw	16.37	15.95	0.17	214	0	84	93	0.17
Chicken, broilers or fryers, leg, meat and skin, cooked, fried, batter	21.77	16.17	8.72	273	0.3	279	90	8.42
Chicken, broilers or fryers, leg, meat and skin, cooked, fried, flour	26.84	14.43	2.5	254	0.1	88	94	2.4
Chicken, broilers or fryers, leg, meat and skin, cooked, roasted	24.03	8.99	0	184	0	98	127	0
Chicken, broilers or fryers, leg, meat and skin, cooked, stewed	24.17	12.92	0	220	0	73	84	0
Chicken, broilers or fryers, leg, meat only, raw	19.16	4.22	0	120	0	96	91	0
Chicken, broilers or fryers, leg, meat only, cooked, fried	28.38	9.32	0.65	208	0	96	99	0.65
Chicken, broilers or fryers, leg, meat only, cooked, roasted	24.22	7.8	0	174	0	99	128	0
Chicken, broilers or fryers, leg, meat only, cooked, stewed	26.26	8.06	0	185	0	78	89	0
Chicken, broilers or fryers, neck, meat and skin, raw	14.07	26.24	0	297	0	64	99	0
Chicken, broilers or fryers, neck, meat and skin, cooked, fried, batter	19.82	23.52	8.7	330	-	276	91	8.7
Chicken, broilers or fryers, neck, meat and skin, cooked, fried, flour	24.01	23.61	4.24	332	-	82	94	4.24
Chicken, broilers or fryers, neck, meat and skin, cooked simmered	19.61	18.1	0	247	0	52	70	0
Chicken, broilers or fryers, neck, meat only, raw	17.55	8.78	0	154	0	81	83	0
Chicken, broilers or fryers, neck, meat only, cooked, fried	26.87	11.88	1.77	229	0	99	105	1.77
Chicken, broilers or fryers, neck, meat only, cooked, simmered	24.56	8.18	0	179	0	64	79	0
Chicken, broilers or fryers, thigh, meat and skin, raw	16.52	16.61	0.25	221	0	81	98	0.25
Chicken, broilers or fryers, thigh, meat and skin, cooked, fried, batter	21.61	16.53	9.08	277	0.3	288	93	8.78
Chicken, broilers or fryers, thigh, meat and skin, cooked, fried, flour	26.75	14.98	3.18	262	0.1	88	97	3.08

Food Name ---> per 100 g	Protein (g)	Fat (g)	Carb (g)	Calories	Fiber (g)	Sodium (mg)	Cholesterol (mg)	Net Carb (g)
Chicken, broilers or fryers, thigh, meat and skin, cooked, roasted	23.26	14.71	0	232	0	102	133	0
Chicken, broilers or fryers, thigh, meat and skin, cooked, stewed	23.26	14.74	0	232	0	71	84	0
Chicken, broilers or fryers, dark meat, thigh, meat only, raw	19.66	4.12	0	121	0	95	94	0
Chicken, broilers or fryers, thigh, meat only, cooked, fried	28.18	10.3	1.18	218	0	95	102	1.18
Chicken, broilers or fryers, thigh, meat only, cooked, roasted	24.76	8.15	0	179	0	106	133	0
Chicken, broilers or fryers, thigh, meat only, cooked, stewed	25	9.79	0	195	0	75	90	0
Chicken, broilers or fryers, wing, meat and skin, raw	17.52	12.85	0	191	0	84	111	0
Chicken, broilers or fryers, wing, meat and skin, cooked, fried, batter	19.87	21.81	10.94	324	0.3	320	79	10.64
Chicken, broilers or fryers, wing, meat and skin, cooked, fried, flour	26.11	22.16	2.39	321	0.1	77	81	2.29
Chicken, broilers or fryers, wing, meat and skin, cooked, roasted	23.79	16.87	0	254	0	98	141	0
Chicken, broilers or fryers, wing, meat and skin, cooked, stewed	22.78	16.82	0	249	0	67	70	0
Chicken, broilers or fryers, wing, meat only, raw	21.97	3.54	0	126	0	81	57	0
Chicken, broilers or fryers, wing, meat only, cooked, fried	30.15	9.15	0	211	0	91	84	0
Chicken, broilers or fryers, wing, meat only, cooked, roasted	30.46	8.13	0	203	0	92	85	0
Chicken, broilers or fryers, wing, meat only, cooked, stewed	27.18	7.18	0	181	0	73	74	0
Chicken, roasting, meat and skin and giblets and neck, raw	17.09	15.46	0.09	213	0	69	86	0.09
Chicken, roasting, meat and skin and giblets and neck, cooked, roasted	23.96	13.07	0.05	220	0	71	94	0.05
Canada Goose, breast meat, skinless, raw	24.31	4.02	0	133	0	50	80	0
Chicken, roasting, meat and skin, cooked, roasted	23.97	13.39	0	223	0	73	76	0
Chicken, roasting, meat only, raw	20.33	2.7	0	111	0	75	65	0
Chicken, roasting, meat only, cooked, roasted	25.01	6.63	0	167	0	75	75	0
Chicken, roasting, giblets, raw	18.14	5.04	1.14	127	0	77	236	1.14
Chicken, roasting, giblets, cooked, simmered	26.77	5.22	0.86	165	0	60	357	0.86
Chicken, roasting, light meat, meat only, raw	22.2	1.63	0	109	0	51	57	0
Chicken, roasting, light meat, meat only, cooked, roasted	27.13	4.07	0	153	0	51	75	0
Chicken, roasting, dark meat, meat only, raw	18.74	3.61	0	113	0	95	72	0
Chicken, roasting, dark meat, meat only, cooked, roasted	23.25	8.75	0	178	0	95	75	0
Chicken, stewing, meat and skin, and giblets and neck, raw	17.48	19.52	0.19	251	0	71	87	0.19
Chicken, stewing, meat and skin, and giblets and neck, cooked, stewed	24.88	11.91	0	214	0	67	107	0
Chicken, stewing, meat and skin, raw	17.55	20.33	0	258	0	71	71	0
Chicken, stewing, meat and skin, cooked, stewed	26.88	18.87	0	285	0	73	79	0
Chicken, stewing, meat only, raw	21.26	6.32	0	148	0	79	63	0
Chicken, stewing, meat only, cooked, stewed	30.42	11.89	0	237	0	78	83	0
Chicken, stewing, giblets, raw	17.89	9.21	2.13	168	0	77	240	2.13
Chicken, stewing, giblets, cooked, simmered	25.73	9.3	0.11	194	0	56	355	0.11
Chicken, stewing, light meat, meat only, raw	23.1	4.21	0	137	0	53	47	0
Chicken, stewing, light meat, meat only, cooked,	33.04	7.98	0	213	0	58	70	0

Food Name ---> per 100 g	Protein (g)	Fat (g)	Carb (g)	Calories	Fiber (g)	Sodium (mg)	Cholesterol (mg)	Net Carb (g)
stewed								
Chicken, stewing, dark meat, meat only, raw	19.7	8.12	0	157	0	101	77	0
Chicken, stewing, dark meat, meat only, cooked, stewed	28.14	15.28	0	258	0	95	95	0
Chicken, capons, meat and skin and giblets and neck, raw	18.51	16.9	0.08	232	0	47	87	0.08
Chicken, capons, meat and skin and giblets and neck, cooked, roasted	28.35	11.67	0.04	226	0	50	103	0.04
Chicken, capons, meat and skin, raw	18.77	17.07	0	234	0	45	75	0
Chicken, capons, meat and skin, cooked, roasted	28.96	11.65	0	229	0	49	86	0
Chicken, capons, giblets, raw	18.28	5.18	1.42	130	0	77	292	1.42
Chicken, capons, giblets, cooked, simmered	26.39	5.4	0.76	164	0	55	434	0.76
Duck, domesticated, meat and skin, raw	11.49	39.34	0	404	0	63	76	0
Duck, domesticated, meat and skin, cooked, roasted	18.99	28.35	0	337	0	59	84	0
Duck, domesticated, meat only, raw	18.28	5.95	0.94	135	0	74	77	0.94
Duck, domesticated, meat only, cooked, roasted	23.48	11.2	0	201	0	65	89	0
Duck, domesticated, liver, raw	18.74	4.64	3.53	136	0	140	515	3.53
Duck, wild, meat and skin, raw	17.42	15.2	0	211	0	56	80	0
Duck, wild, breast, meat only, raw	19.85	4.25	0	123	0	57	77	0
Goose, domesticated, meat and skin, raw	15.86	33.62	0	371	0	73	80	0
Goose, domesticated, meat and skin, cooked, roasted	25.16	21.92	0	305	0	70	91	0
Goose, domesticated, meat only, raw	22.75	7.13	0	161	0	87	84	0
Goose, domesticated, meat only, cooked, roasted	28.97	12.67	0	238	0	76	96	0
Goose, liver, raw	16.37	4.28	6.32	133	0	140	515	6.32
Turkey, whole, giblets, raw	18.18	5.09	0.07	124	0	136	333	0.07
Turkey, whole, giblets, cooked, simmered	26.44	6.61	0	173	0	117	521	0
Turkey, gizzard, all classes, raw	18.8	3.37	0	111	0	147	271	0
Turkey, gizzard, all classes, cooked, simmered	26.45	4.64	0	155	0	127	452	0
Turkey, heart, all classes, raw	16.7	7.44	0.4	140	0	129	225	0.4
Turkey, heart, all classes, cooked, simmered	24.88	7.52	0	174	0	140	359	0
Turkey, liver, all classes, raw	18.26	5.5	0	128	0	131	415	0
Turkey, liver, all classes, cooked, simmered	27	8.18	0	189	0	98	648	0
Turkey from whole, neck, meat only, raw	16.51	6.04	0	125	0	233	115	0
Turkey from whole, neck, meat only, cooked, simmered	22.48	7.36	0	162	0	246	128	0
Turkey from whole, light meat, meat and skin, raw	21.96	7.43	0.15	161	0	105	67	0.15
Turkey from whole, light meat, meat and skin, cooked, roasted	29.55	5.57	0.05	177	0	101	89	0.05
Turkey, dark meat, meat and skin, raw	19.81	8.97	0.15	161	0	113	87	0.15
Turkey, dark meat from whole, meat and skin, cooked, roasted	27.27	9.95	0.07	206	0	105	134	0.07
Turkey from whole, light meat, raw	23.66	1.48	0.14	114	0	113	57	0.14
Turkey, all classes, light meat, cooked, roasted	30.13	2.08	0	147	0	99	80	0
Turkey from whole, dark meat, meat only, raw	21.28	2.5	0.15	108	0	124	79	0.15
Turkey, from whole, dark meat, cooked, roasted	27.71	6.04	0	173	0	104	128	0
Turkey, all classes, back, meat and skin, cooked, roasted	26.59	14.38	0.16	244	0	73	91	0.16
Turkey, all classes, breast, meat and skin, raw	21.89	7.02	0	157	0	59	65	0
Turkey, all classes, breast, meat and skin, cooked, roasted	28.71	7.41	0	189	0	63	74	0
Turkey, all classes, leg, meat and skin, raw	19.54	6.72	0	144	0	74	71	0
Turkey, all classes, leg, meat and skin, cooked, roasted	27.87	9.82	0	208	0	77	85	0

Food Name ---> per 100 g	Protein (g)	Fat (g)	Carb (g)	Calories	Fiber (g)	Sodium (mg)	Cholesterol (mg)	Net Carb (g)
Turkey, all classes, wing, meat and skin, raw	20.22	12.32	0	197	0	55	70	0
Turkey, all classes, wing, meat and skin, cooked, roasted	27.38	12.43	0	229	0	61	81	0
Turkey, fryer-roasters, meat and skin, cooked, roasted	28.26	5.72	0	172	0	66	105	0
Turkey, back from whole bird, meat only, raw	21.28	2.5	0.15	113	0	124	79	0.15
Turkey, back, from whole bird, meat only, roasted	27.71	6.04	0	173	0	104	128	0
Turkey, breast, from whole bird, meat only, raw	23.66	1.48	0.14	114	0	113	57	0.14
Turkey, breast, from whole bird, meat only, roasted	30.13	2.08	0	147	0	99	80	0
Turkey, wing, from whole bird, meat only, raw	23.66	1.48	0.14	114	0	113	57	0.14
Turkey, wing, from whole bird, meat only, roasted	30.13	2.08	0	147	0	99	80	0
Turkey, young hen, skin only, cooked, roasted	19.03	44.45	0	482	0	44	106	0
Chicken, canned, meat only, with broth	21.77	7.95	0	165	0	503	62	0
Pate de foie gras, canned (goose liver pate), smoked	11.4	43.84	4.67	462	0	697	150	4.67
Turkey, canned, meat only, with broth	23.68	6.86	1.47	169	0	518	66	1.47
Turkey, diced, light and dark meat, seasoned	18.7	6	1	138	0	850	55	1
Turkey and gravy, frozen	5.88	2.63	4.61	67	0	554	18	4.61
Turkey breast, pre-basted, meat and skin, cooked, roasted	22.16	3.46	0	126	0	397	42	0
Turkey thigh, pre-basted, meat and skin, cooked, roasted	18.8	8.54	0	157	0	437	62	0
Turkey roast, boneless, frozen, seasoned, light and dark meat, raw	17.6	2.2	6.4	120	0	678	53	6.4
Turkey sticks, breaded, battered, fried	14.2	16.9	17	279	-	838	64	17
Poultry, mechanically deboned, from backs and necks with skin, raw	11.39	24.73	0	272	0	40	130	0
Poultry, mechanically deboned, from backs and necks without skin, raw	13.79	15.48	0	199	0	51	104	0
Poultry, mechanically deboned, from mature hens, raw	14.72	19.98	0	243	0	40	143	0
Turkey, mechanically deboned, from turkey frames, raw	13.29	15.96	0	201	0	48	95	0
Ground turkey, raw	19.66	7.66	0	148	0	58	69	0
Ground turkey, cooked	27.37	10.4	0	203	0	78	93	0
Duck, young duckling, domesticated, White Pekin, breast, meat and skin, boneless, cooked, roasted	24.5	10.85	0	202	-	84	136	0
Duck, young duckling, domesticated, White Pekin, breast, meat only, boneless, cooked without skin, broiled	27.6	2.5	0	140	-	105	143	0
Duck, young duckling, domesticated, White Pekin, leg, meat and skin, bone in, cooked, roasted	26.75	11.4	0	217	-	110	114	0
Duck, young duckling, domesticated, White Pekin, leg, meat only, bone in, cooked without skin, braised	29.1	5.96	0	178	-	108	105	0
Chicken, broiler, rotisserie, BBQ, drumstick, meat only	27.71	6.76	0	172	0	403	155	0
Chicken, wing, frozen, glazed, barbecue flavored, heated (conventional oven)	22.24	14.87	3.36	242	0.5	559	136	2.86
Chicken patty, frozen, uncooked	14.33	20.04	13.61	292	1.2	518	45	12.41
Chicken patty, frozen, cooked	14.85	19.58	12.84	287	0.3	532	43	12.54
Chicken breast tenders, breaded, cooked, microwaved	16.35	12.89	17.56	252	0	446	45	17.56
Chicken breast tenders, breaded, uncooked	14.73	15.75	15.01	263	1.1	536	41	13.91
Chicken, ground, raw	17.44	8.1	0.04	143	0	60	86	0.04
Chicken, ground, crumbles, cooked, pan-browned	23.28	10.92	0	189	0	75	107	0
Chicken, broiler, rotisserie, BBQ, thigh, meat only	24.09	10.74	0	193	0	335	128	0

Food Name ---> per 100 g	Protein (g)	Fat (g)	Carb (g)	Calories	Fiber (g)	Sodium (mg)	Cholesterol (mg)	Net Carb (g)
Chicken, feet, boiled	19.4	14.6	0.2	215	0	67	84	0.2
USDA Commodity Chicken, canned, meat only, drained	27.52	5.72	0	162	0	271	83	0
USDA Commodity, Chicken, canned, meat only, with water	22.02	4.58	0	129	0	251	67	0
USDA Commodity, Chicken, canned, meat only, with broth	22.41	4.69	0.23	133	0	256	67	0.23
Chicken, broiler, rotisserie, BBQ, wing, meat only	28.34	7.79	0.54	184	0	725	134	0.54
Chicken, broilers or fryers, back, meat only, cooked, rotisserie, original seasoning	25.34	11.54	0	205	0	661	123	0
Chicken, broilers or fryers, breast, meat only, cooked, rotisserie, original seasoning	28	2.79	0	137	0	313	86	0
Chicken, broilers or fryers, drumstick, meat only, cooked, rotisserie, original seasoning	28.74	6.81	0	176	0	417	160	0
Chicken, broilers or fryers, skin only, cooked, rotisserie, original seasoning	17.66	37.24	0.11	406	0	381	141	0.11
Chicken, broilers or fryers, thigh, meat only, cooked, rotisserie, original seasoning	24.06	11.09	0	196	0	337	130	0
Chicken, broilers or fryers, wing, meat only, cooked, rotisserie, original seasoning	27.69	9.53	0	197	0	725	140	0
Chicken, broilers or fryers, back, meat and skin, cooked, rotisserie, original seasoning	23.23	18.59	0.03	260	0	584	128	0.03
Chicken, broilers or fryers, breast, meat and skin, cooked, rotisserie, original seasoning	27.48	8.18	0.02	184	0	347	96	0.02
Chicken, broilers or fryers, drumstick, meat and skin, cooked, rotisserie, original seasoning	26.86	11.98	0.02	215	0	411	156	0.02
Chicken, broilers or fryers, thigh, meat and skin, cooked, rotisserie, original seasoning	22.93	15.7	0.02	233	0	345	132	0.02
Chicken, broilers or fryers, wing, meat and skin, cooked, rotisserie, original seasoning	24.34	18.77	0.04	266	0	610	140	0.04
USDA Commodity, chicken fajita strips, frozen	18.56	5.73	2.23	135	0	799	88	2.23
USDA Commodity, turkey taco meat, frozen, cooked	16.8	7.58	3.03	148	0	632	71	3.03
Chicken, broiler, rotisserie, BBQ, skin	15.19	35.15	0.7	378	0	335	120	0.7
Chicken, broiler, rotisserie, BBQ, back meat and skin	20.29	18.86	0.4	251	0	509	118	0.4
Chicken, broiler, rotisserie, BBQ, breast meat and skin	26.37	7.67	0.09	175	0	329	90	0.09
Chicken, broiler, rotisserie, BBQ, drumstick meat and skin	25.65	11.46	0.12	206	0	392	149	0.12
Chicken, broiler, rotisserie, BBQ, thigh meat and skin	22.51	15.08	0.12	226	0	335	127	0.12
Chicken, broiler, rotisserie, BBQ, wing meat and skin	23.42	18.04	0.6	257	0	579	129	0.6
Ruffed Grouse, breast meat, skinless, raw	25.94	0.88	0	112	0	50	40	0
USDA Commodity, turkey ham, dark meat, smoked, frozen	16.3	4	3.1	118	0	909	64	3.1
Chicken, liver, all classes, cooked, pan-fried	25.78	6.43	1.11	172	0	92	564	1.11
Ground turkey, fat free, raw	23.57	1.95	0	112	0	51	55	0
Ground turkey, fat free, pan-broiled crumbles	31.69	2.71	0	151	0	61	71	0
Ground turkey, fat free, patties, broiled	28.99	2.48	0	138	0	59	65	0
Ground turkey, 93% lean, 7% fat, raw	18.73	8.34	0	150	0	69	74	0
Ground turkey, 93% lean, 7% fat, pan-broiled crumbles	27.1	11.6	0	213	0	90	104	0
Ground turkey, 93% lean, 7% fat, patties, broiled	25.86	11.45	0	207	0	91	106	0
Ground turkey, 85% lean, 15% fat, raw	16.9	12.54	0	180	0	54	78	0
Ground turkey, 85% lean, 15% fat, pan-broiled	25.11	17.45	0	258	0	85	106	0

crumbles

Food Name ---> per 100 g	Protein (g)	Fat (g)	Carb (g)	Calories	Fiber (g)	Sodium (mg)	Cholesterol (mg)	Net Carb (g)
Ground turkey, 85% lean, 15% fat, patties, broiled	25.88	16.2	0	249	0	81	105	0
Chicken, broilers or fryers, dark meat, drumstick, meat only, cooked, braised	23.93	5.95	0	149	0	117	132	0
Chicken, broilers or fryers, dark meat, thigh, meat only, cooked, braised	24.55	8.63	0	176	0	77	141	0
Chicken, skin (drumsticks and thighs), cooked, braised	14.61	42.76	0	443	0	75	130	0
Chicken, skin (drumsticks and thighs), raw	9.58	44.23	0.79	440	0	51	105	0.79
Chicken, skin (drumsticks and thighs), cooked, roasted	16.57	43.99	0	462	0	85	132	0
Chicken, broilers or fryers, dark meat, drumstick, meat and skin, cooked, braised	22.72	10.73	0	187	0	111	132	0
Chicken, broilers or fryers, dark meat, thigh, meat and skin, cooked, braised	22.57	15.43	0	229	0	76	139	0
Chicken, dark meat, drumstick, meat only, with added solution, raw	19.19	3.26	0	106	0	152	92	0
Chicken, dark meat, drumstick, meat only, with added solution, cooked, roasted	25.34	5	0	146	0	190	124	0
Chicken, dark meat, drumstick, meat only, with added solution, cooked, braised	22.99	6.33	0	149	0	169	135	0
Chicken, dark meat, thigh, meat only, with added solution, cooked, braised	23	7.96	0	164	0	197	126	0
Chicken, dark meat, thigh, meat only, with added solution, raw	19.11	3.69	0	110	0	156	87	0
Chicken, dark meat, thigh, meat only, with added solution, cooked, roasted	24.23	7.73	0	164	0	177	122	0
Chicken, skin (drumsticks and thighs), with added solution, cooked, braised	12.26	38.94	1	403	0	139	124	1
Chicken, skin (drumsticks and thighs), with added solution, raw	11.11	37.9	0.01	386	0	139	113	0.01
Chicken, skin (drumsticks and thighs), with added solution, cooked, roasted	20.31	37.6	0.44	421	0	162	154	0.44
Chicken, dark meat, drumstick, meat and skin, with added solution, cooked, braised	21.55	10.71	0.13	183	0	165	133	0.13
Chicken, dark meat, drumstick, meat and skin, with added solution, raw	18.03	8.24	0	146	0	150	95	0
Chicken, dark meat, drumstick, meat and skin, with added solution, cooked, roasted	24.72	9	0.05	180	0	186	128	0.05
Chicken, dark meat, thigh, meat and skin, with added solution, cooked, braised	20.7	14.62	0.21	215	0	185	125	0.21
Chicken, dark meat, thigh, meat and skin, with added solution, raw	16.56	14.58	0	197	0	151	95	0
Chicken, dark meat, thigh, meat and skin, with added solution, cooked, roasted	23.47	13.81	0.09	214	0	174	128	0.09
Chicken, broiler, rotisserie, BBQ, back meat only	21.85	13.87	0.31	212	0	563	117	0.31
Turkey, dark meat from whole, meat only, with added solution, raw	19.27	4.12	0.1	115	0	167	79	0.1
Turkey, dark meat, meat only, with added solution, cooked, roasted	26.1	6	0	158	0	201	105	0
Turkey from whole, light meat, meat only, with added solution, raw	21.54	1.66	0	101	0	206	54	0
Turkey from whole, light meat, meat only, with added solution, cooked, roasted	26.97	2.08	0	127	0	238	69	0
Turkey, skin from whole (light and dark), with added solution, raw	12.29	36.8	0.21	381	0	138	94	0.21
Turkey, skin from whole, (light and dark), with added solution, roasted	22.15	40.31	0	451	0	234	144	0
Turkey, dark meat from whole, meat and skin, with	17.84	10.83	0.15	169	0	161	82	0.15

Food Name ---> per 100 g	Protein (g)	Fat (g)	Carb (g)	Calories	Fiber (g)	Sodium (mg)	Cholesterol (mg)	Net Carb (g)
added solution, raw								
Turkey, dark meat from whole, meat and skin, with added solution, cooked, roasted	25.55	10.81	0	199	0	206	110	0
Turkey from whole, light meat, meat and skin, with added solution, raw	20.02	7.42	0.14	147	0	195	60	0.14
Turkey from whole, light meat, meat and skin, with added solution, cooked, roasted	26.52	5.64	0	157	0	237	76	0
Turkey, whole, meat only, with added solution, raw	20.87	2.39	0.14	105	0	194	61	0.14
Turkey, whole, meat only, with added solution, roasted	26.61	3.7	0	140	0	223	84	0
Turkey, whole, meat and skin, with added solution, raw	19.03	9.1	0.15	158	0	180	70	0.15
Turkey, whole, meat and skin, with added solution, roasted	26.09	8.01	0	176	0	224	91	0
Turkey, retail parts, breast, meat only, with added solution, raw	21.99	2.53	0	111	0	124	60	0
Turkey, retail parts, breast, meat only, with added solution, cooked, roasted	27.94	2.08	0	130	0	184	74	0
Turkey, retail parts, breast, meat only, raw	23.34	2.33	0	114	0	74	53	0
Turkey, retail parts, breast, meat only, cooked, roasted	29.51	1.97	0	136	0	114	70	0
Turkey, retail parts, wing, meat only, raw	22.48	2.49	0	112	0	69	66	0
Turkey, retail parts, wing, meat only, cooked, roasted	30.17	5.51	0	170	0	103	97	0
Turkey, skin, from retail parts, from dark meat, raw	14.35	35.83	0	380	0	78	111	0
Turkey, skin, from retail parts, from dark meat, cooked, roasted	24.58	35.03	0	414	0	106	139	0
Turkey, retail parts, drumstick, meat only, raw	20.52	3.97	0	118	0	87	79	0
Turkey, retail parts, thigh, meat only, raw	20.6	3.69	0	116	0	75	78	0
Turkey, breast, from whole bird, meat only, with added solution, roasted	26.97	2.08	0	127	0	238	69	0
Turkey, back, from whole bird, meat only, with added solution, raw	19.27	4.12	0.15	115	0	167	79	0.15
Turkey, back, from whole bird, meat only, with added solution, roasted	26.97	2.08	0	127	0	238	69	0
Turkey, breast, from whole bird, meat only, with added solution, raw	21.54	1.66	0.14	102	0	206	54	0.14
Turkey, retail parts, thigh, meat only, cooked, roasted	25.14	6.25	0.46	159	0	104	116	0.46
Turkey, retail parts, drumstick, meat only, cooked, roasted	28.61	6.52	0	173	0	112	118	0
Turkey, drumstick, from whole bird, meat only, with added solution, raw	19.27	4.12	0.15	115	0	167	79	0.15
Turkey, drumstick, from whole bird, meat only, with added solution, roasted	26.1	6	0	158	0	201	105	0
Turkey, thigh, from whole bird, meat only, with added solution, raw	19.27	4.12	0.15	115	0	167	79	0.15
Turkey, retail parts, breast, meat and skin, with added solution, raw	20.79	6.75	0.03	144	0	126	64	0.03
Turkey, thigh, from whole bird, meat only, with added solution, roasted	26.1	6	0	158	0	201	105	0
Turkey, wing, from whole bird, meat only, with added solution, raw	21.54	1.66	0.14	102	0	206	54	0.14
Turkey, wing, from whole bird, meat only, with added solution, roasted	26.97	2.08	0	127	0	238	69	0
Turkey, retail parts, breast, meat and skin, raw	21.88	7.45	0	155	0	72	63	0
Turkey, retail parts, breast, meat and skin, cooked, roasted	29.01	5.33	0.05	164	0	114	79	0.05

Food Name ---> per 100 g	Protein (g)	Fat (g)	Carb (g)	Calories	Fiber (g)	Sodium (mg)	Cholesterol (mg)	Net Carb (g)
Turkey, retail parts, wing, meat and skin, raw	19.53	13.79	0.05	202	0	67	84	0.05
Turkey, retail parts, wing, meat and skin, cooked, roasted	28.74	13.29	0.13	235	0	106	115	0.13
Turkey, retail parts, drumstick, meat and skin, raw	19.96	6.84	0	141	0	86	82	0
Turkey, retail parts, drumstick, meat and skin, cooked, roasted	28.21	9.37	0	197	0	112	120	0
Turkey, drumstick, from whole bird, meat only, raw	23.66	1.48	0.14	109	0	113	57	0.14
Turkey, drumstick, from whole bird, meat only, roasted	30.13	2.08	0	139	0	99	80	0
Turkey, thigh, from whole bird, meat only, raw	21.28	2.5	0.15	108	0	124	79	0.15
Turkey, thigh, from whole bird, meat only, roasted	27.71	6.04	0	165	0	104	128	0
Turkey, retail parts, thigh, meat and skin, raw	19.54	9.16	0	161	0	75	83	0
Turkey, retail parts, thigh, meat and skin, cooked, roasted	23.95	9.5	0.41	183	0	101	116	0.41
Turkey, back, from whole bird, meat and skin, with added solution, raw	16.86	15.41	0.15	206	0	157	84	0.15
Turkey, back, from whole bird, meat and skin, with added solution, roasted	25.8	11.36	0	205	0	237	87	0
Chicken, broiler or fryers, breast, skinless, boneless, meat only, cooked, braised	32.06	3.24	0	157	0	47	116	0
Chicken, broiler or fryers, breast, skinless, boneless, meat only, cooked, grilled	30.54	3.17	0	151	0	52	104	0
Chicken, broiler or fryers, breast, skinless, boneless, meat only, with added solution, cooked, braised	28.24	3.61	0	145	0	172	99	0
Chicken, broiler or fryers, breast, skinless, boneless, meat only, with added solution, cooked, grilled	29.5	3.39	0	148	0	215	106	0
Quail, cooked, total edible	25.1	14.1	0	227	0	52	86	0
Pheasant, cooked, total edible	32.4	12.1	0	239	0	43	89	0
Dove, cooked (includes squab)	23.9	13	0	213	0	57	116	0
Turkey, wing, smoked, cooked, with skin, bone removed	27.4	12.41	0	221	0	996	81	0
Turkey, drumstick, smoked, cooked, with skin, bone removed	27.9	9.8	0	208	0	996	85	0
Turkey, light or dark meat, smoked, cooked, with skin, bone removed	28.1	9.7	0	208	0	996	82	0
Turkey, light or dark meat, smoked, cooked, skin and bone removed	29.3	5	0	170	0	996	76	0

Sausages and Luncheon Meats

Food Name ---> per 100 g	Protein (g)	Fat (g)	Carbohydrates (g)	Calories	Fiber (g)	Sodium (mg)	Cholesterol (mg)	Net Carbs
Sausage, Berliner, pork, beef	15.27	17.2	2.59	230	0	1297	46	2.59
Blood sausage	14.6	34.5	1.29	379	0	680	120	1.29
Bockwurst, pork, veal, raw	14.03	25.87	2.95	301	1	756	93	1.95
Bologna, beef	10.91	26.13	4.29	299	0	1013	57	4.29
Bologna, beef and pork	15.2	24.59	5.49	308	0	960	60	5.49
Bologna, pork	15.3	19.87	0.73	247	0	907	59	0.73
Bologna, turkey	11.42	16.05	4.68	209	0.5	1071	75	4.18
Bratwurst, pork, cooked	13.72	29.18	2.85	333	0	846	74	2.85
Braunschweiger (a liver sausage), pork	14.5	28.5	3.1	327	0	977	180	3.1
Brotwurst, pork, beef, link	14.3	27.8	2.98	323	0	1112	63	2.98
Cheesefurter, cheese smokie, pork, beef	14.1	29	1.51	328	0	1082	68	1.51
Chicken spread	18.01	17.56	4.05	158	0.3	722	56	3.75
Chorizo, pork and beef	24.1	38.27	1.86	455	0	1235	88	1.86
Corned beef loaf, jellied	22.9	6.1	0	153	0	953	47	0
Dutch brand loaf, chicken, pork and beef	12	22.91	3.93	273	0.3	786	60	3.63
Frankfurter, beef, unheated	11.16	28.3	3.36	316	0	992	55	3.36
Frankfurter, chicken	15.51	16.19	2.74	223	0	1027	96	2.74
Frankfurter, turkey	12.23	17.29	3.81	223	0	911	77	3.81
Ham, chopped, canned	16.06	18.83	0.26	239	0	1280	49	0.26
Ham, chopped, not canned	16.5	10.3	4.2	180	0	1039	59	4.2
Ham, sliced, packaged (96% fat free, water added)	16.9	3.4	0.55	100	0	1279	41	0.55
Ham, sliced, regular (approximately 11% fat)	16.6	8.6	3.83	163	1.3	1143	57	2.53
Ham, minced	16.28	20.68	1.84	263	0	1245	70	1.84
Ham salad spread	8.68	15.53	10.64	216	0	1075	37	10.64
Ham and cheese loaf or roll	13.6	18.7	4	241	0	1000	58	4
Ham and cheese spread	16.18	18.53	2.28	245	0	1197	61	2.28
Headcheese, pork	13.83	10.9	0	157	0	941	69	0
Sausage, Italian, pork, raw	14.25	31.33	0.65	346	0	731	76	0.65
Knackwurst, knockwurst, pork, beef	11.1	27.7	3.2	307	0	930	60	3.2
Lebanon bologna, beef	19.03	10.44	0.44	172	0	1374	55	0.44
Liver cheese, pork	15.2	25.6	2.1	304	0	1225	174	2.1
Liver sausage, liverwurst, pork	14.1	28.5	2.2	326	0	860	158	2.2
Roast beef, deli style, prepackaged, sliced	18.62	3.69	0.64	115	0	853	51	0.64
USDA Commodity, luncheon meat, canned	17.5	12.77	1.04	189	0	820	78	1.04
Luncheon meat, pork, canned	12.5	30.3	2.1	334	0	1289	62	2.1
Turkey breast, low salt, prepackaged or deli, luncheon meat	21.81	0.83	3.51	109	0.5	772	44	3.01
Mortadella, beef, pork	16.37	25.39	3.05	311	0	1246	56	3.05
Olive loaf, pork	11.8	16.5	9.2	235	0	964	38	9.2
Pastrami, turkey	16.3	6.21	3.34	139	0.1	1123	68	3.24
Pate, chicken liver, canned	13.45	13.1	6.55	201	0	386	391	6.55
Pate, goose liver, smoked, canned	11.4	43.84	4.67	462	0	697	150	4.67
Pate, liver, not specified, canned	14.2	28	1.5	319	0	697	255	1.5
Peppered loaf, pork, beef	17.3	6.37	4.53	149	0	732	46	4.53
Pepperoni, beef and pork, sliced	19.25	46.28	1.18	504	0	1582	97	1.18
Pickle and pimiento loaf, pork	11.23	15.95	8.46	225	1.5	1040	58	6.96

Food Name ---> per 100 g	Protein (g)	Fat (g)	Carbohydrates (g)	Calories	Fiber (g)	Sodium (mg)	Cholesterol (mg)	Net Carbs
Polish sausage, pork	14.1	28.72	1.63	326	0	876	70	1.63
Luxury loaf, pork	18.4	4.8	4.9	141	0	1225	36	4.9
Mother's loaf, pork	12.07	22.3	7.53	282	0	1127	45	7.53
Picnic loaf, pork, beef	14.92	16.64	4.76	232	0	1164	38	4.76
Pork sausage, link/patty, unprepared	15.39	24.8	0.93	288	0	739	70	0.93
Pork sausage, link/patty, cooked, pan-fried	18.53	27.25	1.42	325	0	814	86	1.42
Pork and beef sausage, fresh, cooked	13.8	36.25	2.7	396	0	929	71	2.7
Turkey sausage, reduced fat, brown and serve, cooked (include BUTTERBALL breakfast links turkey sausage)	17	10.3	10.92	204	0.3	721	58	10.62
Poultry salad sandwich spread	11.64	13.52	7.41	200	0	653	30	7.41
Salami, cooked, beef	12.6	22.2	1.9	261	0	1140	71	1.9
Salami, cooked, beef and pork	21.85	25.9	2.4	336	0	1740	89	2.4
Salami, cooked, turkey	19.2	9.21	1.55	172	0.1	1107	76	1.45
Salami, dry or hard, pork	22.58	33.72	1.6	407	0	2260	79	1.6
Salami, dry or hard, pork, beef	21.07	31.65	0.72	378	0	1756	108	0.72
Sandwich spread, pork, beef	7.66	17.34	11.94	235	0.2	1013	38	11.74
Smoked link sausage, pork	11.98	28.23	0.94	309	0	827	61	0.94
Sausage, smoked link sausage, pork and beef	12	28.73	2.42	320	0	911	58	2.42
Smoked link sausage, pork and beef, nonfat dry milk added	13.28	27.61	1.92	313	0	1173	65	1.92
Thuringer, cervelat, summer sausage, beef, pork	17.45	30.43	3.33	362	0	1300	74	3.33
Turkey breast, sliced, prepackaged	16.33	2.37	2.34	100	0	922	50	2.34
Sausage, Vienna, canned, chicken, beef, pork	10.5	19.4	2.6	230	0	879	87	2.6
Honey roll sausage, beef	18.58	10.5	2.18	182	0	1322	50	2.18
Sausage, Italian, pork, cooked	19.12	27.31	4.27	344	0.1	743	57	4.17
Luncheon sausage, pork and beef	15.38	20.9	1.58	260	0	1182	64	1.58
New england brand sausage, pork, beef	17.27	7.58	4.83	161	0	1220	49	4.83
Turkey bacon, unprepared	15.94	16.93	1.89	226	-	1069	86	1.89
HORMEL Pillow Pak Sliced Turkey Pepperoni	30.99	11.52	3.78	243	0	1858	123	3.78
Turkey, pork, and beef sausage, low fat, smoked	8	2.5	11.54	101	0.6	796	21	10.94
USDA Commodity, pork, sausage, bulk/links/patties, frozen, cooked	19.76	20.26	0	267	0	540	98	0
Frankfurter, beef, pork, and turkey, fat free	12.5	1.59	11.21	109	0	880	41	11.21
Luncheon meat, pork, ham, and chicken, minced, canned, reduced sodium, added ascorbic acid, includes SPAM, 25% less sodium	12.5	25.1	3.4	293	0	1036	76	3.4
USDA Commodity, pork sausage, bulk/links/patties, frozen, raw	14.95	18.56	0	231	0	507	73	0
Luncheon meat, pork with ham, minced, canned, includes SPAM (Hormel)	13.4	26.6	4.6	315	0	1411	71	4.6
Luncheon meat, pork and chicken, minced, canned, includes SPAM Lite	15.23	13.9	1.35	196	0	1032	75	1.35
Bratwurst, veal, cooked	13.99	31.7	0	341	0	60	79	0
Liverwurst spread	12.38	25.45	5.89	305	2.5	700	118	3.39
Roast beef spread	15.27	16.28	3.73	223	0.2	724	70	3.53
Salami, pork, beef, less sodium	15.01	30.5	15.38	396	0.2	623	90	15.18
Sausage, Italian, sweet, links	16.13	8.42	2.1	149	0	570	30	2.1
Sausage, Polish, beef with chicken, hot	17.6	19.4	3.6	259	0	1540	66	3.6
Sausage, Polish, pork and beef, smoked	12.07	26.56	1.98	301	0	848	71	1.98
Sausage, pork and beef, with cheddar cheese, smoked	12.89	25.84	2.13	296	0	848	63	2.13
Sausage, summer, pork and beef, sticks, with	19.43	37.91	1.82	426	0.2	1483	89	1.62

Food Name ---> per 100 g	Protein (g)	Fat (g)	Carbohydrates (g)	Calories	Fiber (g)	Sodium (mg)	Cholesterol (mg)	Net Carbs
cheddar cheese								
Sausage, turkey, breakfast links, mild	15.42	18.09	1.56	235	0	639	160	1.56
Swisswurst, pork and beef, with swiss cheese, smoked	12.69	27.37	1.6	307	0	827	61	1.6
Bacon and beef sticks	29.1	44.2	0.8	517	0	1420	102	0.8
Bratwurst, beef and pork, smoked	12.2	26.34	2	297	0	848	78	2
Bratwurst, chicken, cooked	19.44	10.35	0	176	0	72	71	0
Bratwurst, pork, beef and turkey, lite, smoked	14.45	13.53	1.62	186	0	982	56	1.62
Pastrami, beef, 98% fat-free	19.6	1.16	1.54	95	0	1010	47	1.54
Salami, Italian, pork	21.7	37	1.2	425	0	1890	80	1.2
Sausage, Italian, turkey, smoked	15.05	8.75	4.65	158	0.9	928	53	3.75
Sausage, chicken, beef, pork, skinless, smoked	13.6	14.3	8.1	216	0	1034	120	8.1
Sausage, turkey, hot, smoked	15.05	8.75	4.65	158	0.3	916	53	4.35
Yachtwurst, with pistachio nuts, cooked	14.8	22.6	1.4	268	0	936	64	1.4
Beerwurst, pork and beef	14	22.53	4.27	276	0.9	732	62	3.37
Chicken breast, fat-free, mesquite flavor, sliced	16.8	0.39	2.25	80	0	1040	36	2.25
Chicken breast, oven-roasted, fat-free, sliced	16.79	0.39	2.17	79	0	1087	36	2.17
Kielbasa, Polish, turkey and beef, smoked	13.1	17.6	3.9	226	0	1200	70	3.9
Oven-roasted chicken breast roll	14.59	7.65	1.79	134	0	883	39	1.79
Bologna, pork and turkey, lite	13.06	16.06	3.45	211	0	716	79	3.45
Bologna, pork, turkey and beef	11.56	29.25	6.66	336	0	1055	75	6.66
Ham, honey, smoked, cooked	17.93	2.37	7.27	122	0	900	22	7.27
Frankfurter, pork	12.81	23.68	0.28	269	0.1	816	66	0.18
Macaroni and cheese loaf, chicken, pork and beef	11.76	14.96	11.63	228	0	3	44	11.63
Salami, Italian, pork and beef, dry, sliced, 50% less sodium	21.8	26.4	6.4	350	0	936	89	6.4
Pate, truffle flavor	11.2	28.5	6.3	327	-	807	105	6.3
Turkey, breast, smoked, lemon pepper flavor, 97% fat-free	20.9	0.69	1.31	95	0	1160	48	1.31
Turkey, white, rotisserie, deli cut	13.5	3	7.7	112	0.4	1200	55	7.3
Frankfurter, beef, heated	11.69	29.36	2.66	322	0	852	58	2.66
Frankfurter, meat, heated	9.77	24.31	4.9	278	0	1013	73	4.9
Frankfurter, meat	10.26	25.76	4.17	290	0	1090	77	4.17
Scrapple, pork	8.06	13.87	14.06	213	0.3	482	49	13.76
Bologna, chicken, turkey, pork	9.88	26.18	5.65	298	0	922	80	5.65
Pork sausage, link/patty, fully cooked, microwaved	15.12	41.66	0.62	438	0	990	79	0.62
Beef sausage, pre-cooked	15.5	37.57	0.03	405	0	822	83	0.03
Turkey sausage, fresh, raw	18.79	8.08	0.47	155	0	593	75	0.47
Beef sausage, fresh, cooked	18.21	27.98	0.35	332	0	813	82	0.35
Pork and turkey sausage, pre-cooked	12.05	30.64	3.63	342	0	876	72	3.63
Turkey sausage, fresh, cooked	23.89	10.44	0	196	0	665	92	0
Bologna, chicken, pork, beef	11.33	22.73	5.61	272	0	1120	83	5.61
Bologna, chicken, pork	10.31	30.61	4.19	336	0	1240	87	4.19
Chicken breast, deli, rotisserie seasoned, sliced, prepackaged	17.4	1.86	2.92	98	0	1032	51	2.92
Frankfurter, meat and poultry, unheated	9.72	24.18	5.02	277	0	976	78	5.02
Frankfurter, meat and poultry, cooked, boiled	10.31	26.28	4.96	298	0	914	84	4.96
Frankfurter, meat and poultry, cooked, grilled	10.67	26.43	5.24	302	0	1079	85	5.24
Pork sausage, link/patty, reduced fat, unprepared	16.75	16.55	0.2	217	0	581	67	0.2
Pork sausage, link/patty, reduced fat, cooked, pan-fried	20.94	20.32	0.15	267	0	698	82	0.15

Food Name ---> per 100 g	Protein (g)	Fat (g)	Carbohydrates (g)	Calories	Fiber (g)	Sodium (mg)	Cholesterol (mg)	Net Carbs
Pork sausage, link/patty, fully cooked, unheated	13.46	37.25	0.69	392	0	810	74	0.69
Kielbasa, fully cooked, grilled	12.45	29.68	5.03	337	0	1062	73	5.03
Kielbasa, fully cooked, pan-fried	12.36	29.43	4.78	333	0	1046	73	4.78
Kielbasa, fully cooked, unheated	10.84	29.63	3.72	325	0	928	61	3.72
Bologna, meat and poultry	10.34	23.77	6.31	281	0	1379	92	6.31
Meatballs, frozen, Italian style	14.4	22.21	8.06	286	2.3	666	66	5.76
Turkey bacon, microwaved	29.5	25.87	4.24	368	0	2021	153	4.24
Bacon, turkey, low sodium	13.33	20	4.8	253	0	900	100	4.8
Sausage, chicken or turkey, Italian style, lower sodium	21.43	4.46	14.25	183	0	446	36	14.25
Ham, smoked, extra lean, low sodium	18.52	2.71	10.7	141	0	1062	50	10.7
Pork sausage, reduced sodium, cooked	9.41	22.35	8.13	271	0	294	59	8.13
Sausage, pork, turkey, and beef, reduced sodium	10.71	26.79	0.11	284	0.1	679	70	0.01
Beef, cured, corned beef, canned	27.1	14.93	0	250	0	897	86	0
Beef, cured, dried	31.1	1.94	2.76	153	0	2790	79	2.76
Beef, cured, luncheon meat, jellied	19	3.3	0	111	0	1322	34	0
Beef, cured, pastrami	21.8	5.82	0.36	147	0	1078	68	0.36
Beef, cured, sausage, cooked, smoked	14.11	26.91	2.42	312	0	1131	67	2.42
Beef, cured, smoked, chopped beef	20.19	4.42	1.86	133	0	1258	46	1.86
Turkey ham, sliced, extra lean, prepackaged or deli-sliced	19.6	3.8	2.93	124	0	1038	67	2.93
Bologna, beef and pork, low fat	11.5	19.3	2.6	230	0	1108	39	2.6
Bologna, beef, low fat	11.8	14.8	5.2	204	0	821	44	5.2
Turkey and pork sausage, fresh, bulk, patty or link, cooked	22.7	23	0.7	307	0	878	84	0.7
Frankfurter, beef, low fat	12	9.5	1.6	233	0	744	40	1.6
Pork sausage rice links, brown and serve, cooked	13.7	37.63	2.36	407	0	689	66	2.36
Frankfurter, meat and poultry, low fat	15.5	2.8	8.4	121	0.1	983	44	8.3
Beef, bologna, reduced sodium	11.7	28.4	2	310	0	682	56	2
Frankfurter, low sodium	12	28.51	1.8	312	0	311	61	1.8

Snacks

Food Name ---> per 100 g	Protein (g)	Fat (g)	Carb (g)	Calories	Fiber (g)	Sodium (mg)	Cholesterol (mg)	Net Carb (g)
Snacks, beef jerky, chopped and formed	33.2	25.6	11	410	1.8	2081	48	9.2
Snacks, corn-based, extruded, chips, plain	6.17	33.36	56.9	538	4	514	0	52.9
Snacks, corn-based, extruded, chips, barbecue-flavor	7	32.7	56.2	523	5.2	763	0	51
Snacks, corn-based, extruded, cones, plain	5.8	26.9	62.9	510	1.1	1022	0	61.8
Snacks, corn-based, extruded, onion-flavor	7.7	22.6	65.1	499	3.9	950	0	61.2
Snacks, corn-based, extruded, puffs or twists, cheese-flavor	5.85	36.01	53.53	560	1.4	942	7	52.13
Snacks, KRAFT, CORNNUTS, plain	8.5	15.64	71.86	446	6.9	564	0	64.96
Snacks, crisped rice bar, chocolate chip	5.1	13.5	73	404	2.2	278	0	70.8
Snacks, granola bars, hard, plain	10.1	19.8	64.4	471	5.3	294	0	59.1
Snacks, granola bars, hard, almond	7.7	25.5	62	495	4.8	256	0	57.2
Snacks, granola bars, hard, chocolate chip	7.3	16.3	72.1	438	4.4	344	0	67.7
Snacks, granola bars, soft, uncoated, plain	7.4	17.2	67.3	443	4.6	278	0	62.7
Snacks, granola bars, soft, uncoated, peanut butter	10.5	15.8	64.4	426	4.3	409	0	60.1
Snacks, granola bars, soft, uncoated, raisin	7.6	17.8	66.4	448	4.2	282	0	62.2
Snacks, granola bars, soft, coated, milk chocolate coating, chocolate chip	5.8	24.9	63.8	466	3.4	200	5	60.4
Snacks, granola bars, soft, coated, milk chocolate coating, peanut butter	10.2	31.1	53.4	508	2.8	193	12	50.6
Snacks, granola bars, soft, uncoated, peanut butter and chocolate chip	9.8	20	62.2	432	4.2	328	1	58
Snacks, oriental mix, rice-based	17.31	25.58	51.62	506	13.2	413	0	38.42
Snacks, GENERAL MILLS, CHEX MIX, traditional flavor	8.83	10	75.69	428	5.8	696	4	69.89
Snacks, popcorn, air-popped	12.94	4.54	77.78	387	14.5	8	0	63.28
Snacks, popcorn, oil-popped, microwave, regular flavor, no trans fat	7.29	43.55	45.06	583	8.1	679	0	36.96
Snacks, popcorn, cakes	9.7	3.1	80.1	384	2.9	288	0	77.2
Snacks, popcorn, caramel-coated, with peanuts	6.4	7.8	80.7	400	3.8	177	0	76.9
Snacks, popcorn, caramel-coated, without peanuts	3.8	12.8	79.1	431	5.2	206	0	73.9
Snacks, popcorn, cheese-flavor	9.3	33.2	51.6	526	9.9	889	11	41.7
Snacks, pork skins, plain	61.3	31.3	0	544	0	1818	95	0
Snacks, potato chips, barbecue-flavor	6.51	31.06	55.92	487	3.8	545	0	52.12
Snacks, potato chips, sour-cream-and-onion-flavor	8.1	33.9	51.5	531	5.2	549	7	46.3
Snacks, potato chips, made from dried potatoes, reduced fat	4.56	26.14	64.76	502	3.2	450	0	61.56
Snacks, potato chips, made from dried potatoes, sour-cream and onion-flavor	6.6	37	51.3	547	1.2	541	3	50.1
Snacks, pretzels, hard, plain, salted	10.04	2.93	80.39	384	3.4	1240	0	76.99
Snacks, pretzels, hard, confectioner's coating, chocolate-flavor	7.5	16.7	70.9	457	2.4	569	0	68.5
Snacks, M&M MARS, COMBOS Snacks Cheddar Cheese Pretzel	9.85	16.92	66.5	463	3.6	1117	5	62.9
Snacks, pretzels, hard, whole-wheat including both salted and unsalted	11.1	2.6	81.3	362	7.7	203	0	73.6
Snacks, rice cracker brown rice, plain	8.2	2.8	81.5	387	4.2	326	0	77.3
Snacks, rice cakes, brown rice, buckwheat	9	3.5	80.1	380	3.8	116	0	76.3

Food Name ---> per 100 g	Protein (g)	Fat (g)	Carb (g)	Calories	Fiber (g)	Sodium (mg)	Cholesterol (mg)	Net Carb (g)
Snacks, rice cakes, brown rice, sesame seed	7.6	3.8	81.5	392	5.4	227	0	76.1
Snacks, tortilla chips, plain, white corn, salted	7.1	20.68	67.78	472	5.4	328	0	62.38
Snacks, tortilla chips, nacho cheese	7.36	27.42	60.81	519	5.1	691	0	55.71
Snacks, tortilla chips, ranch-flavor	7.19	24.63	62.74	501	4	519	-	58.74
Snacks, trail mix, regular	13.8	29.4	44.9	462	-	229	0	44.9
Snacks, trail mix, tropical	6.3	17.1	65.6	442	-	95	0	65.6
Snacks, trail mix, regular, with chocolate chips, salted nuts and seeds	14.2	31.9	44.9	484	5	121	4	39.9
Snacks, tortilla chips, taco-flavor	7.9	24.2	63.1	480	5.3	787	0	57.8
Snacks, GENERAL MILLS, BETTY CROCKER Fruit Roll Ups, berry flavored, with vitamin C	0.1	3.5	85.2	373	-	317	-	85.2
Snacks, FARLEY CANDY, FARLEY Fruit Snacks, with vitamins A, C, and E	4.4	0	80.9	341	-	36	-	80.9
Snacks, SUNKIST, SUNKIST Fruit Roll, strawberry, with vitamins A, C, and E	0.6	1	82.7	342	7.7	111	-	75
Snacks, fruit leather, pieces, with vitamin C	0.1	3.5	85.2	373	3.5	317	0	81.7
Snacks, banana chips	2.3	33.6	58.4	519	7.7	6	0	50.7
Snacks, cornnuts, barbecue-flavor	9	14.3	71.7	436	8.4	600	0	63.3
Snacks, crisped rice bar, almond	7	20.4	64.6	458	3.6	234	0	61
Snacks, granola bars, soft, uncoated, chocolate chip	5.65	16.57	70.2	418	3.8	251	0	66.4
Snacks, granola bars, soft, uncoated, chocolate chip, graham and marshmallow	6.1	15.5	70.8	427	4	316	0	66.8
Snacks, granola bars, soft, uncoated, nut and raisin	8	20.4	63.6	454	5.6	254	0	58
Snacks, beef sticks, smoked	21.5	49.6	5.4	550	-	1531	133	5.4
Snacks, pork skins, barbecue-flavor	57.9	31.8	1.6	538	-	2667	115	1.6
Snack, potato chips, made from dried potatoes, plain	4.62	35.28	55.38	545	2.9	400	0	52.48
Snacks, potato chips, plain, salted	6.39	33.98	53.83	532	3.1	527	0	50.73
Snacks, potato chips, made from dried potatoes, cheese-flavor	7	37	50.6	551	3.4	600	4	47.2
Snacks, rice cakes, brown rice, corn	8.4	3.2	81.2	385	2.9	167	0	78.3
Snacks, rice cakes, brown rice, multigrain	8.5	3.5	80.1	387	3	252	0	77.1
Snacks, potato sticks	6.7	34.4	53.3	522	3.4	633	0	49.9
Snacks, rice cakes, brown rice, rye	8.1	3.8	79.9	386	4	110	0	75.9
Snacks, sesame sticks, wheat-based, salted	10.9	36.7	46.5	541	2.8	1488	0	43.7
Snacks, corn cakes	8.1	2.4	83.4	387	1.9	488	0	81.5
Snacks, granola bars, hard, peanut butter	9.8	23.8	62.3	483	2.9	283	0	59.4
Snacks, potato chips, cheese-flavor	8.5	27.2	57.7	496	5.2	458	4	52.5
Snacks, potato chips, reduced fat	7.1	20.8	66.9	471	5.9	492	0	61
Snacks, potato chips, fat-free, made with olestra	7.74	0.7	65	274	6.8	554	0	58.2
Snacks, tortilla chips, nacho-flavor, reduced fat	8.7	15.2	71.6	445	4.8	1003	3	66.8
Tortilla chips, low fat, baked without fat	11	5.7	80	415	5.3	517	0	74.7
Cheese puffs and twists, corn based, baked, low fat	8.5	12.1	72.35	432	3.6	847	1	68.75
Snacks, granola bar, fruit-filled, nonfat	5.9	0.9	77.6	342	7.4	16	0	70.2
Popcorn, sugar syrup/caramel, fat-free	2	1.4	90.06	381	2.5	286	0	87.56
Snacks, potato chips, fat free, salted	9.64	0.6	83.76	379	7.5	643	0	76.26
Snacks, KELLOGG, KELLOGG'S RICE KRISPIES TREATS Squares	3.4	9	80.5	414	0	351	0	80.5
Snacks, KELLOGG, KELLOGG'S Low Fat Granola Bar, Crunchy Almond/Brown Sugar	8	7.4	78	390	6.2	291	0	71.8

Food Name ---> per 100 g	Protein (g)	Fat (g)	Carb (g)	Calories	Fiber (g)	Sodium (mg)	Cholesterol (mg)	Net Carb (g)
Snacks, M&M MARS, KUDOS Whole Grain Bar, chocolate chip	4.47	13.02	72.31	420	2.6	246	0	69.71
Snacks, KELLOGG'S, NUTRI-GRAIN Cereal Bars, fruit	4.22	8.67	67.61	365	3	354	0	64.61
Snacks, tortilla chips, low fat, made with olestra, nacho cheese	8.44	3.53	65.22	318	6.4	705	2	58.82
Snacks, potato chips, made from dried potatoes, fat-free, made with olestra	5.06	0.93	56	253	7.3	429	0	48.7
Snacks, taro chips	2.3	24.9	68.1	498	7.2	342	0	60.9
Snacks, corn cakes, very low sodium	8.1	2.4	83.4	387	-	28	0	83.4
Snacks, corn-based, extruded, puffs or twists, cheese-flavor, unenriched	5.76	35.76	54.1	558	2.2	896	4	51.9
Snacks, corn-based, extruded, chips, barbecue-flavor, made with enriched masa flour	7	32.7	56.2	523	-	763	0	56.2
Snacks, popcorn, air-popped (Unsalted)	12	4.2	77.9	382	15.1	4	0	62.8
Snacks, popcorn, oil-popped, white popcorn, salt added	9	28.1	57.2	500	10	884	0	47.2
Snacks, potato chips, plain, made with partially hydrogenated soybean oil, salted	7	34.6	52.9	536	4.8	594	0	48.1
Snacks, potato chips, plain, made with partially hydrogenated soybean oil, unsalted	7	34.6	52.9	536	4.8	8	0	48.1
Snacks, potato chips, plain, unsalted	7	34.6	52.9	536	4.8	8	0	48.1
Snacks, pretzels, hard, plain, made with unenriched flour, salted	9.1	3.5	79.2	381	2.8	1715	0	76.4
Snacks, pretzels, hard, plain, made with unenriched flour, unsalted	9.1	3.5	79.2	381	2.8	289	0	76.4
Snacks, pretzels, hard, plain, made with enriched flour, unsalted	9.1	3.5	79.2	381	2.8	250	0	76.4
Snacks, rice cakes, brown rice, plain, unsalted	8.2	2.8	81.5	387	4.2	26	0	77.3
Snacks, rice cakes, brown rice, buckwheat, unsalted	9	3.5	80.1	380	-	4	0	80.1
Snacks, rice cakes, brown rice, multigrain, unsalted	8.5	3.5	80.1	387	-	4	0	80.1
Snacks, rice cakes, brown rice, sesame seed, unsalted	7.6	3.8	81.5	392	-	4	0	81.5
Snacks, sesame sticks, wheat-based, unsalted	10.9	36.7	46.5	541	-	29	0	46.5
Snacks, trail mix, regular, unsalted	13.8	29.4	44.9	462	-	10	0	44.9
Snacks, trail mix, regular, with chocolate chips, unsalted nuts and seeds	14.2	31.9	44.9	484	-	27	0	44.9
Potato chips, without salt, reduced fat	7.1	20.8	67.8	487	6.1	8	0	61.7
Snacks, tortilla chips, low fat, unsalted	11	5.7	80.1	416	5.3	15	0	74.8
Snacks, tortilla chips, nacho-flavor, made with enriched masa flour	7.8	25.6	62.4	498	5.3	708	3	57.1
Snacks, popcorn, microwave, 94% fat free	10.72	6.1	76.04	402	13.6	571	0	62.44
Snacks, popcorn, microwave, low fat	12.6	9.5	72	424	14.2	540	0	57.8
Snacks, candy rolls, yogurt-covered, fruit flavored with high vitamin C	0.46	6.53	74.64	359	3.3	8	0	71.34
Formulated bar, MARS SNACKFOOD US, SNICKERS MARATHON Chewy Chocolate Peanut Bar	24.29	13.12	47.24	396	2.5	462	4	44.74
Formulated bar, MARS SNACKFOOD US, SNICKERS MARATHON MULTIGRAIN CRUNCH BAR	18.49	13.18	57.27	422	2.8	418	3	54.47
Formulated bar, MARS SNACKFOOD US, SNICKERS MARATHON Double Chocolate Nut Bar	22.35	8.99	52.47	343	10.5	333	4	41.97

Food Name ---> per 100 g	Protein (g)	Fat (g)	Carb (g)	Calories	Fiber (g)	Sodium (mg)	Cholesterol (mg)	Net Carb (g)
Snacks, M&M MARS, KUDOS Whole Grain Bars, peanut butter	5.88	20.78	64.69	463	2.6	268	0	62.09
Formulated bar, MARS SNACKFOOD US, SNICKERS MARATHON Honey Nut Oat Bar	22.5	7.87	54.3	378	11	318	-	43.3
Snacks, M&M MARS, KUDOS Whole Grain Bar, M&M's milk chocolate	3.78	11.95	73.01	415	2.4	341	4	70.61
Formulated bar, MARS SNACKFOOD US, COCOAVIA, Chocolate Almond Snack Bar	7.72	14.19	51.68	347	5.2	260	2	46.48
Snacks, sweet potato chips, unsalted	2.94	32.35	56.82	532	8.8	35	0	48.02
Snacks, FRITOLAY, SUNCHIPS, Multigrain Snack, original flavor	7.95	21.11	67.26	491	8.8	423	0	58.46
Snacks, popcorn, microwave, regular (butter) flavor, made with partially hydrogenated oil	7.5	34.02	55.16	557	10	764	0	45.16
Formulated bar, MARS SNACKFOOD US, SNICKERS MARATHON Protein Performance Bar, Caramel Nut Rush	25	12.5	50.5	415	12.5	238	6	38
Formulated bar, MARS SNACKFOOD US, SNICKERS MARATHON Energy Bar, all flavors	21.91	10.79	50.3	386	6.7	383	4	43.6
Formulated bar, POWER BAR, chocolate	14.15	3.11	69.63	363	5.7	308	0	63.93
Formulated bar, MARS SNACKFOOD US, COCOAVIA, Chocolate Blueberry Snack Bar	6.21	9.27	57.87	325	4.6	260	2	53.27
Formulated bar, SLIM-FAST OPTIMA meal bar, milk chocolate peanut	16.19	8.92	60.21	386	5.1	253	7	55.11
Formulated bar, LUNA BAR, NUTZ OVER CHOCOLATE	20.75	12.19	52.49	403	4.3	386	0	48.19
Snacks, FRITOLAY, SUNCHIPS, multigrain, French onion flavor	8.68	22.15	65.49	496	7.8	467	0	57.69
Snacks, FRITOLAY, SUNCHIPS, Multigrain Snack, Harvest Cheddar flavor	8.08	22.22	64.7	491	8.1	705	0	56.6
Pretzels, soft, unsalted	8.2	3.1	71.04	345	1.7	252	0	69.34
Snacks, soy chips or crisps, salted	26.5	7.35	53.15	385	3.5	842	0	49.65
Popcorn, microwave, regular (butter) flavor, made with palm oil	8.38	30.22	57.26	535	10	763	0	47.26
Snacks, plantain chips, salted	2.28	29.59	63.84	531	3.5	202	0	60.34
Tortilla chips, yellow, plain, salted	6.62	22.33	67.38	497	4.7	310	0	62.68
Snacks, vegetable chips, HAIN CELESTIAL GROUP, TERRA CHIPS	4.13	29.81	57.97	517	10.9	246	0	47.07
Formulated bar, ZONE PERFECT CLASSIC CRUNCH BAR, mixed flavors	30	14	45	422	2	520	8	43
Snacks, granola bar, KASHI GOLEAN, chewy, mixed flavors	16.67	7.69	63.42	390	7.7	321	6	55.72
Snacks, granola bar, KASHI TLC Bar, chewy, mixed flavors	18.57	15.71	53.26	429	11.4	293	0	41.86
Snacks, granola bar, KASHI GOLEAN, crunchy, mixed flavors	17.88	9.23	59.58	393	5.9	486	0	53.68
Snacks, granola bar, chewy, reduced sugar, all flavors	5.55	12.5	69.4	412	3.1	312	0	66.3
Snacks, granola bites, mixed flavors	7.17	17.5	66.27	451	5.7	167	0	60.57
Snacks, pita chips, salted	11.79	15.2	68.26	457	3.8	854	0	64.46
Snacks, granola bars, soft, almond, confectioners coating	8.6	20	60.13	455	4.3	486	0	55.83
Snacks, granola bars, QUAKER OATMEAL TO GO, all flavors	6.67	6.67	75.47	389	4.6	367	36	70.87
Snacks, vegetable chips, made from garden vegetables	5.32	23.3	60.43	473	4.7	357	0	55.73

Food Name ---> per 100 g	Protein (g)	Fat (g)	Carb (g)	Calories	Fiber (g)	Sodium (mg)	Cholesterol (mg)	Net Carb (g)
Snacks, granola bar, KASHI TLC Bar, crunchy, mixed flavors	15	15	62.78	446	10	400	0	52.78
Snacks, candy bits, yogurt covered with vitamin C	0	7.5	86.9	415	0.2	75	3	86.7
Formulated bar, high fiber, chewy, oats and chocolate	5	10	69.78	350	22.5	350	0	47.28
Snacks, bagel chips, plain	12.34	15.14	66.36	451	4.1	233	0	62.26
Snacks, NUTRI-GRAIN FRUIT AND NUT BAR	9.38	10.93	66.72	403	7.5	195	0	59.22
Snacks, yucca (cassava) chips, salted	1.34	25.91	69.23	515	3.7	296	-	65.53
Snacks, CLIF BAR, mixed flavors	14.71	5.88	65.44	346	7.4	195	0	58.04
Snacks, granola bar, QUAKER, chewy, 90 Calorie Bar	4.17	8.33	79.17	408	4.2	313	0	74.97
Snacks, granola bar, GENERAL MILLS NATURE VALLEY, SWEET&SALTY NUT, peanut	9.14	22.86	61.14	487	2.9	414	0	58.24
Snacks, granola bar, GENERAL MILLS, NATURE VALLEY, with yogurt coating	5.71	11.43	74.29	423	4.4	271	0	69.89
Snacks, granola bar, GENERAL MILLS, NATURE VALLEY, CHEWY TRAIL MIX	5.71	11.43	72.27	415	3.8	185	0	68.47
Snacks, granola bar, QUAKER, DIPPS, all flavors	7.52	20.42	64.96	480	3.2	269	0	61.76
Snacks, brown rice chips	8.2	2.8	81.5	384	4.2	326	0	77.3
Snack, Pretzel, hard chocolate coated	7.05	17.64	70.07	467	3.5	494	0	66.57
Snack, Mixed Berry Bar	13.16	10.53	58.84	383	7.9	447	0	50.94
Snacks, potato chips, made from dried potatoes (preformed), multigrain	5.3	24.74	65.34	505	2.7	544	0	62.64
Snacks, potato chips, lightly salted	6.72	35.39	53.54	560	4.2	187	0	49.34
Snacks, Pretzels, gluten- free made with cornstarch and potato flour	3.52	6.67	78.62	389	3.3	1567	0	75.32
Snacks, peas, roasted, wasabi-flavored	14.11	14.11	62.2	432	3.8	300	0	58.4
Formulated Bar, SOUTH BEACH protein bar	30.34	15.17	38.4	412	7.3	436	3	31.1
Snack, BALANCE, original bar	28	12	48.73	415	3.1	253	1	45.63
Snacks, shrimp cracker	7.14	17.86	59.09	426	5.6	571	2	53.49
Rice crackers	10	5	82.64	416	0	233	0	82.64
Granola bar, soft, milk chocolate coated, peanut butter	9.6	31.2	54.1	536	3.8	193	12	50.3
Rice cake, cracker (include hain mini rice cakes)	7.1	4.3	81.1	392	4.2	71	0	76.9
Snacks, popcorn, home-prepared, oil-popped, unsalted	9	28.1	58.1	500	10	3	0	48.1
Snacks, granola bar, with coconut, chocolate coated	5.2	32.2	55.2	531	6.2	152	0	49
Snacks, potato chips, white, restructured, baked	5	18.2	71.4	469	4.8	554	0	66.6
Breakfast bars, oats, sugar, raisins, coconut (include granola bar)	9.8	17.6	66.7	464	3.1	251	0	63.6
Pretzels, soft	8.2	3.1	69.39	338	1.7	545	0	67.69
Snacks, tortilla chips, unsalted, white corn	7.79	23.36	65.32	503	5.3	15	0	60.02
Snacks, corn-based, extruded, chips, unsalted	6.6	33.4	57.4	557	4.4	15	0	53
Snacks, tortilla chips, light (baked with less oil)	8.7	15.2	73.4	465	5.7	564	0	67.7
Popcorn, microwave, low fat and sodium	12.6	9.5	73.39	429	14.2	490	0	59.19
Breakfast bar, corn flake crust with fruit	4.4	7.5	72.9	377	2.1	297	0	70.8

Soups, Sauces, and Gravies

Food Name ---> per 100 g	Protein (g)	Fat (g)	Carb (g)	Calories	Fiber (g)	Sodium (mg)	Cholesterol (mg)	Net Carb (g)
Soup, egg drop, Chinese restaurant	1.16	0.61	4.29	27	0.4	370	23	3.89
Soup, hot and sour, Chinese restaurant	2.58	1.21	4.35	39	0.5	376	21	3.85
Soup, wonton, Chinese restaurant	2.08	0.26	5.25	32	0.2	406	4	5.05
CAMPBELL'S CHUNKY Soups, HEALTHY REQUEST Microwavable Bowls, Chicken Noodle Soup	2.86	1.02	6.94	49	0.4	167	6	6.54
CAMPBELL'S CHUNKY Soups, HEALTHY REQUEST Microwavable Bowls, Grilled Chicken & Sausage Gumbo Soup	2.86	1.22	7.35	53	0.8	167	4	6.55
CAMPBELL'S CHUNKY Soups, HEALTHY REQUEST New England Clam Chowder	2.04	1.22	8.16	53	0.8	167	4	7.36
CAMPBELL'S Red and White, Chicken Barley with Mushrooms Soup, condensed	3.17	1.19	12.7	71	2.4	571	4	10.3
CAMPBELL'S Red and White, Italian Style Wedding Soup, condensed	3.17	1.98	9.52	71	2.4	643	8	7.12
CAMPBELL'S Red and White, PHINEAS and FERB Soup, condensed	2.38	1.59	8.73	56	0.8	627	4	7.93
CAMPBELL'S Homestyle Microwaveable Bowls, HEALTHY REQUEST Italian Wedding Soup	2.45	1.02	5.31	41	0.8	167	4	4.51
CAMPBELL'S Homestyle Microwaveable Bowls, HEALTHY REQUEST Mexican Style Tortilla	2.86	1.02	7.76	53	1.2	167	4	6.56
CAMPBELL'S Homestyle Harvest Tomato with Basil Soup	0.82	0.41	9.39	45	0.8	322	2	8.59
CAMPBELL'S Homestyle HEALTHY REQUEST Chicken with Whole Grain Pasta Soup	3.8	0.82	4.28	40	0.7	167	4	3.58
CAMPBELL'S Soup on the GO, HEALTHY REQUEST Chicken with Mini Noodles Soup	0.98	0.66	2.62	20	0.7	134	3	1.92
CAMPBELL'S Soup on the Go, HEALTHY REQUEST Classic Tomato Soup	0.98	0	9.18	39	0.7	134	0	8.48
PACE, Pico De Gallo	0	0	9.38	31	-	469	0	9.38
PACE, Salsa Verde	0	1.56	6.25	47	0	719	0	6.25
PACE, Tequila Lime Salsa	0	0	9.38	47	0	594	0	9.38
PACE, Triple Pepper Salsa	3.13	0	9.38	47	3.1	594	0	6.28
CAMPBELL'S Red and White, Lentil Soup, condensed	6.35	0.79	19.05	111	4	635	0	15.05
PREGO Pasta, Heart Smart- Traditional Sauce, ready-to-serve	1.54	1.15	10	54	2.3	277	0	7.7
CAMPBELL'S, 98% Fat Free Cream of Mushroom Soup, condensed	1.1	1.98	7.63	53	1.2	392	0	6.43
Soup, ramen noodle, dry, any flavor, reduced fat, reduced sodium	10.89	2.5	70.95	350	2.7	1200	0	68.25
Soup, clam chowder, new england, canned, ready-to-serve	2.61	3.94	8.28	79	1	343	-	7.28
Soup, clam chowder, new england, reduced sodium, canned, ready-to-serve	2.33	4.23	5.68	70	0.8	194	3	4.88

Food Name ---> per 100 g	Protein (g)	Fat (g)	Carb (g)	Calories	Fiber (g)	Sodium (mg)	Cholesterol (mg)	Net Carb (g)
Soup, chicken noodle, reduced sodium, canned, ready-to-serve	3.29	1.34	3.84	41	0.8	186	4	3.04
Soup, beef and vegetables, reduced sodium, canned, ready-to-serve	3.26	0.95	4.99	42	0.8	175	-	4.19
Sauce, duck, ready-to-serve	0.36	0.13	60.61	245	0.6	455	0	60.01
Sauce, salsa, verde, ready-to-serve	1.13	0.89	6.36	38	1.9	600	0	4.46
Sauce, steak, tomato based	1.25	0.23	22.04	95	1.5	1647	0	20.54
Sauce, tartar, ready-to-serve	1	16.7	13.3	211	0.5	667	7	12.8
Sauce, sweet and sour, ready-to-serve	0.27	0.02	38.22	150	0.1	371	0	38.12
Sauce, cocktail, ready-to-serve	1.36	1.05	28.22	124	1.8	983	0	26.42
Dip, salsa con queso, cheese and salsa- medium	3.14	9.51	11.14	143	0.7	796	9	10.44
Dip, OLD EL PASO, Cheese 'n Salsa, medium	2.7	8.43	10.65	129	0.6	690	5	10.05
Dip, TOSTITOS, salsa con queso, medium	2.92	8.26	11.72	133	0.6	773	9	11.12
Sauce, barbecue, SWEET BABY RAY'S, original	0.95	0.43	46.08	192	1.3	765	-	44.78
Sauce, barbecue, BULL'S-EYE, original	0.91	0.67	39.95	170	1	1012	-	38.95
Sauce, barbecue, KC MASTERPIECE, original	1	0.52	37.92	160	1.4	613	-	36.52
Sauce, barbecue, OPEN PIT, original	0.44	1.41	29.45	132	0.5	1517	-	28.95
Sauce, peanut, made from peanut butter, water, soy sauce	6.31	16.02	22.02	257	1.8	1338	0	20.22
Soup, chunky vegetable, reduced sodium, canned, ready-to-serve	1.16	0.51	10.28	50	1.1	138	1	9.18
Gravy, HEINZ Home Style, classic chicken	0.67	2.57	5.01	46	-	372	4	5.01
Soup, beef barley, ready to serve	2.81	0.96	7.94	52	0.9	297	4	7.04
Sauce, enchilada, red, mild, ready to serve	0.62	0.91	4.87	30	0.5	547	0	4.37
Wasabi	2.23	10.9	46.13	292	6.1	3390	0	40.03
Dip, bean, original flavor	5.44	3.7	15.89	119	4.9	443	0	10.99
Sauce, horseradish	1.09	50.89	10.05	503	1	730	50	9.05
Sauce, OLD EL PASO, enchilada, red, mild, ready to serve	0.59	0.67	5.04	29	0.6	543	-	4.44
Dip, FRITO'S, bean, original flavor	5.44	3.7	15.89	119	4.9	443	-	10.99

Spices and Herbs

Food Name ---> per 100 g	Protein (g)	Fat (g)	Carb (g)	Calories	Fiber (g)	Sodium (mg)	Cholesterol (mg)	Net Carbs
Spices, allspice, ground	6.09	8.69	72.12	263	21.6	77	0	50.52
Spices, anise seed	17.6	15.9	50.02	337	14.6	16	0	35.42
Spices, basil, dried	22.98	4.07	47.75	233	37.7	76	0	10.05
Spices, bay leaf	7.61	8.36	74.97	313	26.3	23	0	48.67
Spices, caraway seed	19.77	14.59	49.9	333	38	17	0	11.9
Spices, cardamom	10.76	6.7	68.47	311	28	18	0	40.47
Spices, celery seed	18.07	25.27	41.35	392	11.8	160	0	29.55
Spices, chervil, dried	23.2	3.9	49.1	237	11.3	83	0	37.8
Spices, chili powder	13.46	14.28	49.7	282	34.8	2867	0	14.9
Spices, cinnamon, ground	3.99	1.24	80.59	247	53.1	10	0	27.49
Spices, cloves, ground	5.97	13	65.53	274	33.9	277	0	31.63
Spices, coriander leaf, dried	21.93	4.78	52.1	279	10.4	211	0	41.7
Spices, coriander seed	12.37	17.77	54.99	298	41.9	35	0	13.09
Spices, cumin seed	17.81	22.27	44.24	375	10.5	168	0	33.74
Spices, curry powder	14.29	14.01	55.83	325	53.2	52	0	2.63
Spices, dill seed	15.98	14.54	55.17	305	21.1	20	0	34.07
Spices, dill weed, dried	19.96	4.36	55.82	253	13.6	208	0	42.22
Spices, fennel seed	15.8	14.87	52.29	345	39.8	88	0	12.49
Spices, fenugreek seed	23	6.41	58.35	323	24.6	67	0	33.75
Spices, garlic powder	16.55	0.73	72.73	331	9	60	0	63.73
Spices, ginger, ground	8.98	4.24	71.62	335	14.1	27	0	57.52
Spices, mace, ground	6.71	32.38	50.5	475	20.2	80	0	30.3
Spices, marjoram, dried	12.66	7.04	60.56	271	40.3	77	0	20.26
Spices, mustard seed, ground	26.08	36.24	28.09	508	12.2	13	0	15.89
Spices, nutmeg, ground	5.84	36.31	49.29	525	20.8	16	0	28.49
Spices, onion powder	10.41	1.04	79.12	341	15.2	73	0	63.92
Spices, oregano, dried	9	4.28	68.92	265	42.5	25	0	26.42
Spices, paprika	14.14	12.89	53.99	282	34.9	68	0	19.09
Spices, parsley, dried	26.63	5.48	50.64	292	26.7	452	0	23.94
Spices, pepper, black	10.39	3.26	63.95	251	25.3	20	0	38.65
Spices, pepper, red or cayenne	12.01	17.27	56.63	318	27.2	30	0	29.43
Spices, pepper, white	10.4	2.12	68.61	296	26.2	5	0	42.41
Spices, poppy seed	17.99	41.56	28.13	525	19.5	26	0	8.63
Spices, poultry seasoning	9.59	7.53	65.59	307	11.3	27	0	54.29
Spices, pumpkin pie spice	5.76	12.6	69.28	342	14.8	52	0	54.48
Spices, rosemary, dried	4.88	15.22	64.06	331	42.6	50	0	21.46
Spices, saffron	11.43	5.85	65.37	310	3.9	148	0	61.47
Spices, sage, ground	10.63	12.75	60.73	315	40.3	11	0	20.43
Spices, savory, ground	6.73	5.91	68.73	272	45.7	24	0	23.03
Spices, tarragon, dried	22.77	7.24	50.22	295	7.4	62	0	42.82
Spices, thyme, dried	9.11	7.43	63.94	276	37	55	0	26.94
Spices, turmeric, ground	9.68	3.25	67.14	312	22.7	27	0	44.44
Basil, fresh	3.15	0.64	2.65	23	1.6	4	0	1.05
Dill weed, fresh	3.46	1.12	7.02	43	2.1	61	0	4.92
Mustard, prepared, yellow	3.74	3.34	5.83	60	4	1104	0	1.83
Salt, table	0	0	0	0	0	38758	0	0
Vinegar, cider	0	0	0.93	21	0	5	0	0.93

Food Name ---> per 100 g	Protein (g)	Fat (g)	Carb (g)	Calories	Fiber (g)	Sodium (mg)	Cholesterol (mg)	Net Carbs
Thyme, fresh	5.56	1.68	24.45	101	14	9	0	10.45
Vanilla extract	0.06	0.06	12.65	288	0	9	0	12.65
Vanilla extract, imitation, alcohol	0.05	0	2.41	237	0	4	0	2.41
Vanilla extract, imitation, no alcohol	0.03	0	14.4	56	0	3	0	14.4
Vinegar, distilled	0	0	0.04	18	0	2	0	0.04
Capers, canned	2.36	0.86	4.89	23	3.2	2348	0	1.69
Horseradish, prepared	1.18	0.69	11.29	48	3.3	420	0	7.99
Rosemary, fresh	3.31	5.86	20.7	131	14.1	26	0	6.6
Peppermint, fresh	3.75	0.94	14.89	70	8	31	0	6.89
Spearmint, fresh	3.29	0.73	8.41	44	6.8	30	0	1.61
Spearmint, dried	19.93	6.03	52.04	285	29.8	344	0	22.24
Vinegar, red wine	0.04	0	0.27	19	0	8	-	0.27
Vinegar, balsamic	0.49	0	17.03	88	-	23	-	17.03
PACE, Dry Taco Seasoning Mix	0	0	56.29	188	18.8	8068	0	37.49
Seasoning mix, dry, sazon, coriander & annatto	0	0	0	0	0	17000	0	0
Seasoning mix, dry, taco, original	4.5	0	58	322	13.3	7203	0	44.7
Seasoning mix, dry, chili, original	10.82	7.3	56.56	335	10.8	4616	0	45.76

Sweets

Food Name ---> per 100 g	Protein (g)	Fat (g)	Carb (g)	Calories	Fiber (g)	Sodium (mg)	Cholesterol (mg)	Net Carb (g)
SCHIFF, TIGER'S MILK BAR	16.8	14.29	56.46	422	2.3	168	2	54.16
Candies, TOBLERONE, milk chocolate with honey and almond nougat	5.71	28.57	61.21	525	2.5	54	14	58.71
Snacks, fruit leather, pieces	1	2.68	82.82	359	0	403	0	82.82
Snacks, fruit leather, rolls	0.1	3	85.8	371	0	317	0	85.8
Fruit syrup	0	0	85.13	341	0.1	0	0	85.03
Candies, honey-combed, with peanut butter	8.72	20.18	67.41	486	1.9	174	0	65.51
Topping, SMUCKER'S MAGIC SHELL	2.94	44.1	50.07	609	2.9	29	2	47.17
Syrup, fruit flavored	0	0.02	65.1	261	0	0	0	65.1
Candies, TOOTSIE ROLL, chocolate-flavor roll	1.59	3.31	87.73	387	0.1	44	2	87.63
Candies, ALMOND JOY Candy Bar	4.13	26.93	59.51	479	5	142	4	54.51
Candies, TWIZZLERS CHERRY BITES	2.97	1.7	79.38	338	0.1	261	0	79.28
Candies, NESTLE, BIT-O'-HONEY Candy Chews	2	7.5	80.89	375	0.2	295	0	80.69
Candies, NESTLE, BUTTERFINGER Bar	5.4	18.9	72.9	459	2	230	0	70.9
Candies, butterscotch	0.03	3.3	90.4	391	0	391	9	90.4
Candies, carob, unsweetened	8.15	31.36	56.29	540	3.8	107	1	52.49
Candies, caramels	4.6	8.1	77	382	0	245	7	77
Candies, CARAMELLO Candy Bar	6.19	21.19	63.81	462	1.2	122	27	62.61
Candies, caramels, chocolate-flavor roll	1.59	3.31	87.73	387	0.1	44	2	87.63
Baking chocolate, unsweetened, liquid	12.1	47.7	36.2	472	18.1	12	0	18.1
Baking chocolate, unsweetened, squares	14.32	52.31	28.42	642	16.6	24	2	11.82
Candies, confectioner's coating, yogurt	5.87	27	63.94	522	0	88	1	63.94
Candies, semisweet chocolate	4.2	30	63.9	480	5.9	11	0	58
Candies, sweet chocolate	3.9	34.2	60.4	507	5.5	16	0	54.9
Candies, sweet chocolate coated fondant	2.2	9.3	80.4	366	2.1	26	0	78.3
Candies, HERSHEY'S GOLDEN ALMOND SOLITAIRES	11.97	37.13	46.85	569	4.4	52	13	42.45
Candies, confectioner's coating, butterscotch	2.2	29.05	67.1	539	0	89	0	67.1
Candies, confectioner's coating, peanut butter	18.3	29.8	46.88	529	5	250	1	41.88
Candies, white chocolate	5.87	32.09	59.24	539	0.2	90	21	59.04
Ice creams, vanilla, light	4.78	4.83	29.46	180	0.3	74	27	29.16
Ice creams, vanilla, rich	3.5	16.2	22.29	249	0	61	92	22.29
Ice creams, french vanilla, soft-serve	4.1	13	22.2	222	0.7	61	91	21.5
Candies, YORK Peppermint Pattie	2.19	7.17	80.99	384	2	28	1	78.99
Candies, TWIZZLERS NIBS CHERRY BITS	2.3	2.64	79.37	347	0.6	195	0	78.77
Candies, SYMPHONY Milk Chocolate Bar	8.51	30.57	58.01	531	1.7	101	24	56.31
Desserts, flan, caramel custard, prepared-from-recipe	4.53	4.03	22.78	145	0	53	90	22.78
Ice creams, vanilla	3.5	11	23.6	207	0.7	80	44	22.9
Ice creams, vanilla, light, soft-serve	4.9	2.6	21.8	126	0	70	12	21.8
Sherbet, orange	1.1	2	30.4	144	1.3	46	1	29.1
Candies, 5TH AVENUE Candy Bar	8.78	23.98	62.68	482	3.1	225	6	59.58
Candies, fondant, prepared-from-recipe	0	0.02	93.18	373	0	11	0	93.18
Candies, fudge, chocolate, prepared-from-recipe	2.39	10.41	76.44	411	1.7	45	14	74.74
Candies, fudge, chocolate, with nuts, prepared-from-recipe	4.38	18.93	67.93	461	2.5	39	12	65.43
Candies, fudge, peanut butter, prepared-from-recipe	3.78	6.59	77.75	387	0.7	118	3	77.05

Food Name ---> per 100 g	Protein (g)	Fat (g)	Carb (g)	Calories	Fiber (g)	Sodium (mg)	Cholesterol (mg)	Net Carb (g)
Candies, fudge, vanilla, prepared-from-recipe	1.05	5.45	82.15	383	0	47	15	82.15
Candies, fudge, vanilla with nuts	3	13.69	74.61	435	0.9	42	13	73.71
Candies, NESTLE, GOOBERS Chocolate Covered Peanuts	9.7	34	53	512	9.7	36	12	43.3
Candies, gumdrops, starch jelly pieces	0	0	98.9	396	0.1	44	0	98.8
Candies, hard	0	0.2	98	394	0	38	0	98
Candies, jellybeans	0	0.05	93.55	375	0.2	50	0	93.35
Candies, KIT KAT Wafer Bar	6.51	25.99	64.59	518	1	54	11	63.59
Candies, KRACKEL Chocolate Bar	6.62	26.58	63.96	512	2.2	196	11	61.76
Candies, NESTLE, BABY RUTH Bar	5.4	21.6	64.8	459	2	230	0	62.8
Candies, TWIZZLERS Strawberry Twists Candy	2.56	2.32	79.16	348	0	287	0	79.16
Syrups, table blends, pancake, with butter	0	0.09	72.43	291	0	287	0	72.43
Ice creams, chocolate, light	5	7.19	25.7	187	0.8	71	28	24.9
Candies, MARS SNACKFOOD US, MARS Almond Bar	8.1	23	62.7	467	2	170	17	60.7
Candies, marshmallows	1.8	0.2	81.3	318	0.1	80	0	81.2
Candies, halavah, plain	12.49	21.52	60.49	469	4.5	195	0	55.99
Candies, NESTLE, OH HENRY! Bar	7.7	23	65.5	462	1.9	193	7	63.6
Candies, NESTLE, CHUNKY Bar	7.5	27.5	60	475	2.5	38	10	57.5
Candies, milk chocolate	7.65	29.66	59.4	535	3.4	79	23	56
Puddings, banana, dry mix, instant, prepared with 2% milk	2.76	1.7	19.74	105	0	296	6	19.74
Puddings, banana, dry mix, regular, prepared with 2% milk	2.9	1.73	18.43	101	0	164	7	18.43
Puddings, chocolate, dry mix, instant, prepared with 2% milk	3.15	1.92	18.89	105	0.4	284	6	18.49
Baking chocolate, mexican, squares	3.64	15.59	77.41	426	4	3	0	73.41
Chocolate-flavored hazelnut spread	5.41	29.73	62.16	541	5.4	41	0	56.76
Candies, milk chocolate coated peanuts	13.1	33.5	49.7	519	4.7	41	9	45
Candies, milk chocolate coated raisins	4.1	14.8	68.4	390	3.1	36	3	65.3
Syrups, table blends, pancake, reduced-calorie	0	0	44.55	165	0	178	0	44.55
Syrups, table blends, pancake	0	0	61.47	234	0	82	0	61.47
Candies, HERSHEY'S POT OF GOLD Almond Bar	12.82	38.46	44.89	577	3.8	64	13	41.09
Candies, milk chocolate, with almonds	9	34.4	53.4	526	6.2	74	19	47.2
Candies, milk chocolate, with rice cereal	7.64	29.37	59.67	511	3.3	86	23	56.37
Candies, MARS SNACKFOOD US, MILKY WAY Bar	4.01	17.23	71.17	456	1	167	9	70.17
Candies, HERSHEY'S SKOR Toffee Bar	3.13	30.37	63.73	541	1.3	317	53	62.43
Toppings, strawberry	0.2	0.1	66.3	254	0.7	21	0	65.6
Candies, truffles, prepared-from-recipe	6.21	33.76	44.88	510	2.5	68	53	42.38
Baking chocolate, MARS SNACKFOOD US, M&M's Semisweet Chocolate Mini Baking Bits	4.44	26.15	65.96	517	6.7	2	3	59.26
Candies, MARS SNACKFOOD US, M&M's Peanut Chocolate Candies	9.57	26.13	60.48	515	3.7	50	8	56.78
Candies, MARS SNACKFOOD US, M&M's Milk Chocolate Candies	4.33	21.13	71.19	492	2.8	61	14	68.39
Candies, MOUNDS Candy Bar	4.6	26.6	58.59	486	3.7	145	2	54.89
Candies, MR. GOODBAR Chocolate Bar	10.22	33.21	54.34	538	3.8	41	10	50.54
Candies, NESTLE, 100 GRAND Bar	2.5	19.33	70.97	468	1	203	12	69.97
Candies, NESTLE, CRUNCH Bar and Dessert Topping	5	26	67	500	1.9	150	13	65.1
Baking chocolate, MARS SNACKFOOD US,	4.78	23.36	68.4	502	2.7	68	15	65.7

212

Food Name ---> per 100 g	Protein (g)	Fat (g)	Carb (g)	Calories	Fiber (g)	Sodium (mg)	Cholesterol (mg)	Net Carb (g)
M&M's Milk Chocolate Mini Baking Bits Candies, peanut bar	15.5	33.7	47.4	522	4.1	156	0	43.3
Candies, peanut brittle, prepared-from-recipe	7.57	18.98	71.24	486	2.5	445	12	68.74
Candies, NESTLE, RAISINETS Chocolate Covered Raisins	4.4	17	71	422	2.2	33	11	68.8
Candies, REESE'S Peanut Butter Cups	10.24	30.53	55.36	515	3.6	357	6	51.76
Candies, REESE'S PIECES Candy	12.46	24.77	59.86	497	3	194	0	56.86
Candies, ROLO Caramels in Milk Chocolate	5.08	20.93	67.95	474	0.9	188	12	67.05
Candies, NESTLE, AFTER EIGHT Mints	1.67	11.9	79.53	432	2.4	1	0	77.13
Candies, sesame crunch	11.6	33.3	50.3	516	7.7	167	0	42.6
Candies, MARS SNACKFOOD US, SNICKERS Bar	7.53	23.85	61.51	491	2.3	239	13	59.21
Candies, MARS SNACKFOOD US, STARBURST Fruit Chews, Original fruits	0.41	8.21	82.57	408	0	2	0	82.57
Candies, MARS SNACKFOOD US, M&M's MINIs Milk Chocolate Candies	4.78	23.36	68.4	502	2.7	68	15	65.7
Candies, MARS SNACKFOOD US, 3 MUSKETEERS Bar	2.6	12.75	77.77	436	1.5	194	5	76.27
Candies, MARS SNACKFOOD US, TWIX Caramel Cookie Bars	4.91	24.85	64.8	502	1.1	198	7	63.7
Candies, MARS SNACKFOOD US, TWIX Peanut Butter Cookie Bars	9.18	32.67	54.15	536	3.1	226	6	51.05
Candies, WHATCHAMACALLIT Candy Bar	8.04	23.68	63.23	494	1.9	299	12	61.33
Chewing gum	0	0.3	96.7	360	2.4	1	0	94.3
Candies, SPECIAL DARK Chocolate Bar	5.54	32.4	60.49	556	6.5	6	5	53.99
Cocoa, dry powder, unsweetened	19.6	13.7	57.9	228	37	21	0	20.9
Cocoa, dry powder, unsweetened, processed with alkali	18.1	13.1	58.3	220	29.8	19	0	28.5
Desserts, egg custard, baked, prepared-from-recipe	5.02	4.58	11	104	0	61	84	11
Egg custards, dry mix	6.9	6.4	82.8	410	0	281	258	82.8
Egg custards, dry mix, prepared with whole milk	3.99	4	17.6	122	0	84	51	17.6
Cocoa, dry powder, unsweetened, HERSHEY'S European Style Cocoa	20	10	60	410	20	0	0	40
Gelatin desserts, dry mix	7.8	0	90.5	381	0	466	0	90.5
Gelatin desserts, dry mix, prepared with water	1.22	0	14.19	62	0	75	0	14.19
Gelatin desserts, dry mix, reduced calorie, with aspartame	15.67	0	80.21	198	0.1	862	0	80.11
Gelatin desserts, dry mix, reduced calorie, with aspartame, prepared with water	0.83	0	4.22	20	0	48	0	4.22
Gelatins, dry powder, unsweetened	85.6	0.1	0	335	0	196	0	0
Candies, YORK BITES	1.78	7.32	81.64	394	2	46	1	79.64
Desserts, mousse, chocolate, prepared-from-recipe	4.14	16	16.07	225	0.6	38	140	15.47
Puddings, chocolate, ready-to-eat	2.09	4.6	23.01	142	0	152	1	23.01
Puddings, chocolate, dry mix, instant	2.3	1.9	87.9	378	3.6	1771	0	84.3
Puddings, chocolate, dry mix, instant, prepared with whole milk	3.1	3.1	18.8	111	1	284	11	17.8
Desserts, apple crisp, prepared-from-recipe	1.75	3.43	30.84	161	1.4	351	0	29.44
Flan, caramel custard, dry mix	0	0	91.6	348	0	432	0	91.6
Puddings, chocolate, dry mix, regular	2.6	2.1	89.3	362	4.5	479	0	84.8
Puddings, chocolate, dry mix, regular, prepared with whole milk	3.16	3.15	19.64	120	0.8	98	9	18.84
Puddings, chocolate, dry mix, regular, prepared	3.28	2.06	19.76	111	0.8	102	7	18.96

Food Name ---> per 100 g	Protein (g)	Fat (g)	Carb (g)	Calories	Fiber (g)	Sodium (mg)	Cholesterol (mg)	Net Carb (g)
with 2% milk								
Puddings, coconut cream, dry mix, instant, prepared with 2% milk	2.9	2.3	19.2	107	0.1	246	6	19.1
Puddings, rice, ready-to-eat	3.23	2.15	18.39	108	0.3	97	12	18.09
Puddings, rice, dry mix	2.7	0.1	91.2	376	0.7	366	0	90.5
Puddings, rice, dry mix, prepared with whole milk	3.25	2.82	20.68	121	0.1	108	11	20.58
Puddings, tapioca, dry mix	0.1	0.1	94.3	369	0.2	477	0	94.1
Puddings, tapioca, dry mix, prepared with whole milk	2.84	2.89	19.43	115	0	120	12	19.43
Puddings, vanilla, ready-to-eat	1.45	3.78	22.6	130	0	142	1	22.6
Puddings, vanilla, dry mix, instant	0	0.6	92.9	377	0	1441	0	92.9
Puddings, vanilla, dry mix, instant, prepared with whole milk	2.7	2.9	19.7	114	0	286	11	19.7
Puddings, lemon, dry mix, instant, prepared with 2% milk	2.76	1.71	20.2	107	0	268	6	20.2
Egg custards, dry mix, prepared with 2% milk	4.13	2.83	17.61	112	0	87	49	17.61
Puddings, vanilla, dry mix, regular	0.3	0.4	93.5	379	0.6	635	0	92.9
Puddings, vanilla, dry mix, regular, prepared with whole milk	2.8	2.9	18.92	113	0.1	156	9	18.82
Puddings, rice, dry mix, prepared with 2% milk	3.29	1.63	20.81	111	0.1	109	6	20.71
Puddings, tapioca, dry mix, prepared with 2% milk	2.88	1.67	19.56	105	0	121	6	19.56
Puddings, vanilla, dry mix, regular, prepared with 2% milk	2.94	1.73	18.53	101	0	159	7	18.53
Rennin, chocolate, dry mix, prepared with 2% milk	3.24	2.06	13.47	85	0.5	52	7	12.97
Rennin, vanilla, dry mix, prepared with 2% milk	3.06	1.77	12.34	77	0	46	7	12.34
Candies, praline, prepared-from-recipe	3.3	25.9	59.59	485	3.5	48	0	56.09
Frozen novelties, ice type, fruit, no sugar added	0.5	0.1	6.2	24	0	5	0	6.2
Puddings, tapioca, ready-to-eat	1.95	3.88	21.69	130	0	145	1	21.69
Puddings, coconut cream, dry mix, regular, prepared with 2% milk	3.1	2.5	17.8	104	0.2	163	7	17.6
Desserts, rennin, chocolate, dry mix	2.4	3.3	91.5	363	5.1	187	0	86.4
Rennin, chocolate, dry mix, prepared with whole milk	3.2	3.34	13.34	96	0.5	51	12	12.84
Desserts, rennin, vanilla, dry mix	0	0	99	383	0	6	0	99
Rennin, vanilla, dry mix, prepared with whole milk	3.03	3.07	12.21	89	0	46	13	12.21
Desserts, rennin, tablets, unsweetened	1	0.1	19.8	84	0	26050	0	19.8
Frostings, chocolate, creamy, ready-to-eat	1.1	17.6	63.2	397	0.9	183	0	62.3
Frostings, coconut-nut, ready-to-eat	1.5	24	52.7	433	2.5	160	0	50.2
Frostings, cream cheese-flavor, ready-to-eat	0.1	17.3	67.32	415	0	191	0	67.32
Frostings, vanilla, creamy, ready-to-eat	0	16.23	67.89	418	0	184	0	67.89
Flan, caramel custard, dry mix, prepared with 2% milk	2.99	1.72	18.82	103	0	113	7	18.82
Flan, caramel custard, dry mix, prepared with whole milk	2.95	3	18.68	113	0	112	12	18.68
Puddings, vanilla, ready-to-eat, fat free	2.02	0	20.16	89	0	191	0	20.16
Puddings, tapioca, ready-to-eat, fat free	1.44	0.35	21.31	94	0	187	1	21.31
Puddings, chocolate, ready-to-eat, fat free	1.93	0.3	20.87	93	0.3	154	1	20.57
Candies, HERSHEY'S MILK CHOCOLATE WITH ALMOND BITES	9.76	35.73	51.72	568	3.6	74	19	48.12

Food Name ---> per 100 g	Protein (g)	Fat (g)	Carb (g)	Calories	Fiber (g)	Sodium (mg)	Cholesterol (mg)	Net Carb (g)
Candies, REESE'S BITES	11.34	29.85	55.18	521	3.1	179	7	52.08
Candies, REESE'S NUTRAGEOUS Candy Bar	11.28	32.09	52.8	517	3.9	141	3	48.9
Frostings, chocolate, creamy, dry mix	1.3	5.2	92	389	2.4	76	0	89.6
Frostings, chocolate, creamy, dry mix, prepared with butter	1.11	13.06	71.8	408	1.9	124	24	69.9
Candies, HEATH BITES	3.94	30.38	63.39	530	2	245	19	61.39
Frostings, vanilla, creamy, dry mix	0.3	4.9	93.8	410	0.1	13	0	93.7
Frostings, white, fluffy, dry mix	2.3	0	94.9	371	0	234	0	94.9
Frostings, white, fluffy, dry mix, prepared with water	1.5	0	62.6	244	0	156	0	62.6
Candies, HERSHEY'S, ALMOND JOY BITES	5.58	34.5	57.54	563	4.3	39	11	53.24
Candies, HERSHEY, REESESTICKS crispy wafers, peanut butter, milk chocolate	9.53	31.34	55.38	521	3.3	264	6	52.08
Candies, HERSHEY, KIT KAT BIG KAT Bar	6.24	27.84	63.64	520	1.9	64	9	61.74
Candies, REESE'S, FAST BREAK, milk chocolate peanut butter and soft nougats	8.66	23.42	61.6	474	2.9	330	4	58.7
Candies, MARS SNACKFOOD US, DOVE Milk Chocolate	5.94	31.72	59.78	546	2.4	63	18	57.38
Candies, MARS SNACKFOOD US, DOVE Dark Chocolate	5.19	32.45	59.4	520	7.6	4	7	51.8
Candies, MARS SNACKFOOD US, MILKY WAY Caramels, milk chocolate covered	4.28	19.17	68.49	463	0.7	273	20	67.79
Candies, MARS SNACKFOOD US, MILKY WAY Caramels. dark chocolate covered	3.82	20.42	67.56	458	2.8	246	17	64.76
Ice creams, vanilla, light, no sugar added	3.97	7.45	21.42	169	0	96	27	21.42
Frozen novelties, fruit and juice bars	1.2	0.1	20.2	87	1	4	0	19.2
Ice creams, chocolate, light, no sugar added	3.54	5.74	26.79	173	0.9	75	16	25.89
Candies, dark chocolate coated coffee beans	7.5	30	59.95	540	7.5	25	13	52.45
Ice creams, chocolate	3.8	11	28.2	216	1.2	76	34	27
Ice creams, strawberry	3.2	8.4	27.6	192	0.9	60	29	26.7
Candies, milk chocolate coated coffee beans	7.41	33.18	55.25	549	5.7	70	20	49.55
Frozen novelties, ice type, lime	0.4	0	32.6	128	0	22	0	32.6
Frozen novelties, ice type, italian, restaurant-prepared	0.03	0.02	13.5	53	0	4	0	13.5
Frozen novelties, ice type, pop	0	0.24	19.23	79	0	7	0	19.23
Candies, MARS SNACKFOOD US, M&M's Crispy Chocolate Candies	4.28	19.32	72.4	475	2	136	12	70.4
Frozen yogurts, vanilla, soft-serve	4	5.6	24.2	159	0	87	2	24.2
Fruit butters, apple	0.39	0.3	42.47	173	1.5	15	0	40.97
Candies, MARS SNACKFOOD US, SNICKERS MUNCH bar	15.25	36.22	43.64	536	4.7	358	24	38.94
Honey	0.3	0	82.4	304	0.2	4	0	82.2
Jams and preserves	0.37	0.07	68.86	278	1.1	32	0	67.76
Jellies	0.15	0.02	69.95	266	1	30	0	68.95
Candies, fudge, chocolate marshmallow, with nuts, prepared-by-recipe	3.24	21.11	67.69	474	2.1	79	23	65.59
Candies, MARS SNACKFOOD US, SNICKERS Almond bar	5.4	22.4	64.67	472	2.6	156	13	62.07
Marmalade, orange	0.3	0	66.3	246	0.7	56	0	65.6
Molasses	0	0.1	74.73	290	0	37	0	74.73
Candies, MARS SNACKFOOD US, POP'ABLES SNICKERS Brand Bite Size Candies	7.15	24.32	61.07	480	2.3	224	13	58.77
Candies, MARS SNACKFOOD US,	3.3	18	71.85	463	1	146	11	70.85

Food Name ---> per 100 g	Protein (g)	Fat (g)	Carb (g)	Calories	Fiber (g)	Sodium (mg)	Cholesterol (mg)	Net Carb (g)
POP'ABLES MILKY WAY Brand Bite Size Candies								
Candies, MARS SNACKFOOD US, POP'ABLES 3 MUSKETEERS Brand Bite Size Candies	2.59	15.17	75.94	443	1.3	172	7	74.64
Candies, MARS SNACKFOOD US, STARBURST Fruit Chews, Fruit and Creme	0.41	8.36	82.43	408	0	2	0	82.43
Pectin, unsweetened, dry mix	0.3	0.3	90.4	325	8.6	200	0	81.8
Pie fillings, apple, canned	0.1	0.1	26.1	100	1	47	0	25.1
Candies, MARS SNACKFOOD US, STARBURST Fruit Chews, Tropical fruits	0.41	8.31	82.76	409	0	2	0	82.76
Pie fillings, canned, cherry	0.37	0.07	28	115	0.6	18	0	27.4
Candies, MARS SNACKFOOD US, STARBURST Sour Fruit Chews	0.39	7.78	79.73	400	0	89	0	79.73
Puddings, banana, dry mix, instant	0	0.6	92.7	367	0	1499	0	92.7
Puddings, banana, dry mix, instant, prepared with whole milk	2.62	2.8	19.76	115	0	290	9	19.76
Puddings, banana, dry mix, regular	0	0.4	93	366	0.3	788	0	92.7
Puddings, banana, dry mix, regular, prepared with whole milk	2.74	2.89	18.44	111	0	158	9	18.44
Puddings, coconut cream, dry mix, instant	0.9	10	83.5	415	4	1040	0	79.5
Puddings, coconut cream, dry mix, instant, prepared with whole milk	2.9	3.5	19.1	117	0.1	246	11	19
Puddings, coconut cream, dry mix, regular	1	11.36	81.84	434	1.6	682	0	80.24
Puddings, coconut cream, dry mix, regular, prepared with whole milk	3	3.8	17.7	114	0.2	162	12	17.5
Candies, MARS SNACKFOOD US, COCOAVIA Chocolate Bar	5.81	29.3	62.99	539	8.7	7	0	54.29
Candies, MARS SNACKFOOD US, COCOAVIA Blueberry and Almond Chocolate Bar	6.35	28.68	60.37	525	9.1	8	0	51.27
Candies, MARS SNACKFOOD US, COCOAVIA Crispy Chocolate Bar	8.21	26.23	62.06	517	7.8	40	0	54.26
Puddings, lemon, dry mix, instant	0	0.7	95.4	378	0	1332	0	95.4
Puddings, lemon, dry mix, instant, prepared with whole milk	2.7	2.9	20.1	115	0	267	11	20.1
Puddings, lemon, dry mix, regular	0.1	0.5	91.8	363	0.1	506	0	91.7
Pudding, lemon, dry mix, regular, prepared with sugar, egg yolk and water	0.65	1.12	24.2	109	0	63	49	24.2
Sugars, brown	0.12	0	98.09	380	0	28	0	98.09
Sugars, granulated	0	0	99.98	387	0	1	0	99.98
Sugars, powdered	0	0	99.77	389	0	2	0	99.77
Sweeteners, tabletop, aspartame, EQUAL, packets	2.17	0	89.08	365	0	0	0	89.08
Sugars, maple	0.1	0.2	90.9	354	0	11	0	90.9
Syrups, chocolate, HERSHEY'S Genuine Chocolate Flavored Lite Syrup	1.4	0.97	34.56	153	0	100	0	34.56
Syrups, chocolate, fudge-type	4.6	8.9	62.9	350	2.8	346	1	60.1
Syrups, corn, dark	0	0	77.59	286	0	155	0	77.59
Syrups, corn, light	0	0.2	76.79	283	0	62	0	76.79
Syrups, corn, high-fructose	0	0	76	281	0	2	0	76
Syrups, malt	6.2	0	71.3	318	0	35	0	71.3
Syrups, maple	0.04	0.06	67.04	260	0	12	0	67.04
Syrups, sorghum	0	0	74.9	290	0	8	0	74.9
Candies, MARS SNACKFOOD US,	6.86	24.38	62.85	488	1.9	189	9	60.95

SNICKERS CRUNCHER

Food Name ---> per 100 g	Protein (g)	Fat (g)	Carb (g)	Calories	Fiber (g)	Sodium (mg)	Cholesterol (mg)	Net Carb (g)
Syrups, table blends, pancake, with 2% maple	0	0.1	69.6	265	0	61	0	69.6
Syrups, table blends, cane and 15% maple	0	0.1	69.52	278	0.1	104	0	69.42
Syrups, table blends, corn, refiner, and sugar	0	0	83.9	319	0	71	0	83.9
Candies, MARS SNACKFOOD US, SKITTLES Wild Berry Bite Size Candies	0.19	4.25	90.76	402	0	15	0	90.76
Toppings, butterscotch or caramel	1.21	0	57.01	216	0	341	0	57.01
Toppings, marshmallow cream	0.8	0.3	79	322	0.1	80	0	78.9
Toppings, pineapple	0.1	0.1	66.4	253	0.4	42	0	66
Toppings, nuts in syrup	4.5	22	58.08	448	2.3	42	0	55.78
Candies, MARS SNACKFOOD US, SKITTLES Tropical Bite Size Candies	0.19	4.34	90.77	405	0	15	0	90.77
Candies, MARS SNACKFOOD US, SKITTLES Sours Original	0.18	4	91.02	401	0	14	0	91.02
Candies, MARS SNACKFOOD US, SKITTLES Original Bite Size Candies	0.19	4.37	90.78	405	0	15	0	90.78
Frostings, vanilla, creamy, dry mix, prepared with margarine	0.34	12.74	74.28	413	0.1	114	0	74.18
Frostings, chocolate, creamy, dry mix, prepared with margarine	1.1	12.87	71.02	404	1.9	163	0	69.12
Frostings, glaze, prepared-from-recipe	0.44	0.53	83.65	341	0	6	1	83.65
Candies, fudge, chocolate marshmallow, prepared-from-recipe	2.26	17.48	71.34	453	1.7	85	25	69.64
Candies, taffy, prepared-from-recipe	0.03	3.33	91.56	397	0	52	9	91.56
Candies, toffee, prepared-from-recipe	1.07	32.75	64.72	560	0	135	104	64.72
Candies, divinity, prepared-from-recipe	1.32	0.06	89.05	364	0	34	0	89.05
Frozen novelties, ice type, pineapple-coconut	0	2.6	23.9	113	0.7	35	0	23.2
Frozen yogurts, chocolate, soft-serve	4	6	24.9	160	2.2	98	5	22.7
Frostings, glaze, chocolate, prepared-from-recipe, with butter, NFSMI Recipe No. C-32	1.42	7.17	72.18	359	1.1	132	18	71.08
Candies, semisweet chocolate, made with butter	4.2	29.7	63.4	477	5.9	11	18	57.5
Gelatin desserts, dry mix, with added ascorbic acid, sodium-citrate and salt	7.8	0	90.5	381	0	491	0	90.5
Gelatin desserts, dry mix, reduced calorie, with aspartame, added phosphorus, potassium, sodium, vitamin C	55.3	0	33.3	345	0	2751	0	33.3
Gelatin desserts, dry mix, reduced calorie, with aspartame, no added sodium	55.3	0	33.3	345	0	158	0	33.3
Puddings, banana, dry mix, instant, with added oil	0	4.4	89	386	0	1499	0	89
Puddings, banana, dry mix, regular, with added oil	0	5	88.4	387	0.3	788	0	88.1
Puddings, lemon, dry mix, regular, with added oil, potassium, sodium	0.1	1.5	90.3	366	0.1	849	0	90.2
Puddings, tapioca, dry mix, with no added salt	0.1	0.1	94.3	369	0.2	8	0	94.1
Puddings, vanilla, dry mix, regular, with added oil	0.3	1.1	92.4	369	0	754	0	92.4
Jams and preserves, apricot	0.7	0.2	64.4	242	0.3	40	0	64.1
Syrups, table blends, pancake, with 2% maple, with added potassium	0	0.1	69.6	265	0	61	0	69.6
Frozen novelties, juice type, POPSICLE SCRIBBLERS	0	0.24	19.68	81	0	13	-	19.68
Candies, sugar-coated almonds	10	17.93	68.26	474	2.5	13	0	65.76
Cocoa, dry powder, hi-fat or breakfast, plain	16.8	23.71	51.39	486	29.8	20	0	21.59
Cocoa, dry powder, hi-fat or breakfast,	16.8	23.71	49.71	479	33.9	20	0	15.81

Food Name ---> per 100 g	Protein (g)	Fat (g)	Carb (g)	Calories	Fiber (g)	Sodium (mg)	Cholesterol (mg)	Net Carb (g)
processed with alkali								
Candies, soft fruit and nut squares	2.31	9.52	73.81	390	2.4	131	0	71.41
Ice creams, vanilla, fat free	4.48	0	30.06	138	1	97	0	29.06
Sweeteners, tabletop, sucralose, SPLENDA packets	0	0	91.17	336	0	0	0	91.17
Frozen novelties, No Sugar Added, FUDGSICLE pops	3.67	1.87	23.11	124	1.5	96	2	21.61
Frozen novelties, ice type, sugar free, orange, cherry, and grape POPSICLE pops	0	0	5.14	21	0	10	0	5.14
Frozen novelties, KLONDIKE, SLIM-A-BEAR Fudge Bar, 98% fat free, no sugar added	4.31	1.88	30.07	124	6	120	7	24.07
Ice creams, BREYERS, All Natural Light Vanilla	4.84	4.59	25.3	162	0.2	71	15	25.1
Ice creams, BREYERS, All Natural Light French Vanilla	4.82	5.56	26.03	173	0.2	73	53	25.83
Ice creams, BREYERS, 98% Fat Free Vanilla	3.3	2.2	30.51	137	5.4	73	8	25.11
Ice creams, BREYERS, All Natural Light Vanilla Chocolate Strawberry	4.69	4.35	26.06	161	0.4	69	14	25.66
Ice creams, BREYERS, All Natural Light Mint Chocolate Chip	4.69	7.09	28.39	196	0.6	67	15	27.79
Ice creams, BREYERS, No Sugar Added, Butter Pecan	3.99	10.3	21.3	180	0.9	164	18	20.4
Ice creams, BREYERS, No Sugar Added, French Vanilla	4.5	7.05	20.75	154	0.5	87	53	20.25
Ice creams, BREYERS, No Sugar Added, Vanilla	3.68	6.2	21.92	143	0.5	66	18	21.42
Ice creams, BREYERS, No Sugar Added, Vanilla Fudge Twirl	3.53	5.68	25.63	153	0.8	72	16	24.83
Ice creams, BREYERS, No Sugar Added, Vanilla Chocolate Strawberry	3.71	6.26	21.7	143	0.7	68	18	21
Frozen novelties, KLONDIKE, SLIM-A-BEAR Chocolate Cone	4.09	4.1	45.32	224	4.3	159	2	41.02
Frozen novelties, KLONDIKE, SLIM-A-BEAR Vanilla Sandwich	3.9	5.85	42.75	239	4.3	191	4	38.45
Frozen novelties, KLONDIKE, SLIM-A-BEAR, No Sugar Added, Stickless Bar	5.2	13	25.98	242	3.9	86	8	22.08
Frozen novelties, No Sugar Added CREAMSICLE Pops	3.69	0.61	12.88	72	3.6	41	3	9.28
Frozen novelties, Sugar Free, CREAMSICLE Pops	1.37	2.33	11.95	49	7.5	6	0	4.45
Ice creams, BREYERS, All Natural Light French Chocolate	5.3	7.28	29.68	201	1	75	41	28.68
Ice creams, BREYERS, 98% Fat Free Chocolate	3.89	2.17	30.18	136	5.8	75	7	24.38
Ice creams, BREYERS, No Sugar Added, Chocolate Caramel	3.54	5.8	25.17	151	1	77	16	24.17
Candies, REESE's Fast Break, milk chocolate, peanut butter, soft nougats, candy bar	8.93	23.21	63.9	495	3.6	321	9	60.3
Candies, MARS SNACKFOOD US, COCOAVIA Chocolate Covered Almonds	9.51	37.07	50.22	573	10.4	9	0	39.82
Ice creams, regular, low carbohydrate, vanilla	3.17	12.7	22.23	216	4.8	48	32	17.43
Ice creams, regular, low carbohydrate, chocolate	3.8	12.7	26.8	237	4.8	76	34	22
Chocolate, dark, 45- 59% cacao solids	4.88	31.28	61.17	546	7	24	8	54.17
Chocolate, dark, 60-69% cacao solids	6.12	38.31	52.42	579	8	10	6	44.42
Chocolate, dark, 70-85% cacao solids	7.79	42.63	45.9	598	10.9	20	3	35
Candies, chocolate, dark, NFS (45-59% cacao solids 90%; 60-69% cacao solids 5%; 70-85%	5.09	32.2	59.97	550	7.2	23	7	52.77

Food Name ---> per 100 g	Protein (g)	Fat (g)	Carb (g)	Calories	Fiber (g)	Sodium (mg)	Cholesterol (mg)	Net Carb (g)
cacao solids 5%)								
Sweeteners, for baking, brown, contains sugar and sucralose	0	0	97.11	388	-	11	-	97.11
Sweeteners, for baking, contains sugar and sucralose	0	0	99.53	398	-	2	-	99.53
Sugar, turbinado	0	0	99.8	399	-	3	-	99.8
Sweeteners, sugar substitute, granulated, brown	2.06	0	84.77	347	0.6	572	-	84.17
Candies, crispy bar with peanut butter filling	9.53	31.34	55.53	542	3.3	264	5	52.23
Syrup, maple, Canadian	0	0	67.38	270	0	9	0	67.38
Sweetener, syrup, agave	0.09	0.45	76.37	310	0.2	4	0	76.17
Candies, NESTLE, BUTTERFINGER Crisp	6.67	18.33	68.45	465	1.7	13	0	66.75
Candies, M&M MARS 3 MUSKETEERS Truffle Crisp	6.41	28.85	63.15	538	0	63	18	63.15
Syrups, chocolate, HERSHEY'S Sugar free, Genuine Chocolate Flavored, Lite Syrup	2.87	2.03	14.2	43	2.9	343	0	11.3
Candies, M&M MARS Pretzel Chocolate Candies	5	15	72.94	447	2.5	475	13	70.44
Sweetener, herbal extract powder from Stevia leaf	0	0	100	0	0	0	0	100
Candies, fruit snacks, with high vitamin C	0.08	0	87.97	352	0	23	0	87.97
Jams, preserves, marmalades, sweetened with fruit juice	0	0	52.93	212	0.9	0	0	52.03
Candies, Tamarind	0	0	91.96	368	2.5	1643	0	89.46
Candies, coconut bar, not chocolate covered	2.13	27.65	55.87	481	6.4	128	0	49.47
Candies, HERSHEYS, PAYDAY Bar	13.44	25	52.88	490	3.8	231	0	49.08
Syrup, NESTLE, chocolate	0	0	67.21	269	0	150	0	67.21
Syrups, grenadine	0	0	66.91	268	0	27	0	66.91
Pectin, liquid	0	0	2.1	11	2.1	0	0	0
Frozen novelties, ice cream type, vanilla ice cream, light, no sugar added, chocolate coated	6.4	10.1	26.11	221	0.8	104	10	25.31
Milk dessert, frozen, milk-fat free, chocolate	4.3	1	37.7	167	0	97	0	37.7
Candies, MARS SNACKFOOD US, M&M's Peanut Butter Chocolate Candies	10.16	29.32	56.89	529	4	213	7	52.89
Candies, MARS SNACKFOOD US, TWIX chocolate fudge cookie bars	7.3	33.3	56	550	3	266	6	53
Frozen yogurts, chocolate, nonfat milk, sweetened without sugar	4.4	0.8	19.7	107	2	81	4	17.7
Frozen yogurts, chocolate	3	3.6	21.6	127	2.3	63	13	19.3
Frozen yogurts, flavors other than chocolate	3	3.6	21.6	127	0	63	13	21.6
Candies, MARS SNACKFOOD US, MILKY WAY Midnight Bar	3.2	17.5	71.22	443	2.9	168	10	68.32
Candies, MARS SNACKFOOD US, M&M's Almond Chocolate Candies	7.53	27.76	60.5	522	5.6	45	8	54.9
Gums, seed gums (includes locust bean, guar)	4.6	0.5	77.3	332	77.3	125	0	0
Syrups, sugar free	0.8	0	12.13	52	0.7	210	0	11.43
Jellies, no sugar (with sodium saccharin), any flavors	0.55	0	29.6	121	2.2	3	0	27.4
Jams and preserves, no sugar (with sodium saccharin), any flavor	0.3	0.3	53.42	132	2.5	0	0	50.92
Candies, chocolate covered, caramel with nuts	9.5	21	60.67	470	4.3	156	0	56.37
Candies, nougat, with almonds	3.33	1.67	92.39	398	3.3	33	0	89.09
Candies, gum drops, no sugar or low calorie (sorbitol)	0	0.2	88.1	354	0	7	0	88.1
Candies, hard, dietetic or low calorie (sorbitol)	0	0	98.6	394	0	0	0	98.6

Food Name ---> per 100 g	Protein (g)	Fat (g)	Carb (g)	Calories	Fiber (g)	Sodium (mg)	Cholesterol (mg)	Net Carb (g)
Candies, chocolate covered, low sugar or low calorie	12.39	43.27	37.68	590	3.5	111	22	34.18
Chewing gum, sugarless	0	0.4	94.8	268	2.4	7	0	92.4
Pie fillings, cherry, low calorie	0.82	0.16	11.98	53	1.2	12	0	10.78
Sweeteners, tabletop, saccharin (sodium saccharin)	0.94	0	89.11	360	0	428	0	89.11
Sweeteners, tabletop, fructose, dry, powder	0	0	100	368	0	12	0	100
Frozen novelties, ice cream type, sundae, prepackaged	4.3	6	29.4	185	0.3	95	13	29.1
Jams, preserves, marmalade, reduced sugar	0	0.1	37.6	151	1.5	0	0	36.1
Frozen novelties, juice type, orange	0.5	0	23.17	95	0.1	8	0	23.07
Frozen novelties, juice type, juice with cream	1.41	1.41	24.11	115	0.1	42	7	24.01
Frozen novelties, ice cream type, chocolate or caramel covered, with nuts	4.4	20.2	30.9	323	0.6	92	1	30.3
Frozen novelties, ice type, pop, with low calorie sweetener	0	0	5.92	24	0	10	0	5.92
Ice creams, chocolate, rich	4.72	16.98	19.78	251	0.9	57	60	18.88
Sweeteners, tabletop, fructose, liquid	0	0	76.1	279	0.1	2	0	76
Puddings, chocolate flavor, low calorie, instant, dry mix	5.3	2.4	78.2	356	6.1	2838	0	72.1
Jellies, reduced sugar, home preserved	0.3	0.03	46.1	179	0.8	2	0	45.3
Pie fillings, blueberry, canned	0.41	0.2	44.38	181	2.6	12	0	41.78
Puddings, chocolate flavor, low calorie, regular, dry mix	10.08	3	74.42	365	10.1	3326	0	64.32
Puddings, all flavors except chocolate, low calorie, regular, dry mix	1.6	0.1	86.04	351	0.9	1765	0	85.14
Puddings, all flavors except chocolate, low calorie, instant, dry mix	0.81	0.9	84.66	350	0.8	3750	0	83.86
Syrup, Cane	0	0	73.14	269	0	58	0	73.14

Vegetables and Vegetable Products

Food Name ---> per 100 g	Protein (g)	Fat (g)	Carb (g)	Calories	Fiber (g)	Sodium (mg)	Cholesterol (mg)	Net Carb (g)
Alfalfa seeds, sprouted, raw	3.99	0.69	2.1	23	1.9	6	0	0.2
Amaranth leaves, raw	2.46	0.33	4.02	23	-	20	0	4.02
Amaranth leaves, cooked, boiled, drained, without salt	2.11	0.18	4.11	21	-	21	0	4.11
Arrowhead, raw	5.33	0.29	20.23	99	-	22	0	20.23
Arrowhead, cooked, boiled, drained, without salt	4.49	0.1	16.14	78	-	18	0	16.14
Artichokes, (globe or french), raw	3.27	0.15	10.51	47	5.4	94	0	5.11
Artichokes, (globe or french), cooked, boiled, drained, without salt	2.89	0.34	11.95	53	5.7	60	0	6.25
Artichokes, (globe or french), frozen, unprepared	2.63	0.43	7.75	38	3.9	47	0	3.85
Artichokes, (globe or french), frozen, cooked, boiled, drained, without salt	3.11	0.5	9.18	45	4.6	53	0	4.58
Asparagus, raw	2.2	0.12	3.88	20	2.1	2	0	1.78
Asparagus, cooked, boiled, drained	2.4	0.22	4.11	22	2	14	0	2.11
Asparagus, canned, regular pack, solids and liquids	1.8	0.18	2.48	15	1	284	0	1.48
Asparagus, canned, drained solids	2.14	0.65	2.46	19	1.6	287	0	0.86
Asparagus, frozen, unprepared	3.23	0.23	4.1	24	1.9	8	0	2.2
Asparagus, frozen, cooked, boiled, drained, without salt	2.95	0.42	1.92	18	1.6	3	0	0.32
Balsam-pear (bitter gourd), leafy tips, raw	5.3	0.69	3.29	30	-	11	0	3.29
Balsam-pear (bitter gourd), leafy tips, cooked, boiled, drained, without salt	3.6	0.2	6.68	34	1.9	13	0	4.78
Balsam-pear (bitter gourd), pods, raw	1	0.17	3.7	17	2.8	5	0	0.9
Balsam-pear (bitter gourd), pods, cooked, boiled, drained, without salt	0.84	0.18	4.32	19	2	6	0	2.32
Bamboo shoots, raw	2.6	0.3	5.2	27	2.2	4	0	3
Bamboo shoots, cooked, boiled, drained, without salt	1.53	0.22	1.92	12	1	4	0	0.92
Bamboo shoots, canned, drained solids	1.72	0.4	3.22	19	1.4	7	0	1.82
Beans, kidney, mature seeds, sprouted, raw	4.2	0.5	4.1	29	-	6	0	4.1
Beans, kidney, mature seeds, sprouted, cooked, boiled, drained, without salt	4.83	0.58	4.72	33	-	7	0	4.72
Lima beans, immature seeds, raw	6.84	0.86	20.17	113	4.9	8	0	15.27
Lima beans, immature seeds, cooked, boiled, drained, without salt	6.81	0.32	23.64	123	5.4	17	0	18.24
Lima beans, immature seeds, canned, regular pack, solids and liquids	4.07	0.29	13.33	71	3.6	252	0	9.73
Lima beans, immature seeds, frozen, fordhook, unprepared	6.4	0.35	19.83	106	5.5	58	0	14.33
Lima beans, immature seeds, frozen, fordhook, cooked, boiled, drained, without salt	6.07	0.34	19.32	103	5.3	69	0	14.02
Lima beans, immature seeds, frozen, baby, unprepared	7.59	0.44	25.14	132	6	52	0	19.14
Lima beans, immature seeds, frozen, baby, cooked, boiled, drained, without salt	6.65	0.3	19.45	105	4.8	29	0	14.65
Mung beans, mature seeds, sprouted, raw	3.04	0.18	5.94	30	1.8	6	0	4.14
Mung beans, mature seeds, sprouted, cooked, boiled, drained, without salt	2.03	0.09	4.19	21	0.8	10	0	3.39
Mung beans, mature seeds, sprouted, cooked, stir-fried	4.3	0.21	10.59	50	1.9	9	0	8.69
Beans, navy, mature seeds, sprouted, raw	6.15	0.7	13.05	67	-	13	0	13.05
Beans, navy, mature seeds, sprouted, cooked, boiled,	7.07	0.81	15.01	78	-	14	0	15.01

Food Name ---> per 100 g	Protein (g)	Fat (g)	Carb (g)	Calories	Fiber (g)	Sodium (mg)	Cholesterol (mg)	Net Carb (g)
drained, without salt								
Beans, pinto, immature seeds, frozen, unprepared	9.8	0.5	32.5	170	5.7	92	0	26.8
Beans, pinto, immature seeds, frozen, cooked, boiled, drained, without salt	9.31	0.48	30.87	162	5.4	83	0	25.47
Beans, shellie, canned, solids and liquids	1.76	0.19	6.19	30	3.4	334	0	2.79
Beans, snap, green, raw	1.83	0.22	6.97	31	2.7	6	0	4.27
Beans, snap, green, cooked, boiled, drained, without salt	1.89	0.28	7.88	35	3.2	1	0	4.68
Beans, snap, green, canned, regular pack, solids and liquids	0.72	0.17	3.27	15	1.5	192	0	1.77
Beans, snap, green, canned, regular pack, drained solids	1.12	0.46	4.32	22	1.9	230	0	2.42
Beans, snap, canned, all styles, seasoned, solids and liquids	0.83	0.2	3.49	16	1.5	373	0	1.99
Beans, snap, green, frozen, all styles, unprepared	1.79	0.21	7.54	39	2.6	3	0	4.94
Beans, snap, green, frozen, cooked, boiled, drained without salt	1.49	0.17	6.45	28	3	1	0	3.45
Beans, snap, green, frozen, all styles, microwaved	1.98	0.41	6.98	40	3.4	3	-	3.58
Beans, snap, green, microwaved	2.31	0.5	6.41	39	3.4	3	-	3.01
Beets, raw	1.61	0.17	9.56	43	2.8	78	0	6.76
Beets, cooked, boiled, drained	1.68	0.18	9.96	44	2	77	0	7.96
Beets, canned, regular pack, solids and liquids	0.73	0.09	7.14	30	1.2	143	0	5.94
Beets, canned, drained solids	0.91	0.14	7.21	31	1.8	194	0	5.41
Beet greens, raw	2.2	0.13	4.33	22	3.7	226	0	0.63
Beet greens, cooked, boiled, drained, without salt	2.57	0.2	5.46	27	2.9	241	0	2.56
Broadbeans, immature seeds, raw	5.6	0.6	11.7	72	4.2	50	0	7.5
Broadbeans, immature seeds, cooked, boiled, drained, without salt	4.8	0.5	10.1	62	3.6	41	0	6.5
Broccoli, raw	2.82	0.37	6.64	34	2.6	33	0	4.04
Broccoli, cooked, boiled, drained, without salt	2.38	0.41	7.18	35	3.3	41	0	3.88
Broccoli, frozen, chopped, unprepared	2.81	0.29	4.78	26	3	24	0	1.78
Broccoli, frozen, chopped, cooked, boiled, drained, without salt	3.1	0.12	5.35	28	3	11	0	2.35
Broccoli, frozen, spears, unprepared	3.06	0.34	5.35	29	3	17	0	2.35
Broccoli, frozen, spears, cooked, boiled, drained, without salt	3.1	0.11	5.36	28	3	24	0	2.36
Broccoli raab, raw	3.17	0.49	2.85	22	2.7	33	0	0.15
Broccoli raab, cooked	3.83	0.52	3.12	33	2.8	56	0	0.32
Brussels sprouts, raw	3.38	0.3	8.95	43	3.8	25	0	5.15
Brussels sprouts, cooked, boiled, drained, without salt	2.55	0.5	7.1	36	2.6	21	0	4.5
Brussels sprouts, frozen, unprepared	3.78	0.41	7.86	41	3.8	10	0	4.06
Brussels sprouts, frozen, cooked, boiled, drained, without salt	3.64	0.39	8.32	42	4.1	15	0	4.22
Burdock root, raw	1.53	0.15	17.34	72	3.3	5	0	14.04
Burdock root, cooked, boiled, drained, without salt	2.09	0.14	21.15	88	1.8	4	0	19.35
Butterbur, (fuki), raw	0.39	0.04	3.61	14	-	7	0	3.61
Butterbur, cooked, boiled, drained, without salt	0.23	0.02	2.16	8	-	4	0	2.16
Butterbur, canned	0.11	0.13	0.38	3	-	4	0	0.38
Cabbage, raw	1.28	0.1	5.8	25	2.5	18	0	3.3
Cabbage, cooked, boiled, drained, without salt	1.27	0.06	5.51	23	1.9	8	0	3.61
Cabbage, red, raw	1.43	0.16	7.37	31	2.1	27	0	5.27
Cabbage, red, cooked, boiled, drained, without salt	1.51	0.09	6.94	29	2.6	28	0	4.34

Food Name ---> per 100 g	Protein (g)	Fat (g)	Carb (g)	Calories	Fiber (g)	Sodium (mg)	Cholesterol (mg)	Net Carb (g)
Cabbage, savoy, raw	2	0.1	6.1	27	3.1	28	0	3
Cabbage, savoy, cooked, boiled, drained, without salt	1.8	0.09	5.41	24	2.8	24	0	2.61
Cabbage, chinese (pak-choi), raw	1.5	0.2	2.18	13	1	65	0	1.18
Cabbage, chinese (pak-choi), cooked, boiled, drained, without salt	1.56	0.16	1.78	12	1	34	0	0.78
Cabbage, kimchi	1.1	0.5	2.4	15	1.6	498	0	0.8
Cabbage, chinese (pe-tsai), raw	1.2	0.2	3.23	16	1.2	9	0	2.03
Cabbage, chinese (pe-tsai), cooked, boiled, drained, without salt	1.5	0.17	2.41	14	1.7	9	0	0.71
Cardoon, raw	0.7	0.1	4.07	17	1.6	170	0	2.47
Cardoon, cooked, boiled, drained, without salt	0.76	0.11	5.33	22	1.7	176	0	3.63
Carrots, raw	0.93	0.24	9.58	41	2.8	69	0	6.78
Carrots, cooked, boiled, drained, without salt	0.76	0.18	8.22	35	3	58	0	5.22
Carrots, canned, regular pack, solids and liquids	0.58	0.14	5.37	23	1.8	240	0	3.57
Carrots, canned, regular pack, drained solids	0.64	0.19	5.54	25	1.5	242	0	4.04
Carrots, frozen, unprepared	0.78	0.46	7.9	36	3.3	68	0	4.6
Carrots, frozen, cooked, boiled, drained, without salt	0.58	0.68	7.73	37	3.3	59	0	4.43
Cassava, raw	1.36	0.28	38.06	160	1.8	14	0	36.26
Cauliflower, raw	1.92	0.28	4.97	25	2	30	0	2.97
Cauliflower, cooked, boiled, drained, without salt	1.84	0.45	4.11	23	2.3	15	0	1.81
Cauliflower, frozen, unprepared	2.01	0.27	4.68	24	2.3	24	0	2.38
Cauliflower, frozen, cooked, boiled, drained, without salt	1.61	0.22	3.75	19	2.7	18	0	1.05
Celeriac, raw	1.5	0.3	9.2	42	1.8	100	0	7.4
Celeriac, cooked, boiled, drained, without salt	0.96	0.19	5.9	27	1.2	61	0	4.7
Celery, raw	0.69	0.17	2.97	16	1.6	80	0	1.37
Celery, cooked, boiled, drained, without salt	0.83	0.16	4	18	1.6	91	0	2.4
Celtuce, raw	0.85	0.3	3.65	18	1.7	11	0	1.95
Chard, swiss, raw	1.8	0.2	3.74	19	1.6	213	0	2.14
Chard, swiss, cooked, boiled, drained, without salt	1.88	0.08	4.13	20	2.1	179	0	2.03
Chayote, fruit, raw	0.82	0.13	4.51	19	1.7	2	0	2.81
Chayote, fruit, cooked, boiled, drained, without salt	0.62	0.48	5.09	24	2.8	1	0	2.29
Chicory, witloof, raw	0.9	0.1	4	17	3.1	2	0	0.9
Chicory greens, raw	1.7	0.3	4.7	23	4	45	0	0.7
Chicory roots, raw	1.4	0.2	17.51	72	1.5	50	0	16.01
Chives, raw	3.27	0.73	4.35	30	2.5	3	0	1.85
Chrysanthemum, garland, raw	3.36	0.56	3.02	24	3	118	0	0.02
Chrysanthemum, garland, cooked, boiled, drained, without salt	1.64	0.09	4.31	20	2.3	53	0	2.01
Collards, raw	3.02	0.61	5.42	32	4	17	0	1.42
Collards, cooked, boiled, drained, without salt	2.71	0.72	5.65	33	4	15	0	1.65
Collards, frozen, chopped, unprepared	2.69	0.37	6.46	33	3.6	48	0	2.86
Collards, frozen, chopped, cooked, boiled, drained, without salt	2.97	0.41	7.1	36	2.8	50	0	4.3
Coriander (cilantro) leaves, raw	2.13	0.52	3.67	23	2.8	46	0	0.87
Corn, sweet, yellow, raw	3.27	1.35	18.7	86	2	15	0	16.7
Corn, sweet, yellow, cooked, boiled, drained, without salt	3.41	1.5	20.98	96	2.4	1	0	18.58
Corn, sweet, yellow, canned, brine pack, regular pack, solids and liquids	1.95	0.77	13.86	61	1.7	195	0	12.16
Corn, sweet, yellow, canned, whole kernel, drained solids	2.29	1.22	14.34	67	2	205	0	12.34
Corn, sweet, yellow, canned, cream style, regular	1.74	0.42	18.13	72	1.2	261	0	16.93

Food Name ---> per 100 g	Protein (g)	Fat (g)	Carb (g)	Calories	Fiber (g)	Sodium (mg)	Cholesterol (mg)	Net Carb (g)
pack								
Corn, sweet, yellow, canned, vacuum pack, regular pack	2.41	0.5	19.44	79	2	272	0	17.44
Corn, sweet, yellow, canned, drained solids, rinsed with tap water	2.18	1.43	13.02	74	1.7	163	0	11.32
Corn, sweet, yellow, frozen, kernels cut off cob, unprepared	3.02	0.78	20.71	88	2.1	3	0	18.61
Corn, sweet, yellow, frozen, kernels cut off cob, boiled, drained, without salt	2.55	0.67	19.3	81	2.4	1	0	16.9
Corn, sweet, yellow, frozen, kernels on cob, unprepared	3.28	0.78	23.5	98	2.8	5	0	20.7
Corn, sweet, yellow, frozen, kernels on cob, cooked, boiled, drained, without salt	3.11	0.74	22.33	94	2.8	4	0	19.53
Corn, yellow, whole kernel, frozen, microwaved	3.62	1.42	25.87	131	2.6	4	0	23.27
Corn with red and green peppers, canned, solids and liquids	2.33	0.55	18.17	75	-	347	0	18.17
Cornsalad, raw	2	0.4	3.6	21	-	4	0	3.6
Cowpeas (blackeyes), immature seeds, raw	2.95	0.35	18.83	90	5	4	0	13.83
Cowpeas (blackeyes), immature seeds, cooked, boiled, drained, without salt	3.17	0.38	20.32	97	5	4	0	15.32
Cowpeas (blackeyes), immature seeds, frozen, unprepared	8.98	0.7	25.13	139	5	6	0	20.13
Cowpeas (blackeyes), immature seeds, frozen, cooked, boiled, drained, without salt	8.49	0.66	23.76	132	6.4	5	0	17.36
Cowpeas, young pods with seeds, raw	3.3	0.3	9.5	44	3.3	4	0	6.2
Cowpeas, young pods with seeds, cooked, boiled, drained, without salt	2.6	0.3	7	34	-	3	0	7
Yardlong bean, raw	2.8	0.4	8.35	47	-	4	0	8.35
Yardlong bean, cooked, boiled, drained, without salt	2.53	0.1	9.18	47	-	4	0	9.18
Cowpeas, leafy tips, raw	4.1	0.25	4.82	29	-	7	0	4.82
Cowpeas, leafy tips, cooked, boiled, drained, without salt	4.67	0.1	2.8	22	-	6	0	2.8
Cress, garden, raw	2.6	0.7	5.5	32	1.1	14	0	4.4
Cress, garden, cooked, boiled, drained, without salt	1.9	0.6	3.8	23	0.7	8	0	3.1
Cucumber, with peel, raw	0.65	0.11	3.63	15	0.5	2	0	3.13
Cucumber, peeled, raw	0.59	0.16	2.16	12	0.7	2	0	1.46
Dandelion greens, raw	2.7	0.7	9.2	45	3.5	76	0	5.7
Dandelion greens, cooked, boiled, drained, without salt	2	0.6	6.4	33	2.9	44	0	3.5
Eggplant, raw	0.98	0.18	5.88	25	3	2	0	2.88
Eggplant, cooked, boiled, drained, without salt	0.83	0.23	8.73	35	2.5	1	0	6.23
Edamame, frozen, unprepared	11.22	4.73	7.61	109	4.8	6	-	2.81
Edamame, frozen, prepared	11.91	5.2	8.91	121	5.2	6	0	3.71
Endive, raw	1.25	0.2	3.35	17	3.1	22	0	0.25
Escarole, cooked, boiled, drained, no salt added	1.15	0.18	3.07	19	2.8	19	0	0.27
Garlic, raw	6.36	0.5	33.06	149	2.1	17	0	30.96
Ginger root, raw	1.82	0.75	17.77	80	2	13	0	15.77
Gourd, white-flowered (calabash), raw	0.62	0.02	3.39	14	0.5	2	0	2.89
Gourd, white-flowered (calabash), cooked, boiled, drained, without salt	0.6	0.02	3.69	15	1.2	2	0	2.49
Gourd, dishcloth (towelgourd), raw	1.2	0.2	4.35	20	1.1	3	0	3.25
Gourd, dishcloth (towelgourd), cooked, boiled, drained, without salt	0.66	0.34	14.34	56	2.9	21	0	11.44
Drumstick leaves, raw	9.4	1.4	8.28	64	2	9	0	6.28

Food Name ---> per 100 g	Protein (g)	Fat (g)	Carb (g)	Calories	Fiber (g)	Sodium (mg)	Cholesterol (mg)	Net Carb (g)
Drumstick leaves, cooked, boiled, drained, without salt	5.27	0.93	11.15	60	2	9	0	9.15
Hyacinth-beans, immature seeds, raw	2.1	0.2	9.19	46	3.3	2	0	5.89
Hyacinth-beans, immature seeds, cooked, boiled, drained, without salt	2.95	0.27	9.2	50	-	2	0	9.2
Jerusalem-artichokes, raw	2	0.01	17.44	73	1.6	4	0	15.84
Jew's ear, (pepeao), raw	0.48	0.04	6.75	25	-	9	0	6.75
Pepeao, dried	4.82	0.44	81.03	298	-	70	0	81.03
Jute, potherb, raw	4.65	0.25	5.8	34	-	8	0	5.8
Jute, potherb, cooked, boiled, drained, without salt	3.68	0.2	7.29	37	2	11	0	5.29
Kale, raw	4.28	0.93	8.75	49	3.6	38	0	5.15
Kale, cooked, boiled, drained, without salt	1.9	0.4	5.63	28	2	23	0	3.63
Kale, frozen, unprepared	2.66	0.46	4.9	28	2	15	0	2.9
Kale, frozen, cooked, boiled, drained, without salt	2.84	0.49	5.23	30	2	15	0	3.23
Kanpyo, (dried gourd strips)	8.58	0.56	65.03	258	9.8	15	0	55.23
Mushrooms, shiitake, raw	2.24	0.49	6.79	34	2.5	9	-	4.29
Mushrooms, Chanterelle, raw	1.49	0.53	6.86	38	3.8	9	-	3.06
Mushrooms, morel, raw	3.12	0.57	5.1	31	2.8	21	-	2.3
Kohlrabi, raw	1.7	0.1	6.2	27	3.6	20	0	2.6
Kohlrabi, cooked, boiled, drained, without salt	1.8	0.11	6.69	29	1.1	21	0	5.59
Mushrooms, portabella, grilled	3.28	0.58	4.44	29	2.2	11	0	2.24
Lambsquarters, raw	4.2	0.8	7.3	43	4	43	0	3.3
Lambsquarters, cooked, boiled, drained, without salt	3.2	0.7	5	32	2.1	29	0	2.9
Leeks, (bulb and lower leaf-portion), raw	1.5	0.3	14.15	61	1.8	20	0	12.35
Leeks, (bulb and lower leaf-portion), cooked, boiled, drained, without salt	0.81	0.2	7.62	31	1	10	0	6.62
Lentils, sprouted, raw	8.96	0.55	22.14	106	-	11	0	22.14
Lentils, sprouted, cooked, stir-fried, without salt	8.8	0.45	21.25	101	-	10	0	21.25
Lettuce, butterhead (includes boston and bibb types), raw	1.35	0.22	2.23	13	1.1	5	0	1.13
Lettuce, cos or romaine, raw	1.23	0.3	3.29	17	2.1	8	0	1.19
Lettuce, iceberg (includes crisphead types), raw	0.9	0.14	2.97	14	1.2	10	0	1.77
Lettuce, green leaf, raw	1.36	0.15	2.87	15	1.3	28	0	1.57
Lotus root, raw	2.6	0.1	17.23	74	4.9	40	0	12.33
Lotus root, cooked, boiled, drained, without salt	1.58	0.07	16.02	66	3.1	45	0	12.92
Lettuce, red leaf, raw	1.33	0.22	2.26	16	0.9	25	0	1.36
Mountain yam, hawaii, raw	1.34	0.1	16.3	67	2.5	13	0	13.8
Mountain yam, hawaii, cooked, steamed, without salt	1.73	0.08	20	82	-	12	0	20
Mushrooms, white, raw	3.09	0.34	3.26	22	1	5	0	2.26
Mushrooms, white, cooked, boiled, drained, without salt	2.17	0.47	5.29	28	2.2	2	0	3.09
Mushrooms, white, stir-fried	3.58	0.33	4.04	26	1.8	12	0	2.24
Mushrooms, canned, drained solids	1.87	0.29	5.09	25	2.4	425	0	2.69
Mushrooms, portabella, raw	2.11	0.35	3.87	22	1.3	9	0	2.57
Mushrooms, brown, italian, or crimini, raw	2.5	0.1	4.3	22	0.6	6	0	3.7
Mushrooms, shiitake, stir-fried	3.45	0.35	7.68	39	3.6	5	0	4.08
Mushrooms, shiitake, dried	9.58	0.99	75.37	296	11.5	13	0	63.87
Mushrooms, shiitake, cooked, without salt	1.56	0.22	14.39	56	2.1	4	0	12.29
Mustard greens, raw	2.86	0.42	4.67	27	3.2	20	0	1.47
Mustard greens, cooked, boiled, drained, without salt	2.56	0.47	4.51	26	2	9	0	2.51
Mustard greens, frozen, unprepared	2.49	0.27	3.41	20	3.3	29	0	0.11
Mustard greens, frozen, cooked, boiled, drained, without salt	2.27	0.25	3.11	19	2.8	25	0	0.31

Food Name ---> per 100 g	Protein (g)	Fat (g)	Carb (g)	Calories	Fiber (g)	Sodium (mg)	Cholesterol (mg)	Net Carb (g)
Mustard spinach, (tendergreen), raw	2.2	0.3	3.9	22	2.8	21	0	1.1
Mustard spinach, (tendergreen), cooked, boiled, drained, without salt	1.7	0.2	2.8	16	2	14	0	0.8
New Zealand spinach, raw	1.5	0.2	2.5	14	1.5	130	0	1
New Zealand spinach, cooked, boiled, drained, without salt	1.3	0.17	2.13	12	1.4	107	0	0.73
Okra, raw	1.93	0.19	7.45	33	3.2	7	0	4.25
Okra, cooked, boiled, drained, without salt	1.87	0.21	4.51	22	2.5	6	0	2.01
Okra, frozen, unprepared	1.69	0.25	6.63	30	2.2	3	0	4.43
Okra, frozen, cooked, boiled, drained, without salt	1.63	0.24	6.41	29	2.1	3	0	4.31
Onions, raw	1.1	0.1	9.34	40	1.7	4	0	7.64
Onions, cooked, boiled, drained, without salt	1.36	0.19	10.15	44	1.4	3	0	8.75
Onions, dehydrated flakes	8.95	0.46	83.28	349	9.2	21	0	74.08
Onions, canned, solids and liquids	0.85	0.09	4.02	19	1.2	371	0	2.82
Onions, yellow, sauteed	0.95	10.8	7.86	132	1.7	12	-	6.16
Onions, frozen, chopped, unprepared	0.79	0.1	6.82	29	1.8	12	0	5.02
Onions, frozen, chopped, cooked, boiled, drained, without salt	0.77	0.1	6.59	28	1.8	12	0	4.79
Onions, frozen, whole, unprepared	0.89	0.06	8.45	35	1.7	10	0	6.75
Onions, frozen, whole, cooked, boiled, drained, without salt	0.71	0.05	6.7	28	1.4	8	0	5.3
Onions, spring or scallions (includes tops and bulb), raw	1.83	0.19	7.34	32	2.6	16	0	4.74
Onions, young green, tops only	0.97	0.47	5.74	27	1.8	15	0	3.94
Onions, welsh, raw	1.9	0.4	6.5	34	2.4	17	0	4.1
Onions, sweet, raw	0.8	0.08	7.55	32	0.9	8	0	6.65
Onion rings, breaded, par fried, frozen, unprepared	3.15	14.1	30.53	258	1.8	246	0	28.73
Onion rings, breaded, par fried, frozen, prepared, heated in oven	4.14	14.3	33.79	276	2.2	370	0	31.59
Parsley, fresh	2.97	0.79	6.33	36	3.3	56	0	3.03
Parsnips, raw	1.2	0.3	17.99	75	4.9	10	0	13.09
Parsnips, cooked, boiled, drained, without salt	1.32	0.3	17.01	71	3.6	10	0	13.41
Peas, edible-podded, raw	2.8	0.2	7.55	42	2.6	4	0	4.95
Peas, edible-podded, boiled, drained, without salt	3.27	0.23	7.05	42	2.8	4	0	4.25
Peas, edible-podded, frozen, unprepared	2.8	0.3	7.2	42	3.1	4	0	4.1
Peas, edible-podded, frozen, cooked, boiled, drained, without salt	3.5	0.38	9.02	52	3.1	5	0	5.92
Peas, green, raw	5.42	0.4	14.45	81	5.7	5	0	8.75
Peas, green, cooked, boiled, drained, without salt	5.36	0.22	15.63	84	5.5	3	0	10.13
Peas, green, canned, regular pack, solids and liquids	3.01	0.48	10.6	58	3.3	185	0	7.3
Peas, green (includes baby and lesuer types), canned, drained solids, unprepared	4.47	0.8	11.36	68	4.9	273	0	6.46
Peas, green, canned, seasoned, solids and liquids	3.09	0.27	9.25	50	2	254	0	7.25
Peas, green, canned, drained solids, rinsed in tap water	4.33	0.95	11.82	71	-	231	0	11.82
Peas, green, frozen, unprepared	5.22	0.4	13.62	77	4.5	108	0	9.12
Peas, green, frozen, cooked, boiled, drained, without salt	5.15	0.27	14.26	78	4.5	72	0	9.76
Peas, mature seeds, sprouted, raw	8.8	0.68	27.11	124	-	20	0	27.11
Peas, mature seeds, sprouted, cooked, boiled, drained, without salt	7.05	0.51	17.08	98	-	3	0	17.08
Peas and carrots, canned, regular pack, solids and liquids	2.17	0.27	8.48	38	2	260	0	6.48
Peas and carrots, frozen, unprepared	3.4	0.47	11.15	53	3.4	79	0	7.75

Food Name ---> per 100 g	Protein (g)	Fat (g)	Carb (g)	Calories	Fiber (g)	Sodium (mg)	Cholesterol (mg)	Net Carb (g)
Peas and carrots, frozen, cooked, boiled, drained, without salt	3.09	0.42	10.12	48	3.1	68	0	7.02
Peas and onions, canned, solids and liquids	3.28	0.38	8.57	51	2.3	442	0	6.27
Peas and onions, frozen, unprepared	3.98	0.32	13.51	70	3.5	61	0	10.01
Peas and onions, frozen, cooked, boiled, drained, without salt	2.54	0.2	8.63	45	2.2	37	0	6.43
Peppers, hot chili, green, canned, pods, excluding seeds, solids and liquids	0.9	0.1	5.1	21	1.3	1173	0	3.8
Peppers, sweet, green, raw	0.86	0.17	4.64	20	1.7	3	0	2.94
Peppers, sweet, green, cooked, boiled, drained, without salt	0.92	0.2	6.7	28	1.2	2	0	5.5
Peppers, sweet, green, canned, solids and liquids	0.8	0.3	3.9	18	1.2	1369	0	2.7
Peppers, sweet, green, frozen, chopped, unprepared	1.08	0.21	4.45	20	1.6	5	0	2.85
Peppers, sweet, green, frozen, chopped, boiled, drained, without salt	0.95	0.18	3.9	18	0.9	4	0	3
Peppers, sweet, green, sauteed	0.78	11.85	4.22	127	1.8	17	0	2.42
Pigeonpeas, immature seeds, raw	7.2	1.64	23.88	136	5.1	5	0	18.78
Pigeonpeas, immature seeds, cooked, boiled, drained, without salt	5.96	1.36	19.49	111	4.2	5	0	15.29
Poi	0.38	0.14	27.23	112	0.4	12	0	26.83
Pokeberry shoots, (poke), raw	2.6	0.4	3.7	23	1.7	23	0	2
Pokeberry shoots, (poke), cooked, boiled, drained, without salt	2.3	0.4	3.1	20	1.5	18	0	1.6
Potatoes, flesh and skin, raw	2.05	0.09	17.49	77	2.1	6	0	15.39
Potatoes, russet, flesh and skin, raw	2.14	0.08	18.07	79	1.3	5	0	16.77
Potatoes, white, flesh and skin, raw	1.68	0.1	15.71	69	2.4	16	0	13.31
Potatoes, red, flesh and skin, raw	1.89	0.14	15.9	70	1.7	18	0	14.2
Potatoes, Russet, flesh and skin, baked	2.63	0.13	21.44	97	2.3	14	0	19.14
Potatoes, white, flesh and skin, baked	2.1	0.15	21.08	94	2.1	7	0	18.98
Potatoes, red, flesh and skin, baked	2.3	0.15	19.59	89	1.8	12	0	17.79
Potatoes, french fried, crinkle or regular cut, salt added in processing, frozen, as purchased	2.34	4.99	23.96	150	2	349	0	21.96
Potatoes, french fried, crinkle or regular cut, salt added in processing, frozen, oven-heated	2.51	5.13	27.5	166	2.3	391	0	25.2
Potatoes, roasted, salt added in processing, frozen, unprepared	2.22	1.81	26.15	130	2.6	298	0	23.55
Potatoes, raw, skin	2.57	0.1	12.44	58	2.5	10	0	9.94
Potatoes, baked, flesh, without salt	1.96	0.1	21.55	93	1.5	5	0	20.05
Potatoes, baked, skin, without salt	4.29	0.1	46.06	198	7.9	21	0	38.16
Potatoes, boiled, cooked in skin, flesh, without salt	1.87	0.1	20.13	87	1.8	4	0	18.33
Potatoes, boiled, cooked in skin, skin, without salt	2.86	0.1	17.21	78	3.3	14	0	13.91
Potatoes, boiled, cooked without skin, flesh, without salt	1.71	0.1	20.01	86	1.8	5	0	18.21
Potatoes, microwaved, cooked in skin, flesh, without salt	2.1	0.1	23.28	100	1.6	7	0	21.68
Potatoes, microwaved, cooked in skin, skin, without salt	4.39	0.1	29.63	132	5.5	16	0	24.13
Potatoes, hash brown, home-prepared	3	12.52	35.11	265	3.2	342	0	31.91
Potatoes, mashed, home-prepared, whole milk and margarine added	1.96	4.2	16.94	113	1.5	333	1	15.44
Potatoes, scalloped, home-prepared with butter	2.87	3.68	10.78	88	1.9	335	12	8.88
Potatoes, au gratin, home-prepared from recipe using butter	5.06	7.59	11.27	132	1.8	433	23	9.47
Potatoes, canned, solids and liquids	1.2	0.11	9.89	44	1.4	217	0	8.49

Food Name ---> per 100 g	Protein (g)	Fat (g)	Carb (g)	Calories	Fiber (g)	Sodium (mg)	Cholesterol (mg)	Net Carb (g)
Potatoes, canned, drained solids	1.41	0.21	13.61	60	2.3	219	0	11.31
Potatoes, mashed, dehydrated, flakes without milk, dry form	8.34	0.41	81.17	354	6.6	77	0	74.57
Potatoes, mashed, dehydrated, prepared from flakes without milk, whole milk and butter added	1.77	5.13	10.87	97	0.8	164	14	10.07
Potatoes, mashed, dehydrated, granules without milk, dry form	8.22	0.54	85.51	372	7.1	67	0	78.41
Potatoes, mashed, dehydrated, prepared from granules without milk, whole milk and butter added	2.05	4.96	14.36	108	2.2	257	14	12.16
Potatoes, mashed, dehydrated, granules with milk, dry form	10.9	1.1	77.7	357	6.6	82	2	71.1
Potatoes, mashed, dehydrated, prepared from granules with milk, water and margarine added	2.13	4.8	16.13	116	1.3	172	2	14.83
Potatoes, au gratin, dry mix, unprepared	8.9	3.7	74.31	314	4.1	2095	-	70.21
Potatoes, au gratin, dry mix, prepared with water, whole milk and butter	2.3	4.12	12.84	93	0.9	439	15	11.94
Potatoes, scalloped, dry mix, unprepared	7.77	4.59	73.93	358	8.6	1578	5	65.33
Potatoes, scalloped, dry mix, prepared with water, whole milk and butter	2.12	4.3	12.77	93	1.1	341	11	11.67
Potatoes, hash brown, frozen, plain, unprepared	2.06	0.62	17.72	82	1.4	22	-	16.32
Potatoes, hash brown, frozen, plain, prepared, pan fried in canola oil	2.65	11.59	28.51	219	3.2	15	0	25.31
Potatoes, hash brown, frozen, with butter sauce, unprepared	1.87	6.66	18.28	135	2.9	77	-	15.38
Potatoes, hash brown, frozen, with butter sauce, prepared	2.46	8.79	24.13	178	3.8	101	23	20.33
Potatoes, french fried, shoestring, salt added in processing, frozen, as purchased	2.16	6.24	25.59	167	2.3	323	0	23.29
Potatoes, french fried, shoestring, salt added in processing, frozen, oven-heated	2.9	6.76	31.66	199	2.8	400	0	28.86
Potatoes, o'brien, frozen, unprepared	1.83	0.14	17.47	76	1.9	33	-	15.57
Potatoes, o'brien, frozen, prepared	2.22	13.21	21.86	204	1.7	43	0	20.16
Potato puffs, frozen, unprepared	1.93	8.71	24.8	178	2.3	428	0	22.5
Potato puffs, frozen, oven-heated	2.13	9.05	27.29	192	2	463	0	25.29
Potatoes, frozen, whole, unprepared	2.38	0.16	17.47	78	1.2	25	0	16.27
Potatoes, frozen, whole, cooked, boiled, drained, without salt	1.98	0.13	14.52	65	1.4	20	0	13.12
Potatoes, french fried, all types, salt added in processing, frozen, unprepared	2.24	4.66	24.81	147	1.9	332	0	22.91
Potatoes, french fried, all types, salt added in processing, frozen, home-prepared, oven heated	2.75	5.48	25.55	158	2	324	0	23.55
Potatoes, french fried, cottage-cut, salt not added in processing, frozen, as purchased	2.42	5.78	23.98	153	3	32	0	20.98
Potatoes, french fried, cottage-cut, salt not added in processing, frozen, oven-heated	3.44	8.2	34.03	218	3.2	45	0	30.83
Potatoes, frozen, french fried, par fried, extruded, unprepared	2.83	14.95	30.15	260	2.9	490	0	27.25
Potatoes, frozen, french fried, par fried, extruded, prepared, heated in oven, without salt	3.55	18.71	39.68	333	3.2	613	0	36.48
USDA Commodity, Potato wedges, frozen	2.7	2.2	25.5	123	2	49	0	23.5
Potatoes, french fried, steak fries, salt added in processing, frozen, as purchased	2.19	3.39	23.51	133	1.9	317	0	21.61
Potatoes, french fried, steak fries, salt added in processing, frozen, oven-heated	2.57	3.76	26.98	152	2.6	373	0	24.38
Potato flour	6.9	0.34	83.1	357	5.9	55	0	77.2

Food Name ---> per 100 g	Protein (g)	Fat (g)	Carb (g)	Calories	Fiber (g)	Sodium (mg)	Cholesterol (mg)	Net Carb (g)
Potato salad, home-prepared	2.68	8.2	11.17	143	1.3	529	68	9.87
Pumpkin flowers, raw	1.03	0.07	3.28	15	-	5	0	3.28
Pumpkin flowers, cooked, boiled, drained, without salt	1.09	0.08	3.3	15	0.9	6	0	2.4
Pumpkin leaves, raw	3.15	0.4	2.33	19	-	11	0	2.33
Pumpkin leaves, cooked, boiled, drained, without salt	2.72	0.22	3.39	21	2.7	8	0	0.69
Pumpkin, raw	1	0.1	6.5	26	0.5	1	0	6
Pumpkin, cooked, boiled, drained, without salt	0.72	0.07	4.9	20	1.1	1	0	3.8
Pumpkin, canned, without salt	1.1	0.28	8.09	34	2.9	5	0	5.19
Pumpkin pie mix, canned	1.09	0.13	26.39	104	8.3	208	0	18.09
Purslane, raw	2.03	0.36	3.39	20	-	45	0	3.39
Purslane, cooked, boiled, drained, without salt	1.49	0.19	3.55	18	-	44	0	3.55
Radishes, raw	0.68	0.1	3.4	16	1.6	39	0	1.8
Radishes, oriental, raw	0.6	0.1	4.1	18	1.6	21	0	2.5
Radishes, oriental, cooked, boiled, drained, without salt	0.67	0.24	3.43	17	1.6	13	0	1.83
Radishes, oriental, dried	7.9	0.72	63.37	271	23.9	278	0	39.47
Rutabagas, raw	1.08	0.16	8.62	37	2.3	12	0	6.32
Rutabagas, cooked, boiled, drained, without salt	0.93	0.18	6.84	30	1.8	5	0	5.04
Salsify, (vegetable oyster), raw	3.3	0.2	18.6	82	3.3	20	0	15.3
Salsify, cooked, boiled, drained, without salt	2.73	0.17	15.36	68	3.1	16	0	12.26
Sauerkraut, canned, solids and liquids	0.91	0.14	4.28	19	2.9	661	0	1.38
Seaweed, agar, raw	0.54	0.03	6.75	26	0.5	9	0	6.25
Seaweed, irishmoss, raw	1.51	0.16	12.29	49	1.3	67	0	10.99
Seaweed, kelp, raw	1.68	0.56	9.57	43	1.3	233	0	8.27
Seaweed, laver, raw	5.81	0.28	5.11	35	0.3	48	0	4.81
Sesbania flower, raw	1.28	0.04	6.73	27	-	15	0	6.73
Sesbania flower, cooked, steamed, without salt	1.14	0.05	5.23	22	-	11	0	5.23
Soybeans, green, raw	12.95	6.8	11.05	147	4.2	15	0	6.85
Soybeans, green, cooked, boiled, drained, without salt	12.35	6.4	11.05	141	4.2	14	0	6.85
Soybeans, mature seeds, sprouted, raw	13.09	6.7	9.57	122	1.1	14	0	8.47
Soybeans, mature seeds, sprouted, cooked, steamed	8.47	4.45	6.53	81	0.8	10	0	5.73
Soybeans, mature seeds, sprouted, cooked, stir-fried	13.1	7.1	9.4	125	0.8	14	0	8.6
Spinach, raw	2.86	0.39	3.63	23	2.2	79	0	1.43
Spinach, cooked, boiled, drained, without salt	2.97	0.26	3.75	23	2.4	70	0	1.35
Spinach, canned, regular pack, solids and liquids	2.11	0.37	2.92	19	1.6	319	0	1.32
Spinach, canned, regular pack, drained solids	2.81	0.5	3.4	23	2.4	322	0	1
Spinach, frozen, chopped or leaf, unprepared	3.63	0.57	4.21	29	2.9	74	0	1.31
Spinach, frozen, chopped or leaf, cooked, boiled, drained, without salt	4.01	0.87	4.8	34	3.7	97	0	1.1
Squash, summer, crookneck and straightneck, raw	1.01	0.27	3.88	19	1	2	0	2.88
Squash, summer, crookneck and straightneck, cooked, boiled, drained, without salt	1.04	0.39	3.79	23	1.1	1	0	2.69
Squash, summer, crookneck and straightneck, canned, drained, solid, without salt	0.61	0.07	2.96	13	1.4	5	0	1.56
Squash, summer, crookneck and straightneck, frozen, unprepared	0.83	0.14	4.8	20	1.2	5	0	3.6
Squash, summer, crookneck and straightneck, frozen, cooked, boiled, drained, without salt	1.28	0.2	5.54	25	1.4	6	0	4.14
Squash, summer, scallop, raw	1.2	0.2	3.84	18	1.2	1	0	2.64
Squash, summer, scallop, cooked, boiled, drained, without salt	1.03	0.17	3.3	16	1.9	1	0	1.4

Food Name ---> per 100 g	Protein (g)	Fat (g)	Carb (g)	Calories	Fiber (g)	Sodium (mg)	Cholesterol (mg)	Net Carb (g)
Squash, summer, zucchini, includes skin, raw	1.21	0.32	3.11	17	1	8	0	2.11
Squash, summer, zucchini, includes skin, cooked, boiled, drained, without salt	1.14	0.36	2.69	15	1	3	0	1.69
Squash, summer, zucchini, includes skin, frozen, unprepared	1.16	0.13	3.58	17	1.3	2	0	2.28
Squash, summer, zucchini, includes skin, frozen, cooked, boiled, drained, without salt	1.15	0.13	3.56	17	1.3	2	0	2.26
Squash, summer, zucchini, italian style, canned	1.03	0.11	6.85	29	-	374	0	6.85
Squash, winter, acorn, raw	0.8	0.1	10.42	40	1.5	3	0	8.92
Squash, winter, acorn, cooked, baked, without salt	1.12	0.14	14.58	56	4.4	4	0	10.18
Squash, winter, acorn, cooked, boiled, mashed, without salt	0.67	0.08	8.79	34	2.6	3	0	6.19
Squash, winter, butternut, raw	1	0.1	11.69	45	2	4	0	9.69
Squash, winter, butternut, cooked, baked, without salt	0.9	0.09	10.49	40	3.2	4	0	7.29
Squash, winter, butternut, frozen, unprepared	1.76	0.1	14.41	57	1.3	2	0	13.11
Squash, winter, butternut, frozen, cooked, boiled, without salt	1.23	0.07	10.05	39	-	2	0	10.05
Squash, winter, hubbard, raw	2	0.5	8.7	40	3.9	7	0	4.8
Squash, winter, hubbard, baked, without salt	2.48	0.62	10.81	50	4.9	8	0	5.91
Squash, winter, hubbard, cooked, boiled, mashed, without salt	1.48	0.37	6.46	30	2.9	5	0	3.56
Squash, winter, spaghetti, raw	0.64	0.57	6.91	31	1.5	17	0	5.41
Squash, winter, spaghetti, cooked, boiled, drained, or baked, without salt	0.66	0.26	6.46	27	1.4	18	0	5.06
Succotash, (corn and limas), raw	5.03	1.02	19.59	99	3.8	4	0	15.79
Succotash, (corn and limas), cooked, boiled, drained, without salt	5.07	0.8	24.38	115	4.5	17	0	19.88
Succotash, (corn and limas), canned, with cream style corn	2.64	0.54	17.61	77	3	245	0	14.61
Succotash, (corn and limas), canned, with whole kernel corn, solids and liquids	2.6	0.49	13.98	63	2.6	221	0	11.38
Succotash, (corn and limas), frozen, unprepared	4.31	0.89	19.94	93	4	45	0	15.94
Succotash, (corn and limas), frozen, cooked, boiled, drained, without salt	4.31	0.89	19.95	93	4.1	45	0	15.85
Swamp cabbage, (skunk cabbage), raw	2.6	0.2	3.14	19	2.1	113	0	1.04
Swamp cabbage (skunk cabbage), cooked, boiled, drained, without salt	2.08	0.24	3.7	20	1.9	122	0	1.8
Sweet potato leaves, raw	2.49	0.51	8.82	42	5.3	6	0	3.52
Sweet potato leaves, cooked, steamed, without salt	2.18	0.34	7.38	41	1.9	7	0	5.48
Sweet potato, raw, unprepared	1.57	0.05	20.12	86	3	55	0	17.12
Sweet potato, cooked, baked in skin, flesh, without salt	2.01	0.15	20.71	90	3.3	36	0	17.41
Sweet potato, cooked, boiled, without skin	1.37	0.14	17.72	76	2.5	27	0	15.22
Sweet potato, canned, vacuum pack	1.65	0.2	21.12	91	1.8	53	0	19.32
Sweet potato, canned, mashed	1.98	0.2	23.19	101	1.7	75	0	21.49
Sweet potato, frozen, unprepared	1.71	0.18	22.22	96	1.7	6	0	20.52
Sweet potato, frozen, cooked, baked, without salt	1.71	0.12	23.4	100	1.8	8	0	21.6
Taro, raw	1.5	0.2	26.46	112	4.1	11	0	22.36
Taro, cooked, without salt	0.52	0.11	34.6	142	5.1	15	0	29.5
Taro leaves, raw	4.98	0.74	6.7	42	3.7	3	0	3
Taro leaves, cooked, steamed, without salt	2.72	0.41	4.02	24	2	2	0	2.02
Taro shoots, raw	0.92	0.09	2.32	11	-	1	0	2.32
Taro shoots, cooked, without salt	0.73	0.08	3.2	14	-	2	0	3.2
Taro, tahitian, raw	2.79	0.97	6.91	44	-	50	0	6.91

Food Name ---> per 100 g	Protein (g)	Fat (g)	Carb (g)	Calories	Fiber (g)	Sodium (mg)	Cholesterol (mg)	Net Carb (g)
Taro, tahitian, cooked, without salt	4.16	0.68	6.85	44	-	54	0	6.85
Tomatoes, green, raw	1.2	0.2	5.1	23	1.1	13	0	4
Tomatoes, red, ripe, raw, year round average	0.88	0.2	3.89	18	1.2	5	0	2.69
Tomatoes, red, ripe, cooked	0.95	0.11	4.01	18	0.7	11	0	3.31
Tomatoes, red, ripe, canned, packed in tomato juice	0.79	0.25	3.47	16	1.9	115	0	1.57
Tomatoes, red, ripe, canned, stewed	0.91	0.19	6.19	26	1	221	0	5.19
Tomatoes, red, ripe, canned, with green chilies	0.69	0.08	3.62	15	-	401	0	3.62
Tomato juice, canned, with salt added	0.85	0.29	3.53	17	0.4	253	0	3.13
Tomato products, canned, paste, without salt added	4.32	0.47	18.91	82	4.1	59	0	14.81
Tomato products, canned, puree, without salt added	1.65	0.21	8.98	38	1.9	28	0	7.08
Tomato powder	12.91	0.44	74.68	302	16.5	134	0	58.18
Tomato products, canned, sauce	1.2	0.3	5.31	24	1.5	474	0	3.81
Tomato products, canned, sauce, with mushrooms	1.45	0.13	8.43	35	1.5	452	0	6.93
Tomato products, canned, sauce, with onions	1.56	0.19	9.94	42	1.8	551	0	8.14
Tomato products, canned, sauce, with herbs and cheese	2.13	1.93	10.24	59	2.2	543	3	8.04
Tomato products, canned, sauce, with onions, green peppers, and celery	0.94	0.74	8.77	41	1.4	368	0	7.37
Tomato products, canned, sauce, with tomato tidbits	1.32	0.39	7.09	32	1.4	15	0	5.69
Tree fern, cooked, without salt	0.29	0.07	10.98	40	3.7	5	0	7.28
Turnips, raw	0.9	0.1	6.43	28	1.8	67	0	4.63
Turnips, cooked, boiled, drained, without salt	0.71	0.08	5.06	22	2	16	0	3.06
Turnips, frozen, unprepared	1.04	0.16	2.94	16	1.8	25	0	1.14
Turnips, frozen, cooked, boiled, drained, without salt	1.53	0.24	4.35	23	2	36	0	2.35
Turnip greens, raw	1.5	0.3	7.13	32	3.2	40	0	3.93
Turnip greens, cooked, boiled, drained, without salt	1.14	0.23	4.36	20	3.5	29	0	0.86
Turnip greens, canned, solids and liquids	1.36	0.3	2.42	14	1.7	277	0	0.72
Turnip greens, frozen, unprepared	2.47	0.31	3.67	22	2.5	12	0	1.17
Turnip greens, frozen, cooked, boiled, drained, without salt	3.35	0.42	4.98	29	3.4	15	0	1.58
Turnip greens and turnips, frozen, unprepared	2.46	0.19	3.39	21	2.4	18	0	0.99
Turnip greens and turnips, frozen, cooked, boiled, drained, without salt	2.99	0.38	4.85	35	3.1	19	0	1.75
Vegetable juice cocktail, canned	0.93	0.31	3.87	22	0.5	169	0	3.37
Vegetables, mixed, canned, solids and liquids	1.42	0.25	7.13	36	3.8	224	0	3.33
Vegetables, mixed, canned, drained solids	2.59	0.25	9.26	49	3	214	0	6.26
Vegetables, mixed, frozen, unprepared	3.33	0.52	13.47	72	4	47	0	9.47
Vegetables, mixed, frozen, cooked, boiled, drained, without salt	2.86	0.15	13.09	65	4.4	35	0	8.69
Vegetable juice cocktail, low sodium, canned	0.91	0.32	3.83	19	0.5	55	0	3.33
Vinespinach, (basella), raw	1.8	0.3	3.4	19	-	24	0	3.4
Waterchestnuts, chinese, (matai), raw	1.4	0.1	23.94	97	3	14	0	20.94
Waterchestnuts, chinese, canned, solids and liquids	0.88	0.06	12.3	50	2.5	8	0	9.8
Watercress, raw	2.3	0.1	1.29	11	0.5	41	0	0.79
Waxgourd, (chinese preserving melon), raw	0.4	0.2	3	13	2.9	111	0	0.1
Waxgourd, (chinese preserving melon), cooked, boiled, drained, without salt	0.4	0.2	3.04	14	1	107	0	2.04
Winged beans, immature seeds, raw	6.95	0.87	4.31	49	-	4	0	4.31
Winged beans, immature seeds, cooked, boiled, drained, without salt	5.31	0.66	3.21	38	-	4	0	3.21
Winged bean leaves, raw	5.85	1.1	14.1	74	-	9	0	14.1
Winged bean tuber, raw	11.6	0.9	28.1	148	-	35	0	28.1
Yam, raw	1.53	0.17	27.88	118	4.1	9	0	23.78

Food Name ---> per 100 g	Protein (g)	Fat (g)	Carb (g)	Calories	Fiber (g)	Sodium (mg)	Cholesterol (mg)	Net Carb (g)
Yam, cooked, boiled, drained, or baked, without salt	1.49	0.14	27.48	116	3.9	8	0	23.58
Yambean (jicama), raw	0.72	0.09	8.82	38	4.9	4	0	3.92
Yambean (jicama), cooked, boiled, drained, without salt	0.72	0.09	8.82	38	-	4	0	8.82
Beets, harvard, canned, solids and liquids	0.84	0.06	18.18	73	2.5	162	0	15.68
Beets, pickled, canned, solids and liquids	0.8	0.08	16.28	65	0.8	149	0	15.48
Borage, raw	1.8	0.7	3.06	21	-	80	0	3.06
Borage, cooked, boiled, drained, without salt	2.09	0.81	3.55	25	-	88	0	3.55
Chives, freeze-dried	21.2	3.5	64.29	311	26.2	70	0	38.09
Dock, raw	2	0.7	3.2	22	2.9	4	0	0.3
Dock, cooked, boiled, drained, without salt	1.83	0.64	2.93	20	2.6	3	0	0.33
Eppaw, raw	4.6	1.8	31.68	150	-	12	0	31.68
Drumstick pods, raw	2.1	0.2	8.53	37	3.2	42	0	5.33
Drumstick pods, cooked, boiled, drained, without salt	2.09	0.19	8.18	36	4.2	43	0	3.98
Kale, scotch, raw	2.8	0.6	8.32	42	1.7	70	0	6.62
Kale, scotch, cooked, boiled, drained, without salt	1.9	0.41	5.63	28	1.2	45	0	4.43
Leeks, (bulb and lower-leaf portion), freeze-dried	15.2	2.1	74.65	321	10.4	35	0	64.25
Parsley, freeze-dried	31.3	5.2	42.38	271	32.7	391	0	9.68
Beans, mung, mature seeds, sprouted, canned, drained solids	1.4	0.06	2.14	12	0.8	42	0	1.34
Peppers, jalapeno, canned, solids and liquids	0.92	0.94	4.74	27	2.6	1671	0	2.14
Peppers, sweet, green, freeze-dried	17.9	3	68.7	314	21.3	193	0	47.4
Radishes, white icicle, raw	1.1	0.1	2.63	14	1.4	16	0	1.23
Shallots, freeze-dried	12.3	0.5	80.7	348	15.7	59	0	65
Squash, summer, all varieties, raw	1.21	0.18	3.35	16	1.1	2	0	2.25
Squash, summer, all varieties, cooked, boiled, drained, without salt	0.91	0.31	4.31	20	1.4	1	0	2.91
Squash, winter, all varieties, raw	0.95	0.13	8.59	34	1.5	4	0	7.09
Squash, winter, all varieties, cooked, baked, without salt	0.89	0.35	8.85	37	2.8	1	0	6.05
Sweet potato, canned, syrup pack, solids and liquids	0.98	0.2	20.93	89	2.5	29	0	18.43
Sweet potato, canned, syrup pack, drained solids	1.28	0.32	25.36	108	3	39	0	22.36
Tomato products, canned, sauce, spanish style	1.44	0.27	7.24	33	1.4	472	0	5.84
Beans, pinto, mature seeds, sprouted, raw	5.25	0.9	11.6	62	-	153	0	11.6
Beans, pinto, mature seeds, sprouted, cooked, boiled, drained, without salt	1.86	0.32	4.1	22	-	51	0	4.1
Carrot juice, canned	0.95	0.15	9.28	40	0.8	66	0	8.48
Corn pudding, home prepared	4.42	5.04	16.97	131	1.2	282	72	15.77
Potatoes, mashed, home-prepared, whole milk added	1.91	0.57	17.57	83	1.5	302	2	16.07
Spinach souffle	7.89	12.95	5.9	172	0.7	566	118	5.2
Sweet potato, cooked, candied, home-prepared	0.89	3.54	32.12	164	2.1	119	9	30.02
Tomatoes, red, ripe, cooked, stewed	1.96	2.68	13.05	79	1.7	455	0	11.35
Seaweed, agar, dried	6.21	0.3	80.88	306	7.7	102	0	73.18
Seaweed, spirulina, raw	5.92	0.39	2.42	26	0.4	98	0	2.02
Seaweed, spirulina, dried	57.47	7.72	23.9	290	3.6	1048	0	20.3
Seaweed, wakame, raw	3.03	0.64	9.14	45	0.5	872	0	8.64
Peppers, hot chili, green, raw	2	0.2	9.46	40	1.5	7	0	7.96
Potatoes, o'brien, home-prepared	2.35	1.28	15.47	81	-	217	4	15.47
Potato pancakes	6.08	14.76	27.81	268	3.3	764	95	24.51
Potatoes, baked, flesh and skin, without salt	2.5	0.13	21.15	93	2.2	10	0	18.95
Potatoes, microwaved, cooked in skin, flesh and skin, without salt	2.44	0.1	24.24	105	2.3	8	0	21.94
Radish seeds, sprouted, raw	3.81	2.53	3.6	43	-	6	0	3.6

Food Name ---> per 100 g	Protein (g)	Fat (g)	Carb (g)	Calories	Fiber (g)	Sodium (mg)	Cholesterol (mg)	Net Carb (g)
Shallots, raw	2.5	0.1	16.8	72	3.2	12	0	13.6
Carrot, dehydrated	8.1	1.49	79.57	341	23.6	275	0	55.97
Tomatoes, crushed, canned	1.64	0.28	7.29	32	1.9	186	0	5.39
Tomatoes, orange, raw	1.16	0.19	3.18	16	0.9	42	0	2.28
Tomatoes, yellow, raw	0.98	0.26	2.98	15	0.7	23	0	2.28
Arrowroot, raw	4.24	0.2	13.39	65	1.3	26	0	12.09
Chrysanthemum leaves, raw	3.36	0.56	3.01	24	3	118	0	0.01
Amaranth leaves, cooked, boiled, drained, with salt	2.11	0.18	4.11	21	-	257	0	4.11
Arrowhead, cooked, boiled, drained, with salt	4.49	0.1	16.14	78	-	254	0	16.14
Artichokes, (globe or french), cooked, boiled, drained, with salt	2.89	0.34	11.39	51	5.7	296	0	5.69
Artichokes, (globe or french), frozen, cooked, boiled, drained, with salt	3.11	0.5	9.18	45	4.6	289	0	4.58
Asparagus, cooked, boiled, drained, with salt	2.4	0.22	4.11	22	2	240	0	2.11
Asparagus, canned, no salt added, solids and liquids	1.8	0.18	2.48	15	1	26	0	1.48
Asparagus, frozen, cooked, boiled, drained, with salt	2.95	0.42	1.92	18	1.6	240	0	0.32
Balsam-pear (bitter gourd), leafy tips, cooked, boiled, drained, with salt	3.6	0.2	6.16	32	1.9	249	0	4.26
Balsam-pear (bitter gourd), pods, cooked, boiled, drained, with salt	0.84	0.18	4.32	19	2	242	0	2.32
Bamboo shoots, cooked, boiled, drained, with salt	1.53	0.22	1.52	11	1	240	0	0.52
Beans, kidney, mature seeds, sprouted, cooked, boiled, drained, with salt	4.83	0.58	4.72	33	-	243	0	4.72
Lima beans, immature seeds, cooked, boiled, drained, with salt	6.81	0.32	23.64	123	5.3	253	0	18.34
Lima beans, immature seeds, canned, no salt added, solids and liquids	4.07	0.29	13.33	71	3.6	4	0	9.73
Lima beans, immature seeds, frozen, baby, cooked, boiled, drained, with salt	6.65	0.3	19.45	105	4.8	265	0	14.65
Lima beans, immature seeds, frozen, fordhook, cooked, boiled, drained, with salt	6.07	0.34	19.32	103	5.3	289	0	14.02
Mung beans, mature seeds, sprouted, cooked, boiled, drained, with salt	2.03	0.09	3.6	19	0.8	246	0	2.8
Beans, navy, mature seeds, sprouted, cooked, boiled, drained, with salt	7.07	0.81	15.01	78	-	250	0	15.01
Beans, pinto, immature seeds, frozen, cooked, boiled, drained, with salt	9.31	0.48	30.87	162	5.4	319	0	25.47
Beans, pinto, mature seeds, sprouted, cooked, boiled, drained, with salt	1.86	0.32	3.5	20	-	287	0	3.5
Beans, snap, yellow, raw	1.82	0.12	7.13	31	3.4	6	0	3.73
Beans, snap, green, cooked, boiled, drained, with salt	1.89	0.28	7.88	35	3.2	239	0	4.68
Beans, snap, yellow, cooked, boiled, drained, without salt	1.89	0.28	7.88	35	3.3	3	0	4.58
Beans, snap, yellow, cooked, boiled, drained, with salt	1.89	0.28	7.88	35	3.3	239	0	4.58
Beans, snap, green, canned, no salt added, solids and liquids	0.8	0.1	3.5	15	1.5	14	0	2
Beans, snap, yellow, canned, regular pack, solids and liquids	0.8	0.1	3.5	15	1.5	259	0	2
Beans, snap, yellow, canned, no salt added, solids and liquids	0.8	0.1	3.5	15	1.5	14	0	2
Beans, snap, green, canned, no salt added, drained solids	1.12	0.46	4.32	22	1.9	2	0	2.42
Beans, snap, yellow, frozen, all styles, unprepared	1.8	0.21	7.58	33	2.8	3	0	4.78
Beans, snap, green, frozen, cooked, boiled, drained,	1.49	0.17	6.45	28	3	245	0	3.45

Food Name ---> per 100 g	Protein (g)	Fat (g)	Carb (g)	Calories	Fiber (g)	Sodium (mg)	Cholesterol (mg)	Net Carb (g)
with salt								
Beans, snap, yellow, frozen, cooked, boiled, drained, without salt	1.49	0.17	6.45	28	3	9	0	3.45
Beans, snap, yellow, frozen, cooked, boiled, drained, with salt	1.49	0.17	6.45	28	3	245	0	3.45
Beets, cooked, boiled. drained, with salt	1.68	0.18	9.96	44	2	285	0	7.96
Beets, canned, no salt added, solids and liquids	0.8	0.07	6.57	28	1.2	21	0	5.37
Beet greens, cooked, boiled, drained, with salt	2.57	0.2	5.46	27	2.9	477	0	2.56
Borage, cooked, boiled, drained, with salt	2.09	0.81	3.55	25	-	324	0	3.55
Broadbeans, immature seeds, cooked, boiled, drained, with salt	4.8	0.5	10.1	62	-	277	0	10.1
Broccoli, leaves, raw	2.98	0.35	5.06	28	2.3	27	0	2.76
Broccoli, flower clusters, raw	2.98	0.35	5.06	28	2.3	27	0	2.76
Broccoli, stalks, raw	2.98	0.35	5.24	28		27	0	5.24
Broccoli, cooked, boiled, drained, with salt	2.38	0.41	7.18	35	3.3	262	0	3.88
Broccoli, frozen, chopped, cooked, boiled, drained, with salt	3.1	0.12	5.35	28	3	260	0	2.35
Broccoli, frozen, spears, cooked, boiled, drained, with salt	3.1	0.11	5.35	28	3	260	0	2.35
Brussels sprouts, cooked, boiled, drained, with salt	2.55	0.5	7.1	36	2.6	257	0	4.5
Brussels sprouts, frozen, cooked, boiled, drained, with salt	3.64	0.39	8.32	42	4.1	259	0	4.22
Burdock root, cooked, boiled, drained, with salt	2.09	0.14	21.15	88	1.8	240	0	19.35
Butterbur, cooked, boiled, drained, with salt	0.23	0.02	2.16	8	-	240	0	2.16
Cabbage, common (danish, domestic, and pointed types), freshly harvest, raw	1.21	0.18	5.37	24	2.3	18	0	3.07
Cabbage, common (danish, domestic, and pointed types), stored, raw	1.21	0.18	5.37	24	2.3	18	0	3.07
Cabbage, common, cooked, boiled, drained, with salt	1.27	0.06	5.51	23	1.9	255	0	3.61
Cabbage, red, cooked, boiled, drained, with salt	1.51	0.09	6.94	29	2.6	244	0	4.34
Cabbage, savoy, cooked, boiled, drained, with salt	1.8	0.09	5.41	24	2.8	260	0	2.61
Cabbage, chinese (pak-choi), cooked, boiled, drained, with salt	1.56	0.16	1.78	12	1	270	0	0.78
Cabbage, chinese (pe-tsai), cooked, boiled, drained, with salt	1.5	0.17	2.41	14	1.7	245	0	0.71
Cardoon, cooked, boiled, drained, with salt	0.76	0.11	4.74	20	1.7	412	0	3.04
Carrots, cooked, boiled, drained, with salt	0.76	0.18	8.22	35	3	302	0	5.22
Carrots, canned, no salt added, solids and liquids	0.59	0.14	5.36	23	1.8	34	0	3.56
Carrots, canned, no salt added, drained solids	0.64	0.19	5.54	25	1.5	42	0	4.04
Carrots, frozen, cooked, boiled, drained, with salt	0.58	0.68	7.73	37	3.3	295	0	4.43
Cauliflower, cooked, boiled, drained, with salt	1.84	0.45	4.11	23	2.3	242	0	1.81
Cauliflower, frozen, cooked, boiled, drained, with salt	1.61	0.22	3.16	17	2.7	254	0	0.46
Celeriac, cooked, boiled, drained, with salt	0.96	0.19	5.9	27	-	297	0	5.9
Celery, cooked, boiled, drained, with salt	0.83	0.16	4	18	1.6	327	0	2.4
Chard, swiss, cooked, boiled, drained, with salt	1.88	0.08	4.13	20	2.1	415	0	2.03
Chayote, fruit, cooked, boiled, drained, with salt	0.62	0.48	4.5	22	2.8	237	0	1.7
Chrysanthemum, garland, cooked, boiled, drained, with salt	1.64	0.09	4.31	20	2.3	289	0	2.01
Collards, cooked, boiled, drained, with salt	2.71	0.72	5.65	33	4	252	0	1.65
Collards, frozen, chopped, cooked, boiled, drained, with salt	2.97	0.41	7.1	36	2.8	286	0	4.3
Corn, sweet, yellow, cooked, boiled, drained, with salt	3.41	1.5	20.98	96	2.4	253	0	18.58

Food Name ---> per 100 g	Protein (g)	Fat (g)	Carb (g)	Calories	Fiber (g)	Sodium (mg)	Cholesterol (mg)	Net Carb (g)
Corn, sweet, yellow, canned, no salt added, solids and liquids	1.95	0.77	13.86	61	1.7	12	0	12.16
Corn, sweet, yellow, canned, cream style, no salt added	1.74	0.42	18.13	72	1.2	3	0	16.93
Corn, sweet, yellow, canned, vacuum pack, no salt added	2.41	0.5	19.44	79	2	3	0	17.44
Corn, sweet, yellow, frozen, kernels, cut off cob, boiled, drained, with salt	2.55	0.67	18.71	79	2.4	245	0	16.31
Corn, sweet, yellow, frozen, kernels on cob, cooked, boiled, drained, with salt	3.11	0.74	22.33	94	2.8	240	0	19.53
Cowpeas (blackeyes), immature seeds, cooked, boiled, drained, with salt	3.17	0.38	19.73	94	5	240	0	14.73
Cowpeas (blackeyes), immature seeds, frozen, cooked, boiled, drained, with salt	8.49	0.66	23.5	131	6.4	241	0	17.1
Cowpeas, young pods with seeds, cooked, boiled, drained, with salt	2.6	0.3	7	34	-	239	0	7
Cowpeas, leafy tips, cooked, boiled, drained, with salt	4.67	0.1	2.8	22	-	242	0	2.8
Cress, garden, cooked, boiled, drained, with salt	1.9	0.6	3.8	23	0.7	244	0	3.1
Dandelion greens, cooked, boiled, drained, with salt	2	0.6	6.4	33	2.9	280	0	3.5
Eggplant, cooked, boiled, drained, with salt	0.83	0.23	8.14	33	2.5	239	0	5.64
Gourd, white-flowered (calabash), cooked, boiled, drained, with salt	0.6	0.02	3.1	13	1.2	238	0	1.9
Gourd, dishcloth (towelgourd), cooked, boiled, drained, with salt	0.66	0.34	13.75	54	2.9	257	0	10.85
Drumstick leaves, cooked, boiled, drained, with salt	5.27	0.93	11.15	60	2	245	0	9.15
Drumstick pods, cooked, boiled, drained, with salt	2.09	0.19	8.18	36	4.2	279	0	3.98
Hyacinth-beans, immature seeds, cooked, boiled, drained, with salt	2.95	0.27	9.2	50	-	238	0	9.2
Jute, potherb, cooked, boiled, drained, with salt	3.68	0.2	7.29	37	2	247	0	5.29
Kale, cooked, boiled, drained, with salt	1.9	0.4	5.63	28	2	259	0	3.63
Kale, frozen, cooked, boiled, drained, with salt	2.84	0.49	5.23	30	2	251	0	3.23
Kale, scotch, cooked, boiled, drained, with salt	1.9	0.41	5.62	28	-	281	0	5.62
Kohlrabi, cooked, boiled, drained, with salt	1.8	0.11	6.69	29	1.1	257	0	5.59
Lambsquarters, cooked, boiled, drained, with salt	3.2	0.7	5	32	2.1	265	0	2.9
Leeks, (bulb and lower leaf-portion), cooked, boiled, drained, with salt	0.81	0.2	7.62	31	1	246	0	6.62
Lotus root, cooked, boiled, drained, with salt	1.58	0.07	16.02	66	3.1	281	0	12.92
Mushrooms, white, cooked, boiled, drained, with salt	2.17	0.47	5.29	28	2.2	238	0	3.09
Mushrooms, shiitake, cooked, with salt	1.56	0.22	14.39	56	2.1	240	0	12.29
Mustard greens, cooked, boiled, drained, with salt	2.56	0.47	4.51	26	2	252	0	2.51
Mustard greens, frozen, cooked, boiled, drained, with salt	2.27	0.25	3.11	19	2.8	261	0	0.31
Mustard spinach, (tendergreen), cooked, boiled, drained, with salt	1.7	0.2	2.8	16	2	250	0	0.8
New zealand spinach, cooked, boiled, drained, with salt	1.3	0.17	2.13	12	1.4	343	0	0.73
Okra, cooked, boiled, drained, with salt	1.87	0.21	4.51	22	2.5	241	0	2.01
Okra, frozen, cooked, boiled, drained, with salt	1.63	0.24	6.41	34	2.1	239	0	4.31
Onions, cooked, boiled, drained, with salt	1.36	0.19	9.56	42	1.4	239	0	8.16
Onions, frozen, chopped, cooked, boiled, drained, with salt	0.77	0.1	6	26	1.7	248	0	4.3
Onions, frozen, whole, cooked, boiled, drained, with salt	0.71	0.05	6.11	26	1.4	244	0	4.71
Parsnips, cooked, boiled, drained, with salt	1.32	0.3	17.01	71	4	246	0	13.01

Food Name ---> per 100 g	Protein (g)	Fat (g)	Carb (g)	Calories	Fiber (g)	Sodium (mg)	Cholesterol (mg)	Net Carb (g)
Peas, edible-podded, cooked, boiled, drained, with salt	3.27	0.23	6.46	40	2.8	240	0	3.66
Peas, edible-podded, frozen, cooked, boiled, drained, with salt	3.5	0.38	8.43	50	3.1	241	0	5.33
Peas, green, cooked, boiled, drained, with salt	5.36	0.22	15.63	84	5.5	239	0	10.13
Peas, green, canned, no salt added, solids and liquids	3.19	0.3	9.75	53	3.3	9	0	6.45
Peas, green, canned, no salt added, drained solids	4.42	0.35	12.58	69	4.1	2	0	8.48
Peas, green, frozen, cooked, boiled, drained, with salt	5.15	0.27	14.26	78	4.5	323	0	9.76
Peas, mature seeds, sprouted, cooked, boiled, drained, with salt	7.05	0.51	17.08	98	-	239	0	17.08
Peas and carrots, canned, no salt added, solids and liquids	2.17	0.27	8.48	38	3.3	4	0	5.18
Peas and carrots, frozen, cooked, boiled, drained, with salt	3.09	0.42	10.12	48	3.1	304	0	7.02
Peas and onions, frozen, cooked, boiled, drained, with salt	2.54	0.2	8.63	45	2.2	273	0	6.43
Peppers, hot chili, red, raw	1.87	0.44	8.81	40	1.5	9	0	7.31
Peppers, hot chili, red, canned, excluding seeds, solids and liquids	0.9	0.1	5.1	21	1.3	1173	0	3.8
Peppers, sweet, red, raw	0.99	0.3	6.03	31	2.1	4	0	3.93
Peppers, sweet, green, cooked, boiled, drained, with salt	0.92	0.2	6.11	26	1.2	238	0	4.91
Peppers, sweet, red, cooked, boiled, drained, without salt	0.92	0.2	6.7	28	1.2	2	0	5.5
Peppers, sweet, red, cooked, boiled, drained, with salt	0.92	0.2	6.11	26	1.2	238	0	4.91
Peppers, sweet, green, frozen, chopped, cooked, boiled, drained, with salt	0.95	0.18	3.31	16	0.9	240	0	2.41
Pigeonpeas, immature seeds, cooked, boiled, drained, with salt	5.96	1.36	19.49	111	4.2	240	0	15.29
Pokeberry shoots, (poke), cooked, boiled, drained, with salt	2.3	0.4	3.1	20	1.5	254	0	1.6
Potatoes, baked, flesh and skin, with salt	2.5	0.13	21.15	93	2.2	10	0	18.95
Potatoes, baked, flesh, with salt	1.96	0.1	21.55	93	1.5	241	0	20.05
Potatoes, baked, skin only, with salt	4.29	0.1	46.06	198	7.9	257	0	38.16
Potatoes, boiled, cooked in skin, flesh, with salt	1.87	0.1	20.13	87	2	240	0	18.13
Potatoes, boiled, cooked in skin, skin, with salt	2.86	0.1	17.2	78	3.3	250	0	13.9
Potatoes, boiled, cooked without skin, flesh, with salt	1.71	0.1	20.01	86	2	241	0	18.01
Potatoes, microwaved, cooked, in skin, flesh and skin, with salt	2.44	0.1	24.24	105	2.3	244	0	21.94
Potatoes, microwaved, cooked in skin, flesh, with salt	2.1	0.1	23.28	100	1.6	243	0	21.68
Potatoes, microwaved, cooked, in skin, skin with salt	4.39	0.1	29.63	132	5.5	252	0	24.13
Potatoes, frozen, whole, cooked, boiled, drained, with salt	1.98	0.13	13.93	63	1.4	256	0	12.53
Potatoes, frozen, french fried, par fried, cottage-cut, prepared, heated in oven, with salt	3.44	8.2	34.03	218	3.2	281	0	30.83
Potatoes, french fried, all types, salt not added in processing, frozen, oven-heated	2.66	5.22	28.71	172	2.6	32	0	26.11
Potatoes, french fried, all types, salt not added in processing, frozen, as purchased	2.24	4.66	24.81	150	1.9	23	0	22.91
Potatoes, au gratin, home-prepared from recipe using margarine	5.06	7.59	11.27	132	1.8	433	15	9.47
Potatoes, scalloped, home-prepared with margarine	2.87	3.68	10.78	88	1.9	335	6	8.88
Pumpkin, cooked, boiled, drained, with salt	0.72	0.07	4.31	18	1.1	237	0	3.21
Pumpkin, canned, with salt	1.1	0.28	8.09	34	2.9	241	0	5.19
Pumpkin, flowers, cooked, boiled, drained, with salt	1.09	0.08	3.18	15	0.9	242	0	2.28

Food Name ---> per 100 g	Protein (g)	Fat (g)	Carb (g)	Calories	Fiber (g)	Sodium (mg)	Cholesterol (mg)	Net Carb (g)
Pumpkin leaves, cooked, boiled, drained, with salt	2.72	0.22	3.39	21	2.7	244	0	0.69
Purslane, cooked, boiled, drained, with salt	1.49	0.19	3.55	18	-	280	0	3.55
Radishes, oriental, cooked, boiled, drained, with salt	0.67	0.24	3.43	17	1.6	249	0	1.83
Rutabagas, cooked, boiled, drained, with salt	0.93	0.18	6.84	30	1.8	254	0	5.04
Salsify, cooked, boiled, drained, with salt	2.73	0.17	15.36	68	3.1	252	0	12.26
Soybeans, green, cooked, boiled, drained, with salt	12.35	6.4	11.05	141	4.2	250	0	6.85
Spinach, cooked, boiled, drained, with salt	2.97	0.26	3.75	23	2.4	306	0	1.35
Spinach, canned, no salt added, solids and liquids	2.11	0.37	2.92	19	2.2	75	0	0.72
Spinach, frozen, chopped or leaf, cooked, boiled, drained, with salt	4.01	0.87	4.8	34	3.7	322	0	1.1
Squash, summer, all varieties, cooked, boiled, drained, with salt	0.91	0.31	4.31	20	1.4	237	0	2.91
Squash, summer, crookneck and straightneck, cooked, boiled, drained, with salt	1.04	0.39	3.79	19	1.1	237	0	2.69
Squash, summer, crookneck and straightneck, frozen, cooked, boiled, drained, with salt	1.28	0.2	5.54	25	1.4	242	0	4.14
Squash, summer, scallop, cooked, boiled, drained, with salt	1.03	0.17	3.3	16	1.9	237	0	1.4
Squash, summer, zucchini, includes skin, cooked, boiled, drained, with salt	1.14	0.36	2.69	15	1	239	0	1.69
Squash, summer, zucchini, includes skin, frozen, cooked, boiled, drained, with salt	1.15	0.13	2.97	14	1.3	238	0	1.67
Squash, winter, all varieties, cooked, baked, with salt	0.89	0.35	8.85	37	2.8	237	0	6.05
Squash, winter, acorn, cooked, baked, with salt	1.12	0.14	14.58	56	4.4	240	0	10.18
Squash, winter, acorn, cooked, boiled, mashed, with salt	0.67	0.08	8.79	34	2.6	239	0	6.19
Squash, winter, butternut, cooked, baked, with salt	0.9	0.09	10.49	40	3.2	240	0	7.29
Squash, winter, butternut, frozen, cooked, boiled, with salt	1.23	0.07	10.04	39	-	238	0	10.04
Squash, winter, hubbard, baked, with salt	2.48	0.62	10.81	50	4.9	244	0	5.91
Squash, winter, hubbard, cooked, boiled, mashed, with salt	1.48	0.37	6.46	30	2.9	241	0	3.56
Squash, winter, spaghetti, cooked, boiled, drained, or baked, with salt	0.66	0.26	6.46	27	1.4	254	0	5.06
Succotash, (corn and limas), cooked, boiled, drained, with salt	5.07	0.8	24.37	111	-	253	0	24.37
Succotash, (corn and limas), frozen, cooked, boiled, drained, with salt	4.31	0.89	19.95	93	4.1	281	0	15.85
Swamp cabbage (skunk cabbage), cooked, boiled, drained, with salt	2.08	0.24	3.7	20	1.9	358	0	1.8
Sweet potato leaves, cooked, steamed, with salt	2.18	0.34	7.38	35	1.9	249	0	5.48
Sweet potato, cooked, baked in skin, flesh, with salt	2.01	0.15	20.71	92	3.3	246	0	17.41
Sweet potato, cooked, boiled, without skin, with salt	1.37	0.14	17.72	76	2.5	263	0	15.22
Sweet potato, frozen, cooked, baked, with salt	1.71	0.12	23.4	100	1.8	244	0	21.6
Taro, cooked, with salt	0.52	0.11	34.6	142	5.1	251	0	29.5
Taro, leaves, cooked, steamed, with salt	2.72	0.41	3.89	24	2	238	0	1.89
Taro, shoots, cooked, with salt	0.73	0.08	3.19	14	-	238	0	3.19
Taro, tahitian, cooked, with salt	4.16	0.68	6.85	44	-	290	0	6.85
Tomatoes, red, ripe, cooked, with salt	0.95	0.11	4.01	18	0.7	247	0	3.31
Tomatoes, red, ripe, canned, packed in tomato juice, no salt added	0.79	0.25	3.47	16	1.9	10	0	1.57
Tomato juice, canned, without salt added	0.85	0.29	3.53	17	0.4	10	0	3.13
Tomato products, canned, puree, with salt added	1.65	0.21	8.98	38	1.9	202	0	7.08
Turnips, cooked, boiled, drained, with salt	0.71	0.08	5.06	22	2	286	0	3.06

Food Name ---> per 100 g	Protein (g)	Fat (g)	Carb (g)	Calories	Fiber (g)	Sodium (mg)	Cholesterol (mg)	Net Carb (g)
Turnips, frozen, cooked, boiled, drained, with salt	1.53	0.24	3.73	21	2	272	0	1.73
Turnip greens, cooked, boiled, drained, with salt	1.14	0.23	4.36	20	3.5	265	0	0.86
Turnip greens, frozen, cooked, boiled, drained, with salt	3.35	0.42	4.98	29	3.4	251	0	1.58
Turnip greens and turnips, frozen, cooked, boiled, drained, with salt	2.99	0.38	4.74	34	3.1	255	0	1.64
Vegetables, mixed, frozen, cooked, boiled, drained, with salt	2.86	0.15	13.09	60	4.4	271	0	8.69
Waxgourd, (chinese preserving melon), cooked, boiled, drained, with salt	0.4	0.2	2.45	11	1	343	0	1.45
Winged bean, immature seeds, cooked, boiled, drained, with salt	5.31	0.66	3.21	37	-	240	0	3.21
Yam, cooked, boiled, drained, or baked, with salt	1.49	0.14	26.99	114	3.9	244	0	23.09
Yambean (jicama), cooked, boiled, drained, with salt	0.72	0.09	8.23	36	-	242	0	8.23
Yardlong bean, cooked, boiled, drained, with salt	2.53	0.1	9.17	47	-	240	0	9.17
Corn, sweet, white, raw	3.22	1.18	19.02	86	2.7	15	0	16.32
Corn, sweet, white, cooked, boiled, drained, without salt	3.34	1.41	21.71	97	2.7	3	0	19.01
Corn, sweet, white, cooked, boiled, drained, with salt	3.34	1.41	21.71	97	2.7	253	0	19.01
Corn, sweet, white, canned, whole kernel, regular pack, solids and liquids	1.95	0.5	15.41	64	1.7	213	0	13.71
Corn, sweet, white, canned, whole kernel, no salt added, solids and liquids	1.95	0.5	15.41	64	0.7	12	0	14.71
Corn, sweet, white, canned, whole kernel, drained solids	2.32	1.37	15.06	71	2.3	185	0	12.76
Corn, sweet, white, canned, cream style, regular pack	1.74	0.42	18.62	74	1.2	261	0	17.42
Corn, sweet, white, canned, cream style, no salt added	1.74	0.42	18.13	72	1.2	3	0	16.93
Corn, sweet, white, canned, vacuum pack, regular pack	2.41	0.5	19.44	79	2	272	0	17.44
Corn, sweet, white, canned, vacuum pack, no salt added	2.41	0.5	19.44	79	2	3	0	17.44
Corn, sweet, white, frozen, kernels cut off cob, unprepared	3.02	0.77	20.73	88	2.9	3	0	17.83
Corn, sweet, white, frozen, kernels cut off cob, boiled, drained, without salt	2.75	0.43	19.56	80	2.4	5	0	17.16
Corn, sweet, white, frozen, kernels cut off cob, boiled, drained, with salt	2.75	0.43	19.56	80	2.4	245	0	17.16
Corn, sweet, white, frozen, kernels on cob, unprepared	3.28	0.78	23.5	98	2.8	5	0	20.7
Corn, sweet, white, frozen, kernels on cob, cooked, boiled, drained, without salt	3.11	0.74	22.33	94	2.1	4	0	20.23
Corn, sweet, white, frozen, kernels on cob, cooked, boiled, drained, with salt	3.11	0.74	22.33	94	2.8	240	0	19.53
Peppers, sweet, red, canned, solids and liquids	0.8	0.3	3.9	18	1.2	1369	0	2.7
Peppers, sweet, red, frozen, chopped, unprepared	1.08	0.21	4.45	20	1.6	5	0	2.85
Peppers, sweet, red, frozen, chopped, boiled, drained, without salt	0.95	0.18	3.31	16	0.8	4	0	2.51
Peppers, sweet, red, frozen, chopped, boiled, drained, with salt	0.95	0.18	3.31	16	0.8	240	0	2.51
Peppers, sweet, red, sauteed	1.04	12.75	6.57	133	1.8	21	0	4.77
Sesbania flower, cooked, steamed, with salt	1.14	0.05	5.1	21	-	247	0	5.1
Soybeans, mature seeds, sprouted, cooked, steamed, with salt	8.47	4.45	6.53	81	0.8	246	0	5.73
Soybeans, mature seeds, sprouted, cooked, stir-fried,	13.1	7.1	9.4	125	0.8	250	0	8.6

with salt

Food Name ---> per 100 g	Protein (g)	Fat (g)	Carb (g)	Calories	Fiber (g)	Sodium (mg)	Cholesterol (mg)	Net Carb (g)
Dock, cooked, boiled, drained, with salt	1.83	0.64	2.93	20	-	239	0	2.93
Lentils, sprouted, cooked, stir-fried, with salt	8.8	0.45	21.25	101	-	246	0	21.25
Mountain yam, hawaii, cooked, steamed, with salt	1.73	0.08	19.99	82	-	248	0	19.99
Tree fern, cooked, with salt	0.29	0.07	10.78	40	3.7	241	0	7.08
Potatoes, mashed, prepared from granules, without milk, whole milk and margarine	2.05	4.93	14.4	108	2.2	263	3	12.2
Potatoes, mashed, dehydrated, prepared from flakes without milk, whole milk and margarine added	1.9	5.6	15.02	113	2.3	332	4	12.72
Peppers, sweet, red, freeze-dried	17.9	3	68.7	314	21.3	193	0	47.4
Beans, snap, yellow, canned, regular pack, drained solids	1.15	0.1	4.5	20	1.3	251	0	3.2
Beans, snap, yellow, canned, no salt added, drained solids	1.15	0.1	4.5	20	1.3	2	0	3.2
Potatoes, mashed, home-prepared, whole milk and butter added	1.86	4.22	16.81	113	1.5	317	11	15.31
Catsup	1.04	0.1	27.4	101	0.3	907	0	27.1
Mushrooms, brown, italian, or crimini, exposed to ultraviolet light, raw	2.5	0.1	4.3	22	0.6	6	0	3.7
Pickles, cucumber, dill or kosher dill	0.5	0.3	2.41	12	1	809	0	1.41
Mushroom, white, exposed to ultraviolet light, raw	3.09	0.34	3.26	22	1	5	0	2.26
Mushrooms, portabella, exposed to ultraviolet light, grilled	3.28	0.58	4.44	29	2.2	11	-	2.24
Pickles, cucumber, sweet (includes bread and butter pickles)	0.58	0.41	21.15	91	1	457	0	20.15
Pickles, cucumber, sour	0.33	0.2	2.26	11	1.2	1208	0	1.06
Pimento, canned	1.1	0.3	5.1	23	1.9	14	0	3.2
Pickle relish, hot dog	1.5	0.46	23.35	91	1.5	1091	0	21.85
Pickle relish, sweet	0.37	0.47	35.06	130	1.1	811	0	33.96
Pickles, cucumber, sour, low sodium	0.33	0.2	2.26	11	1.2	18	0	1.06
Pickles, cucumber, dill, reduced sodium	0.5	0.3	2.41	12	1	18	0	1.41
Pickles, cucumber, sweet, low sodium (includes bread and butter pickles)	0.37	0.26	33.73	122	1.1	18	0	32.63
Catsup, low sodium	1.04	0.1	27.4	101	0.3	20	0	27.1
Mushrooms, enoki, raw	2.66	0.29	7.81	37	2.7	3	0	5.11
Peppers, sweet, yellow, raw	1	0.21	6.32	27	0.9	2	0	5.42
Radicchio, raw	1.43	0.25	4.48	23	0.9	22	0	3.58
Squash, zucchini, baby, raw	2.71	0.4	3.11	21	1.1	3	0	2.01
Tomatillos, raw	0.96	1.02	5.84	32	1.9	1	0	3.94
Tomatoes, sun-dried	14.11	2.97	55.76	258	12.3	107	0	43.46
Tomatoes, sun-dried, packed in oil, drained	5.06	14.08	23.33	213	5.8	266	0	17.53
Fennel, bulb, raw	1.24	0.2	7.3	31	3.1	52	0	4.2
Pickle relish, hamburger	0.63	0.54	34.48	129	3.2	1096	0	31.28
Arugula, raw	2.58	0.66	3.65	25	1.6	27	0	2.05
Carrots, baby, raw	0.64	0.13	8.24	35	2.9	78	0	5.34
Hearts of palm, canned	2.52	0.62	4.62	28	2.4	426	0	2.22
Peppers, hot chile, sun-dried	10.58	5.81	69.86	324	28.7	91	0	41.16
Nopales, raw	1.32	0.09	3.33	16	2.2	21	0	1.13
Nopales, cooked, without salt	1.35	0.05	3.28	15	2	20	0	1.28
Cauliflower, green, raw	2.95	0.3	6.09	31	3.2	23	0	2.89
Cauliflower, green, cooked, no salt added	3.04	0.31	6.28	32	3.3	23	0	2.98
Cauliflower, green, cooked, with salt	3.04	0.31	6.28	32	3.3	259	0	2.98
Broccoli, chinese, cooked	1.14	0.72	3.81	22	2.5	7	0	1.31

Food Name ---> per 100 g	Protein (g)	Fat (g)	Carb (g)	Calories	Fiber (g)	Sodium (mg)	Cholesterol (mg)	Net Carb (g)
Cabbage, napa, cooked	1.1	0.17	2.23	12	-	11	0	2.23
Lemon grass (citronella), raw	1.82	0.49	25.31	99	-	6	0	25.31
Beans, fava, in pod, raw	7.92	0.73	17.63	88	7.5	25	0	10.13
Grape leaves, raw	5.6	2.12	17.31	93	11	9	0	6.31
Grape leaves, canned	4.27	1.97	11.71	69	9.9	2853	0	1.81
Pepper, banana, raw	1.66	0.45	5.35	27	3.4	13	0	1.95
Peppers, serrano, raw	1.74	0.44	6.7	32	3.7	10	0	3
Peppers, ancho, dried	11.86	8.2	51.42	281	21.6	43	0	29.82
Peppers, jalapeno, raw	0.91	0.37	6.5	29	2.8	3	0	3.7
Peppers, chili, green, canned	0.72	0.27	4.6	21	1.7	397	0	2.9
Peppers, hungarian, raw	0.8	0.41	6.7	29	1	1	0	5.7
Peppers, pasilla, dried	12.35	15.85	51.13	345	26.8	89	0	24.33
Pickles, chowchow, with cauliflower onion mustard, sweet	1.5	0.9	26.64	121	1.5	527	0	25.14
Epazote, raw	0.33	0.52	7.44	32	3.8	43	0	3.64
Fireweed, leaves, raw	4.71	2.75	19.22	103	10.6	34	0	8.62
Malabar spinach, cooked	2.98	0.78	2.71	23	2.1	55	0	0.61
Mushrooms, oyster, raw	3.31	0.41	6.09	33	2.3	18	0	3.79
Fungi, Cloud ears, dried	9.25	0.73	73.01	284	70.1	35	0	2.91
Mushrooms, straw, canned, drained solids	3.83	0.68	4.64	32	2.5	384	0	2.14
Wasabi, root, raw	4.8	0.63	23.54	109	7.8	17	0	15.74
Yautia (tannier), raw	1.46	0.4	23.63	98	1.5	21	0	22.13
Mushrooms, white, microwaved	3.91	0.46	6.04	35	2.5	17	0	3.54
Mushrooms, maitake, raw	1.94	0.19	6.97	31	2.7	1	0	4.27
Broccoli, chinese, raw	1.2	0.76	4.67	30	2.6	7	0	2.07
Fiddlehead ferns, raw	4.55	0.4	5.54	34	-	1	0	5.54
Fiddlehead ferns, frozen, unprepared	4.31	0.35	5.74	34	-	0	0	5.74
Mushrooms, portabella, exposed to ultraviolet light, raw	2.11	0.35	3.87	22	1.3	9	0	2.57
CAMPBELL'S, Tomato juice	0.82	0	4.12	21	0.8	280	0	3.32
CAMPBELL'S, Tomato juice, low sodium	0.82	0	4.12	21	0.8	58	0	3.32
CAMPBELL'S, V8 Vegetable Juice, Organic V8	0.41	0	4.53	20	0.8	198	0	3.73
CAMPBELL'S, Organic Tomato juice	0.82	0	4.12	21	0.8	280	0	3.32
HEALTHY REQUEST Tomato juice	0.82	0	4.53	21	0.8	198	0	3.73
CAMPBELL'S, V8 100% Vegetable Juice	0.82	0	4.12	21	0.8	173	0	3.32
CAMPBELL'S, V8 Vegetable Juice, Essential Antioxidants V8	0.82	0	4.53	21	0.8	198	0	3.73
CAMPBELL'S, V8 Vegetable Juice, Calcium Enriched V8	0.82	0	4.53	21	0.8	198	0	3.73
CAMPBELL'S, V8 Vegetable Juice, Low Sodium V8	0.82	0	4.12	21	0.8	58	0	3.32
CAMPBELL'S, V8 Vegetable Juice, Spicy Hot V8	0.82	0	4.12	21	0.8	198	0	3.32
PACE, Jalapenos Nacho Sliced Peppers	0	0	3.33	13	3.3	1000	0	0.03
PACE, Diced Green Chilies	0	0	6.67	27	3.3	333	0	3.37
CAMPBELL'S, V8 60% Vegetable Juice, V8 V-Lite	0.41	0	2.88	14	0.4	148	0	2.48
CAMPBELL'S, V8 Vegetable Juice, Low Sodium Spicy Hot	0.82	0	4.53	21	0.8	58	-	3.73
CAMPBELL'S, V8 Vegetable Juice, High Fiber V8	0.82	0	5.39	25	2.1	198	0	3.29
Seaweed, Canadian Cultivated EMI-TSUNOMATA, dry	15.34	1.39	46.24	259	36.7	4331	33	9.54
Seaweed, Canadian Cultivated EMI-TSUNOMATA, rehydrated	1.86	0.17	5.62	31	4.5	526	-	1.12
Potatoes, hash brown, refrigerated, unprepared	1.75	0.08	19.16	84	1.8	42	0	17.36

Food Name ---> per 100 g	Protein (g)	Fat (g)	Carb (g)	Calories	Fiber (g)	Sodium (mg)	Cholesterol (mg)	Net Carb (g)
Potatoes, hash brown, refrigerated, prepared, pan-fried in canola oil	3.24	10.3	33.99	242	3.6	77	0	30.39
Sweet Potatoes, french fried, frozen as packaged, salt added in processing	2.16	8.92	35.58	182	5.7	146	0	29.88
Sweet Potatoes, french fried, crosscut, frozen, unprepared	1.7	11.1	25.52	209	3.4	214	0	22.12
Sweet Potato puffs, frozen, unprepared	1.36	3.58	30.72	161	1.9	250	0	28.82
Potatoes, yellow fleshed, roasted, salt added in processing, frozen, unprepared	1.99	1.85	23.44	119	2.6	338	0	20.84
Potatoes, yellow fleshed, french fried, frozen, unprepared	2.47	5.84	25.01	162	2.2	300	0	22.81
Potatoes, yellow fleshed, hash brown, shredded, salt added in processing, frozen, unprepared	2.04	0.07	17.98	81	2	330	0	15.98
Potatoes, french fried, wedge cut, frozen, unprepared	2.56	7.47	22.22	166	2.4	380	0	19.82
Potatoes, french fried, steak cut, salt not added in processing, frozen, unprepared	2.4	3.42	24.31	138	2.4	30	0	21.91
Potatoes, french fried, cross cut, frozen, unprepared	2.7	10	22.95	193	2.3	393	0	20.65
Vegetable smoothie, NAKED JUICE, KALE BLAZER	0.8	0.07	7	28	0.7	13	0	6.3
Ginger root, pickled, canned, with artificial sweetener	0.33	0.1	4.83	20	2.6	906	0	2.23
Peppers, hot pickled, canned	0.8	0.4	4.56	22	2.6	1430	0	1.96
Vegetable juice, BOLTHOUSE FARMS, DAILY GREENS	0.49	0.04	8.13	31	1.2	15	0	6.93
Potatoes, mashed, ready-to-eat	1.97	5.01	13.29	106	1.9	298	13	11.39
Radishes, hawaiian style, pickled	1.1	0.3	5.2	28	2.2	789	0	3
Cabbage, japanese style, fresh, pickled	1.6	0.1	5.67	30	3.1	277	0	2.57
Cabbage, mustard, salted	1.1	0.1	5.63	28	3.1	717	0	2.53
Eggplant, pickled	0.9	0.7	9.77	49	2.5	1674	0	7.27
Tomato sauce, canned, no salt added	1.2	0.3	5.31	24	1.5	11	0	3.81
Potatoes, canned, drained solids, no salt added	1.4	0.2	13.6	62	2.4	5	0	11.2
Vegetables, mixed (corn, lima beans, peas, green beans, carrots) canned, no salt added	1.4	0.2	7.31	37	3.1	26	0	4.21
Tomato and vegetable juice, low sodium	0.6	0.1	4.59	22	0.8	58	0	3.79
Turnip greens, canned, no salt added	1.36	0.3	2.81	19	1.3	29	0	1.51
Hearts of palm, raw	2.7	0.2	25.61	115	1.5	14	0	24.11
Yeast extract spread	23.88	0.9	20.42	185	6.5	3380	0	13.92
Celery flakes, dried	11.3	2.1	63.7	319	27.8	1435	0	35.9

PART III: Glycemic Index and Glycemic Load

Glycemic index and glycemic load: Overview

Carbohydrate is an essential part of our diets, but not all carbs are equal. The Glycemic Index is an experimental ranking of carbohydrate in foods to measure how slowly or how quickly foods induce rises in blood glucose levels.
There are three classifications for GI:
Individual food portion:
Low: 55 or less
Mid: 56 – 69
High: 70+

Carbohydrates with a low GI value (55 or less) are more slowly digested, absorbed, and metabolized and cause a smaller and slower rise in blood glucose and, therefore, usually, insulin levels.

Low glycemic diet or foods are associated with reduced risk of chronic disease. Foods that have low glycemic index are known for their property to release glucose in the blood slowly and regularly. Conversely, Foods that have a high glycemic index are known for their property to release glucose rapidly. Researches suggest that foods with a low glycemic index (LGI foods) are ideal for weight loss diets and foster lasting weight loss, in addition to their positive effect on the pancreas (insulin release), eyes, and kidney.

The glycemic index (GI) is formed by scale from 1 to 100. Each food gets a score on this scale according to experimental data. **A lower score indicates that food takes longer time to raise the blood sugar levels.**

Glycemic Load is another critical tool to track carbohydrates quality and quantity. Glycemic Load (GL) combines both the quality and amount of carbohydrates following a simple formula:

Glycemic Load (GL) = GI x Carbohydrate (grams) content per portion ÷ 100

For example, an apple has a GI of 32 and contains 13 grams of carbohydrates.
GL= 32 x 13/100 = 3

Sweet potato has a GL of 11. So, We can predict that sweet potato will have the more glycemic effect of an apple (approximately four times).
Like the glycemic index, the glycemic load (GL) of a food can be classified as:
- **Low:** 10 or less
- **Medium:** 11 – 19
- **High:** 20 or more

For an effective Glycemic Index / Glycemic load diet, we recommend you to eat daily the equivalent of 100 in glycemic load. However, following this target can be struggling and sometimes impossible due to the lack of data. The Process of measuring the glycemic index is expensive, time-consuming, and complicated.

To bypass this difficulty, you must mainly use the Net carb grams tables provided for 7000 foods covering the majority of foods we eat. Thus, you can easily monitor your daily carb intake to keep it within the strict limits recommended by your diet.

The data provided in this book comes mainly from the international database of the glycemic index. This database is managed by the team of Dr Jennie Brand-Miller, the Australian researcher who has been since 1981 at the forefront of the glycemic index science.

The International database of the glycemic index is hosted by the University of Sydney and gathers all the data published in the scientific journals and the measurements carried out by the Australian researchers within the Department of Human Nutrition of the University of Sydney. This table is available on the Internet at http://www.glycemicindex.com/.

Low Glycemic Index Foods Tables

Food Name	GI	Serving (g)	Tot Carb (g)	GL
3 Grain Bread, sprouted grains	55	30	10	5
45% oat bran and 50% wheat flour bread	50	30	18	9
50% oat bran bread	44	30	18	8
9-Grain Multi-Grain bread	43	30	14	6
American, easy-cook rice, consumed with 10 g margarine	49	150	46	22
Apple and blackcurrant juice, no added sugar	45	250	25	11
Apple and cherry juice, pure, unsweetened	43	250	33	14
Apple and mango juice, pure, unsweetened	47	250	34	16
Apple blueberry muffin	49	60	25	12
Apple juice, Granny Smith, unsweetened	44	250	30	13
Apple juice, pure, clear, unsweetened	44	250	30	13
Apple juice, pure, cloudy, unsweetened	37	250	28	11
Apple juice, unsweetened, reconstituted	39	250	25	10
Apple muffin, made with rolled oats and sugar	44	60	29	13
Apple muffin, made with rolled oats and without sugar	48	60	19	9
Apple, raw	36 ± 4	120	16	5
Apple, raw, Golden Delicious	39 ± 2	120	16	6
Apricot & apple fruit strips, gluten-free	29 ± 4	20	16	5
Apricot 100% Pure Fruit spread, no added sugar	43 ± 3	30	16	7
Apricot dried fruit snack	42 ± 4	15	12	5
Apricot fruit spread, reduced sugar	55 ± 2	30	13	7
Apricot halves canned in fruit juice	51 ± 4	120	12	6
Apricot, raw	34 ± 2	120	9	3
Apricots, dried	30 ± 2	60	27	8
Arepa, made from white corn meal flour	53 ± 2	100	35	19
Aussie Bodies Start the Day UHT, Choc Banana flavored drink	24 ± 3	250	15	4
Aussie Bodies Start the Day UHT, Chocolate flavored drink	26 ± 3	250	15	4
Aussie Bodies Trim Protein Shake, Chocolate flavoured beverage	39 ± 3	250	12	5
Aussie Bodies Trim Protein Shake, French Vanilla flavoured beverage	41 ± 2	250	12	5
Bakers Delight™ Hi Fibre Lo GI white bread	52 ± 2	30	15	8
Bakers Delight™ Wholemeal Country Grain bread	53 ± 2	30	12	6
Banana cake, made with sugar	47 ± 2	60	29	14
Banana cake, made without sugar	55 ± 2	60	22	12
Banana, over-ripe	52 ± 2	120	20	11
Banana, over-ripe (yellow flecked with brown)	48 ± 3	120	25	12
Banana, raw	47 ± 2	120	24	11
Banana, ripe (all yellow)	51 ± 2	120	25	13
Banana, slightly under-ripe (yellow with green sections)	42 ± 2	120	25	11
Banana, under-ripe	30 ± 2	120	21	6
Barley	23 ± 4	150	42	11
Barley kernels, high-amylose (covered), boiled in water for 25 min (kernel:water = 1:2)	26 ± 2	150	42	11
Barley kernels, high-amylose (hull-less) boiled in water for 25 min	20 ± 2	150	42	8
Barley kernels, waxy (hull-less), boiled in water for 25 min	22 ± 3	150	42	9
Barley, cracked (Malthouth, Tunisia)	50 ± 2	150	42	21
Barley, pearled	22 ± 3	150	41	9
Barley, pearled	29 ± 3	150	42	12
Barley, pearled, boiled 60 min	35 ± 2	150	42	15
Basmati, white rice, boiled 12 min	52 ± 2	150	28	15

Food Name	GI	Serving (g)	Tot Carb (g)	GL
Basmati, white rice, boiled, with 10 g margarine	43 ± 2	150	43	18
Blueberry muffin	50 ± 2	60	31	15
Breakfast Marmalade 100% Fruit Spread, Cottees™ brand	55 ± 3	30	18	10
Brown & Wild rice, Uncle Ben's® Ready Whole Grain Medley™ (pouch)	45 ± 3	150	39	18
Brown & Wild rice, Uncle Ben's® Ready Whole Grain Medley™ (pouch)	45 ± 2	150	39	18
Brown rice, steamed	50 ± 1	150	33	16
Brown Rice, Uncle Ben's® Ready Whole Grain (pouch)	48 ± 2	150	42	20
Buckwheat groats, hydrothermally treated, dehusked, boiled 12 min	45 ± 3	150	30	13
Buckwheat noodles, instant	53 ± 2	180	42	22
Build-Up™ nutrient-fortified drink, vanilla with fibre	41 ± 3	250	33	13
Butternut pumpkin, boiled	51 ± 2	80	6	3
Capellini pasta	45 ± 3	180	45	20
Capilano Premium Honey, blend of eucalypt & floral honeys	51 ± 2	25	21	11
Carrot cake, prepared with coconut flour	36 ± 2	60	23	8
Carrot juice, freshly made	43 ± 2	250	23	10
Carrot soup, President's Choice® Blue Menu™ Soupreme	35 ± 3	250	13	5
Carrots, peeled, boiled	33 ± 2	80	5	2
Carrots, raw, diced	35 ± 2	80	6	2
Carrots, raw, ground	39 ± 4	80	6	2
Cashew nut halves	27 ± 2	50	10	3
Cashew nuts	25 ± 2	50	12	3
Cashew nuts, organic, roasted and salted	25 ± 2	50	12	3
Cashew nuts, roasted and salted	27 ± 2	50	10	3
Cereal bar, cranberry flavor	42 ± 3	30	15	6
Cereal bar, hazelnut flavor	33 ± 3	30	11	4
Cereal bar, orange flavor	33 ± 3	30	14	5
Cereal biscuit (30 g), cocoa flavor wheat biscuits consumed with 125 mL skim milk	46 ± 3	155	27	12
Cereal biscuit (30 g), honey flavor wheat biscuits consumed with 125 mL skim milk	52 ± 3	155	27	14
Cereal biscuit (30 g), wheat based biscuits consumed with 125 mL skim milk	47 ± 3	155	26	12
Cherries, raw, sour	22 ± 2	120	12	3
Chicken Flavored Brown Rice, Uncle Ben's® Ready Whole Grain (pouch)	46 ± 3	150	39	18
Chicken Flavored Brown Rice, Uncle Ben's® Ready Whole Grain (pouch)	46 ± 3	150	39	18
Chicken McNuggets™ consumed with sweet Thai chilli sauce	55 ± 3	100	21	12
Chicken nuggets, frozen, reheated in microwave oven 5 min	46 ± 3	100	16	7
Chicken tikka masala and rice, convenience meal	34 ± 3	300	60	21
Chilli beef noodles, prepared convenience meal	42 ± 3	300	46	19
Chilli con carne, made from haricot beans	34 ± 3	300	36	12
Chocolate butterscotch muffin	53 ± 2	50	28	15
Chocolate cake made from packet mix with chocolate frosting	38 ± 3	111	52	20
Chocolate candy, sugar free, artificially sweetened, Dove®	23 ± 2	50	15	3
Chocolate chip muffin	52 ± 3	60	32	17
Chocolate crinkles, containing coconut flour	43 ± 3	50	23	10
Chocolate Daydream™ shake, fructose, Revival Soy®	33 ± 3	250	18	6
Chocolate Daydream™ shake, sucralose, Revival Soy®	25 ± 3	250	4	1
Chocolate pudding, instant, made from powder and whole milk	47 ± 2	100	16	7
Chocolate, dark with raisins, peanuts and jam	44 ± 3	50	27	12
Chocolate, dark, Dove®	23 ± 4	50	26	6
Chocolate, plain	42 ± 4	50	31	13

Food Name	GI	Serving (g)	Tot Carb (g)	GL
Chocolate, plain with sucrose	34 ± 3	50	22	7
Citrus, reduced-fat mousse, prepared from commercial mousse mix with water	47 ± 2	50	30	14
Coarse rye kernel bread, 80% intact kernels and 20% white wheat flour	41 ± 3	30	12	5
Coarse wheat kernel bread, 80% intact kernels and 20% white wheat flour	52 ± 2	30	20	10
Cocoavia™ Chocolate Covered Almonds, artificially sweetened	21 ± 3	30	10	2
Coconut sugar	54 ± 1	5	5	3
Continental fruit loaf, wheat bread with dried fruit	47 ± 2	30	15	7
Corn granules	52 ± 1	150	28	15
Corn tortilla	52 ± 1	50	24	12
Corn tortilla, made from white corn, Diego's brand	49 ± 3	50	22	11
Corn tortilla, served with refried mashed pinto beans and tomato sauce	39 ± 2	100	23	9
Country Grain Organic Rye bread	53 ± 2	30	10	5
Cranberry & Orange Soy muffin, President's Choice® Blue Menu™	48 ± 2	70	29	14
Cranberry juice cocktail	52 ± 1	250	31	16
Crème fraiche dessert, peach	28 ± 1	150	23	7
Crème fraiche dessert, raspberry	30 ± 1	150	17	5
Crusty malted wheat bread	52 ± 1	30	13	7
Double chocolate muffin	46 ± 2	60	34	16
English Muffin bread, Whole Grain Multigrain, President's Choice® Blue Menu™	45 ± 3	30	11	5
Fettucine, egg	32 ± 1	180	46	15
Fish fingers	38 ± 1	100	19	7
Fromage Frais, red fruit: blackcurrant	22 ± 1	100	7	2
Fromage Frais, red fruit: raspberry	31 ± 1	100	13	2
Fromage Frais, red fruit: red cherry	25 ± 1	100	7	2
Fructose, 25 g portion, Sweeten Less	11	10	10	1
Fructose, 50 g portion	20	10	10	2
Fructose, 50 g portion	23	10	10	2
Fructose, 50 g portion, Sweeten Less	12	10	10	1
Fruit and Spice Loaf bread, thick sliced	54 ± 1	30	15	8
Fusilli pasta twists, boiled 10 min in salted water, served with cheddar cheese	27 ± 2	0	0	0
Fusilli pasta twists, boiled 10 min in salted water, served with canned tuna	28 ± 2	0	0	0
Fusilli pasta twists, boiled 10 min in salted water, served with chilli con carne	40 ± 3	0	0	0
Fusilli pasta twists, dry pasta, boiled in 10 min in unsalted water	54 ± 1	180	48	26
Fusilli pasta twists, tricolour, dry pasta, boiled 10 min in unsalted water	51 ± 1	180	45	23
Fusilli pasta twists, wholewheat, dry pasta, boiled 10 min in unsalted water	55 ± 1	180	41	23
Gluten Free Low GI White bread	53	30	8	4
Gluten-free pasta, maize starch, boiled 8 min	54 ± 1	180	42	23
Gluten-free pasta, maize starch, boiled 8 min	54 ± 1	180	42	23
Golden Hearth™ Organic Heavy Wholegrain bread	53 ± 1	30	12	7
Grapefruit, raw	25 ± 2	120	11	3
Grapefruit, ruby red segments, canned in juice	47 ± 2	120	21	10
Grapes, raw	45 ± 4	120	17	7
Green banana, peeled, boiled 10 min	37 ± 2	120	27	10
Ground beef served with rice and an orange	31 ± 2	300	76	24
Haricot beans, home-cooked, soaked overnight, boiled 1h in water,	23 ± 2	150	30	7

Food Name	GI	Serving (g)	Tot Carb (g)	GL
baked in tomato sauce 2h				
Haricot/Navy beans	39 ± 2	150	30	12
Haricot/Navy beans, boiled	31 ± 2	150	30	9
Hazelnut, 2.4% fat mousse, prepared from commercial mousse mix with water	36 ± 2	50	10	4
Healthy Choice™ Hearty 7 Grain bread	55 ± 1	30	14	8
Honey Crunch cereal (30 g), consumed with 125 mL skim milk	54 ± 2	155	30	16
Honey, Iron Bark (34% fructose)	48 ± 1	25	15	7
Honey, Red Gum (35% fructose)	46 ± 1	25	18	8
Honey, Stringy Bark (52% fructose)	44 ± 1	25	21	9
Honey, Yapunya (42 % fructose)	52 ± 1	25	17	9
Honey, Yellow box (46% fructose)	35 ± 1	25	18	6
Hot oat cereal (30 g) prepared with 125 mL skim milk	47 ± 1	155	23	11
Hot oat cereal (30 g), berry flavor prepared with 125 mL skim milk	43 ± 1	155	26	11
Hot oat cereal (30 g), cocoa flavor prepared with 125 mL skim milk	40 ± 1	155	23	9
Hot oat cereal (30 g), fruit flavor prepared with 125 mL skim milk	47 ± 1	155	25	12
Hot oat cereal (30 g), honey flavor prepared with 125 mL skim milk	47 ± 1	155	26	12
Hot oat cereal (30 g), orchard fruit flavor prepared with 125 mL skim milk	50 ± 1	155	25	12
Ice cream, low-fat, Bulla Light Creamy vanilla	36 ± 1	50	13	7
Ice cream, low-fat, Bulla Light Real Dairy chocolate	27 ± 1	50	13	3
Ice cream, low-fat, Bulla Light Real Dairy mango	30	50	13	4
Ice cream, low-fat, Light & Creamy, Raspberry Ripple	55 ± 1	50	16	9
Ice cream, low-fat, vanilla, 'Light'	46 ± 2	50	15	7
Instant 'two-minute' noodles, Maggi® (Nestlé, Auckland, New Zealand)	48 ± 2	180	26	12
Instant 'two-minute' noodles, Maggi® (Nestlé, Australia) (1995)	46 ± 2	180	23	11
Instant 'two-minute' noodles, Maggi®, all flavors (Nestlé Australia) (2005)	52 ± 2	180	25	13
Instant noodles, all flavors (Woolworths Limited, Australia)	52 ± 2	180	22	11
Instant rice, white, cooked 3 min	46 ± 3	150	42	19
Kidney beans	29 ± 2	150	25	7
Kiwi fruit, Hayward	47 ± 2	120	12	6
Lasagne sheets, dry pasta, boiled in unsalted water for 10 min	55 ± 2	180	47	26
Lasagne, egg, dry pasta, boiled in unsalted water for 10 min	53 ± 2	180	43	23
Lasagne, egg, verdi, dry pasta, boiled in unsalted water for 10 min	52 ± 2	180	45	23
Lemonade, Scheweppes®, lemon soft drink	54 ± 4	250	27	15
Lentils, brown, canned, drained, Edgell's™ brand	42 ± 2	150	21	9
Lentils, green, dried, boiled	37 ± 2	150	14	5
Lentils, red, split, dried, boiled 25 min	21 ± 2	150	18	4
Lentils, raw	29 ± 2	150	18	5
Long Grain and Wild, Jasmine rice, Uncle Ben's® Ready Rice (pouch)	49 ± 3	150	42	21
Long Grain and Wild, Jasmine rice, Uncle Ben's® Ready Rice (pouch)	49 ± 3	150	42	21
Long grain rice quick-cooking variety, white, pre-cooked, microwaved 2 min, Express Rice, plain	52 ± 3	150	37	19
Long grain rice quick-cooking variety, white, pre-cooked, microwaved 2 min, Express Rice, plain	52 ± 3	150	37	19
Low-fat yoghurt, apricot	42 ± 1	200	28	12
Low-fat yoghurt, black cherry	41 ± 1	200	28	11
Low-fat yoghurt, hazelnut	53 ± 1	200	29	15
Low-fat yoghurt, Nestlé Diet Mixed Berry	28 ± 1	200	11	3
Low-fat yoghurt, Nestlé Diet Peaches & Cream	28 ± 1	200	11	3
Low-fat yoghurt, raspberry	34 ± 1	200	28	10

Food Name	GI	Serving (g)	Tot Carb (g)	GL
LU P'tit Déjeuner Chocolat cookies	42 ± 3	50	34	14
LU P'tit Déjeuner Miel et Pépites Chocolat cookies	45 ± 3	50	35	16
LU P'tit Déjeuner Miel et Pépites Chocolat cookies	49 ± 3	50	35	18
LU P'tit Déjeuner Miel et Pépites Chocolat cookies	52 ± 3	50	35	18
LU Petit Dejeuner Cereals & Chocolate Chips, low in sugar cookies	37 ± 3	50	35	13
LU Petit Dejeuner Chocolate & Cereals cookies	46 ± 3	50	35	16
LU Petit Dejeuner Coconut, nuts and chocolate cookies	51 ± 3	50	34	17
LU Petit Dejeuner Coconut, nuts and chocolate cookies	55 ± 3	50	34	19
LU Petit Dejeuner Fruits and Muesli cookies	45 ± 3	50	36	16
LU Petit Dejeuner Fruits and Muesli cookies	47 ± 3	50	36	17
LU Petit Dejeuner Fruits and Muesli cookies	49 ± 3	50	36	18
LU Petit Dejeuner Honey & Chocolate chips cookies	46 ± 3	50	35	16
LU Petit Dejeuner Honey & Chocolate chips cookies	47 ± 3	50	35	17
LU Petit Dejeuner Milk and Cereals cookies	39 ± 3	50	34	13
LU Petit Dejeuner Milk and Cereals cookies	55 ± 3	50	34	19
LU Petit Dejeuner Multicereals cookies	46 ± 3	50	35	16
LU Petit Dejeuner with Fruits and Figs cookies	41 ± 3	50	35	14
LU Petit Dejeuner with Prunes cookies	51 ± 3	50	34	17
LU Petit Dejeuner, Chocolate, low in sugar cookies	51 ± 3	50	36	18
Mandarin segments, canned in juice	47 ± 2	120	12	6
Mango, raw	41 ± 2	120	20	8
Mango, 1.8% fat mousse, prepared from commercial mousse mix with water	33 ± 2	50	11	4
Mango, low-fat frozen fruit dessert, Frutia™	42 ± 2	100	23	10
Marmalade, orange	48 ± 2	30	20	9
Marmalade, orange 100% Pure Fruit spread, no added sugar	27 ± 2	30	16	4
Mars Active® Energy Drink, flavored milk	46 ± 3	250	33	15
Milk, full-fat/whole	36 ± 4	250	12	4
Milk, reduced fat	30 ± 4	250	13	4
Milk, semi-skimmed	32 ± 2	250	13	4
Milk, skim	32 ± 2	250	13	4
Mixed berry, 2.2% fat mousse, prepared from commercial mousse mix with water	36 ± 2	50	10	4
Mixed nuts and raisins	21 ± 2	50	16	3
Mixed nuts, roasted and salted	24 ± 2	50	17	4
Moolgiri white rice	54 ± 2	150	32	17
Muesli, gluten-free with 1.5% fat milk (125 mL)	39 ± 2	30	19	7
Muesli, toasted	43 ± 2	30	17	7
Muesli, Wheat free, consumed with 150 mL semi-skimmed milk	49 ± 2	30	19	9
Muesli, yeast & wheat free	45 ± 2	30	10	4
Muffin, plain, made from wheat flour	46 ± 2	50	23	11
Muffin, reduced-fat, low-calorie, made from high-amylose corn starch and maltitol	37 ± 3	50	25	9
Multigrain (50% kibbled wheat grain) bread	43 ± 2	30	14	6
Multigrain Loaf bread, spelt wheat flour	54 ± 2	30	15	8
Multigrain porridge, containing rolled oats, wheat, triticale, rye, barley and rice, cooked with water	55 ± 2	250	35	19
Multiseed bread	54 ± 2	30	12	7
Nectarines, raw	43 ± 2	120	9	4
Oat porridge made from roasted thick (1.0 mm)	50 ± 1	250	27	14
Oat porridge made from steamed thick (1.0 mm) dehulled oat flakes	53 ± 1	250	27	14
Orange & Grapefruit segments, canned in juice	53 ± 2	120	19	10
Orange Delight Cocktail beverage with pulp, President's Choice® Blue Menu™	44 ± 2	250	16	7
Orange juice	46 ± 2	250	26	12

Food Name	GI	Serving (g)	Tot Carb (g)	GL
Orange juice, unsweetened, reconstituted concentrate, Commercial brand	54 ± 2	250	21	11
Orange, raw	38 ± 7	120	12	7
Original Long Grain, Jasmine rice, Uncle Ben's® Ready Rice (pouch)	48 ± 3	150	46	22
Original Long Grain, Jasmine rice, Uncle Ben's® Ready Rice (pouch)	48 ± 3	150	46	22
Pancakes, prepared with coconut flour	46 ± 3	80	22	10
Pasta bake, tomato and mozzarella	23 ± 3	300	43	10
Peach & Grapes, canned in natural fruit juice	46 ± 2	120	12	6
Peach & pear fruit strips, gluten-free	29 ± 2	20	11	3
Peach & Pineapple, canned in natural fruit juice	45 ± 2	120	13	6
Peach, canned in light syrup	52 ± 2	120	18	9
Peach, canned in natural juice	45 ± 2	120	11	5
Peach, dried	35 ± 2	60	22	8
Peach, raw	28 ± 2	120	13	4
Peanuts, crushed	7 ± 2	50	4	0
Pear halves, canned in natural juice	43 ± 2	120	13	5
Pear, dried	43 ± 2	60	27	12
Pear, raw	33 ± 4	120	13	4
Pineapple, raw	51 ± 2	120	16	8
Pineapple & Papaya pieces, canned in natural juice	53 ± 2	120	17	9
Pineapple pieces, canned in natural fruit juice	55 ± 2	120	17	10
Ploughman's™ Wholegrain bread, original recipe	47 ± 2	30	14	6
Plum, raw	40 ± 2	120	14	7
Popcorn	55 ± 2	20	10	6
Porridge oats, made from rolled oats	50 ± 2	250	19	10
Porridge, jumbo oats, consumed with 150 mL semi-skimmed milk	40 ± 2	250	22	9
Porridge, made from rolled oats	55 ± 2	250	23	13
Potato crisps, plain, salted	51 ± 2	50	24	12
Pound cake	38 ± 2	60	25	9
Proti pasta, protein-enriched, boiled in water	28 ± 2	180	49	14
Prune juice	43 ± 2	250	36	15
Prunes, pitted	29 ± 2	60	33	10
Quinoa, cooked, refrigerated, reheated in microwave for 1.5 min	53 ± 2	150	25	13
Raisin Bran Flax muffin, President's Choice® Blue Menu™	52 ± 3	70	33	17
Raisins	49 ± 2	28	20	10
Raspberry 100% Pure Fruit spread, no added sugar	26 ± 2	25	13	3
Seeded bread	49 ± 2	30	11	6
Sliced Apples, canned, solid packed without juice	42 ± 2	120	10	4
Slim Fast™ French Vanilla ready-to-drink shake	37 ± 2	250	27	10
Smoothie drink soy, banana	30 ± 4	250	22	7
Smoothie drink, banana	30 ± 4	250	26	8
Smoothie drink, banana and strawberry, V8 Splash®	44 ± 4	250	26	11
Smoothie drink, mango	32 ± 4	250	27	9
Smoothie drink, raspberry	33 ± 4	250	41	14
Soy Crunch Multi-Grain Cereal, President's Choice® Blue Menu™	47 ± 3	30	20	9
Soy milk, full-fat (3%), 120 mg calcium, Calciforte	41 ± 3	250	15	6
Soy milk, full-fat (3%), Calciforte, 120 mg calcium, with maltodextrin	36 ± 3	250	18	6
Soy milk, full-fat (3%), Original, 0 mg calcium, with maltodextrin	44 ± 3	250	17	8
Spaghetti bolognaise, home made	52 ± 2	360	48	25
Spaghetti, white, boiled	42 ± 3	180	46	18
Strawberries, fresh, raw	40 ± 3	120	3	1

Food Name	GI	Serving (g)	Tot Carb (g)	GL
Strawberry & wildberry dried fruit leather, Sunripe School Straps	40 ± 3	30	20	8
Strawberry & wildberry dried fruit leather, Sunripe School Straps	40 ± 3	30	20	8
Strawberry fruit leather	29 ± 3	30	24	7
SuperJuice Kickstart, containing apple juice, blueberry puree and banana puree	39 ± 3	250	28	11
Sushi, roasted sea algae, vinegar and rice	55 ± 3	100	37	20
Sushi, salmon	48 ± 3	100	36	17
Sweet and sour chicken with noodles, prepared convenience meal	41 ± 3	300	52	21
Sweet corn	55 ± 3	80	16	9
Sweet corn on the cob, boiled 20 min	48 ± 3	80	16	8
Sweet corn, cooked	52 ± 3	150	33	17
Sweet corn, frozen, reheated in microwave	47 ± 3	150	33	16
Sweet potato, boiled	44 ± 3	150	25	11
Tagliatelle, egg pasta, boiled in water for 7 min	46 ± 3	180	44	20
Tandoori chicken masala & rice convenience meal	45 ± 2	300	61	27
Tomato juice, no added sugar	33 ± 5	250	8	3
Tomato soup	38 ± 2	250	17	6
Tropical dried fruit snack	41 ± 4	15	11	5
Tuna fish bun	46 ± 4	87	32	14
V8 Splash®, tropical blend fruit drink	47 ± 3	250	28	13
V8® 100% vegetable juice	43 ± 3	250	9	4
Vanilla cake, made from packet mix with vanilla frosting	42 ± 3	111	58	24
Vanilla pudding, instant, made from powder and whole milk	40 ± 3	100	16	6
Vermicelli pasta, white, boiled	35 ± 3	180	44	16
White bread, homemade, frozen, defrosted and toasted	52 ± 2	30	13	7
White rice, boiled	43 ± 4	150	38	16
White wheat flour bread, butter, cheese, regular milk and fresh cucumber	55 ± 3	200	68	37
Whole-wheat bread with dried fruit	47 ± 3	30	14	7
Wholegrain water crackers with sesame seeds and rosemary	53 ± 3	25	16	8
Wholemeal (whole wheat) bread	50 ± 3	30	12	6
Wild berry dried fruit snack	35 ± 2	15	12	4
Wild Oats Cluster Crunch Hazelnut Chocolate breakfast cereal	43 ± 3	30	19	8
Xpress beverage, chocolate (soy bean, cereal and legume extract drink with fructose)	39 ± 3	250	34	13
Yam	51 ± 3	150	36	18

Moderate Glycemic Index Foods Tables

Food Name	GI	Serving (g)	Tot Carb (g)	GL
100% Whole wheat Burger Buns	62 ± 2	30	12	7
100% Whole wheat Hot Dog Rolls	62 ± 3	30	12	7
All-Bran Wheat Flakes™ breakfast cereal	60 ± 2	30	21	12
Apricot, coconut and honey muffin	60 ± 3	50	26	16
Apricot, raw	57 ± 2	120	9	5
Apricots, canned in light syrup	64 ± 3	120	19	12
Bagel, white bread	69 ± 3	70	35	24
Baked Beans in Tomato sauce, canned, reheated in microwave for 1.5 min	57 ± 2	150	23	13
Banana, oat and honey muffin	65 ± 2	50	26	17
Banana, raw	58 ± 2	120	23	13
Barley flakes breakfast cereal	69 ± 4	30	20	14
Barley flour bread, 100% barley flour	67 ± 3	30	13	9
Barley, rolled	66 ± 3	50	38	25
Basmati, easy cook white rice, boiled 9 min	67 ± 3	150	42	28
Basmati, easy-cook white rice, consumed with 10 g margarine	68 ± 3	150	41	28
Basmati, white rice, organic, boiled 10 min	57 ± 3	150	40	23
Beer, Toohey's New	66 ± 3	250	8	5
Blueberry (Wild) 10-Grain muffin, President's Choice® Blue Menu™	57 ± 3	70	39	22
Blueberry muffin	59 ± 3	57	29	17
Bran Flakes breakfast cereal	65 ± 3	30	19	12
Bran muffin	60 ± 3	57	24	14
Bread, flax, made from flax meal & wheat flour	67 ± 3	30	12	8
Breadfruit, raw	68 ± 2	120	27	18
Brown rice	66 ± 3	150	33	22
Buckwheat bread	67 ± 3	30	19	13
Carrot muffin	62 ± 3	57	32	20
Cereal biscuit (30 g), fruit flavor wheat biscuits consumed with 125 mL skim milk	56 ± 2	155	27	15
Cherries, dark, raw, pitted	63 ± 3	120	14	9
Chicken and mushroom soup	69 ± 2	250	19	13
Chickpea flour bread, made from extruded chickpea flour	67 ± 2	30	12	8
Classic French baguette bread with 10 g butter and 2 slices of ham (25 g)	59 ± 3	100	42	25
Clover honey, ratio of fructose: glucose, 1.09	69 ± 2	25	21	15
Coarse oat kernel bread, 80% intact oat kernels and 20% white wheat flour	65 ± 3	30	19	13
Coca Cola®, soft drink	63 ± 3	250	26	16
Coco yam (Xanthosoma spp.), peeled, cubed, boiled 30 min	61 ± 3	150	46	28
Cocoa Crunch cereal (30 g), consumed with 125 mL skim milk	58 ± 3	155	28	16
Cordial, orange, reconstituted	66 ± 2	250	20	13
Corn pasta, gluten-free, Orgran brand	68 ± 3	180	46	31
Cornmeal + margarine	69 ± 3	150	12	8
Cornmeal porridge	68 ± 3	150	13	9
Cornmeal, boiled in salted water 2 min	68 ± 2	150	13	9
Cottage pie	65 ± 2	300	34	22
Couscous, boiled 5 min	63 ± 4	150	35	21
Cranberry juice cocktail	68 ± 3	250	35	24

Food Name	GI	Serving (g)	Tot Carb (g)	GL
Cranberry juice drink	56 ± 3	250	29	16
Creamed rice porridge	59 ± 3	75	9	5
Dates	62 ± 3	60	33	21
Digestives, cookies	59 ± 2	25	16	9
Fanta®, orange soft drink	68 ± 3	250	34	23
Fibre First Multi-Bran Cereal, President's Choice® Blue Menu™	56 ± 3	30	10	6
Figs, dried, tenderised, Dessert Maid brand	61 ± 3	60	26	16
Fillet-O-Fish™ burger (fish patty, cheese and tartare sauce on a burger bun)	66 ± 3	128	30	20
Flan cake (Weston's Bakery, Toronto, Canada)	65 ± 3	70	48	31
French baguette bread with butter and strawberry jam	62 ± 3	70	41	26
Fruit and Fibre breakfast cereal	68 ± 3	30	20	13
Fruit loaf bread, sliced	57 ± 3	30	16	9
Fruit punch beverage	67 ± 3	250	29	19
Fruity-Bix™ bar, wheat biscuit cereal with dried fruit and nuts with yoghurt coating	56 ± 3	30	19	11
Fusilli pasta twists, boiled 10 min in salted water	61 ± 3	180	48	29
Glucose, 50 g portion, consumed with 14.5 g guar gum	62	10	10	6
Gnocchi, type not specified (Latina, Pillsbury Australia Ltd, Mt. Waverley, Australia)	68 ± 4	180	48	33
Granola Clusters breakfast cereal, Original, low fat, President's Choice® Blue Menu™	63 ± 2	30	22	14
Grany Rush Apricot, digestive cookies	62 ± 2	30	20	12
Grapes, black, Waltham Cross	59 ± 2	120	18	11
Hamburger (beef patty, ketchup, pickle, onion and mustard on a burger bun)	66 ± 4	95	25	17
Hamburger bun	61 ± 3	30	15	9
Happiness™ bread, cinnamon, raisin, pecan bread	63 ± 2	30	14	9
Healthwise™ for bowel health breakfast cereal	66 ± 2	30	18	12
Honey, Commercial Blend (38% fructose)	62 ± 2	25	18	11
Honey, Pure	58 ± 3	25	21	12
Honey, Pure	58 ± 3	25	21	12
Honey, Salvation Jane (32% fructose)	64 ± 3	25	15	10
Hunger Filler™, whole grain bread	59 ± 2	30	13	7
Ice cream (half vanilla, half chocolate), regular/type not specified	57 ± 2	50	10	6
Instant porridge	69 ± 2	250	20	14
Kiwi fruit	58 ± 2	120	12	7
Lean beef burger (lean beef patty, tomato, mixed lettuce, cheese, onion and sauce on a burger bun)	66 ± 4	164	26	17
Lentil and cauliflower cury with rice	60 ± 2	300	42	25
Low-fat yoghurt, peach melba	56 ± 2	200	28	16
Low-fat yoghurt, strawberry	61 ± 2	200	30	18
LU Petit Dejeuner Chocolate & Cereals cookies	58 ± 3	50	35	20
Macaroni, boiled	56 ± 2	180	48	27
Mars Bar® (M&M/Mars, USA)	68 ± 3	60	40	27
Marshmallows	62 ± 2	30	24	15
McChicken™ burger (chicken patty, lettuce, mayonnaise on a burger bun)	66 ± 2	186	40	26
Oro cookies	61 ± 3	40	34	21
Pastry	59 ± 3	57	26	15
Peach, canned in heavy syrup	64 ± 3	120	19	12
Peach, raw	56 ± 2	120	8	5
Pineapple, raw	66 ± 2	120	10	6
Pita bread, white	67 ± 2	30	17	10
Pita bread, white (Sainsbury's, UK), with 5 g margarine	67 ± 2	30	15	10

Food Name	GI	Serving (g)	Tot Carb (g)	GL
Pita bread, wholemeal	56 ± 2	30	14	8
Pizza, cheese	60 ± 2	100	27	16
Porridge, made from rolled oats	63 ± 2	250	30	19
Potato, type not specified, boiled	66 ± 2	150	19	13
Potato, white with skin, baked, consumed with 10 g margarine	69 ± 2	150	27	19
Potato, white, cooked	61 ± 2	150	26	16
Probiotic yoghurt drink, cranberry	56 ± 2	250	31	17
Raisins	66 ± 2	60	43	28
Soy Tasty™ breakfast cereal (flaked grains, soy nuts, dried fruit)	60 ± 2	30	20	12
Spaghetti, white, durum wheat, boiled 20 min	58 ± 3	180	44	26
Special K™ breakfast cereal	69 ± 3	30	21	14
Sugar (Sucrose), 100 g portion	65	10	10	7
Sunflower and barley bread	57 ± 2	30	11	6
Sweet corn	62 ± 2	80	18	11
Sweet corn, boiled	60 ± 2	80	18	11
Traditional French baguette (prepared with wheat flour, water, salt and 20 g yeast)	69 ± 2	30	18	12
Vegetable soup	60 ± 2	250	18	11
White bread with added wheatgerm and fiber	59 ± 2	30	12	6
White bread with butter	59 ± 2	100	48	28
White bread, fresh, toasted	63 ± 2	30	12	8
White bread, homemade, fresh, toasted	66 ± 2	30	13	9
White bread, wheat flour	69 ± 2	30	14	10
White bread, wheat flour, frozen, defrosted and toasted	64 ± 2	30	12	8
Wholemeal bread, stoneground flour	59 ± 1	30	11	7
Yoghurt, black cherry	67 ± 3	200	12	8
Yoghurt, bourbon vanilla	64 ± 3	200	32	20
Yoghurt, lemon curd	67 ± 3	200	45	30
Yoghurt, peach melba	57 ± 3	200	32	18

High Glycemic Index Foods Tables

Food Name	GI	Serving (g)	Tot Carb (g)	GL
15 g Oat bran (containing 2 g ß-glucan), consumed as a drink mixed with 41g glucose and water	84 ± 3	10	3	2
Bagel, white, frozen (Lender's Bakery, Montreal, Canada)	72 ± 3	70	35	25
Baguette, white, plain	95 ± 2	30	15	14
Barley flour bread, made from 50% wheat flour and 50% coarse sieved barley flour	74 ± 3	30	16	12
Barquette Abricot cookies	71 ± 4	40	32	23
Blackbread, Riga	76 ± 3	30	13	10
Bran Flakes™ breakfast cereal	74 ± 4	30	18	13
Bread stuffing, Paxo	74 ± 3	30	21	16
Breadfruit roasted on preheated charcoal	72 ± 3	120	27	20
Broken rice, white, cooked in rice cooker	86 ± 3	150	43	37
Brown rice	87 ± 2	150	33	29
Brown rice, boiled in excess water for 25 min, SunRice brand	72 ± 3	150	40	29
Brown rice, boiled in excess water for 25 min, SunRice brand	72 ± 3	150	40	29
Cheerios™ breakfast cereal	74 ± 4	30	20	15
Chicken Tandoori Deli Choice white French roll white bread	78 ± 3	270	56	44
Chocapic™ breakfast cereal, wheat-based flaked cereal	70 ± 4	30	25	17
Coco Pops™ breakfast cereal (cocoa flavored puffed rice)	77 ± 4	30	26	20
Corn Bran™ breakfast cereal	75 ± 4	30	20	15
Corn Chex™ breakfast cereal	83 ± 4	30	25	21
Corn pasta, gluten-free, Orgran brand	78 ± 2	180	42	32
Corn Pops™ breakfast cereal	80 ± 4	30	26	21
Cornflakes breakfast cereal	79 ± 4	30	25	20
Cornflakes breakfast cereal (Kellogg's, France)	93 ± 4	30	27	25
Cornflakes breakfast cereal consumed with 150 mL semi-skimmed milk	93 ± 4	30	25	23
Cornflakes, Crunchy Nut™ breakfast cereal	72 ± 4	30	24	17
Cornflakes™ breakfast cereal	77 ± 4	30	25	19
Cornflakes™ breakfast cereal	80 ± 4	30	26	21
Cornflakes™ breakfast cereal (Kellogg's Inc., Canada)	86 ± 4	30	26	22
Cornflakes™ breakfast cereal (Kellogg's, USA)	92 ± 4	30	26	24
Cotton honey, ratio of fructose:glucose, 1.03	74 ± 2	25	22	16
Crunchy Nut Cornflakes™ bar	72 ± 4	30	26	19
Crunchy Nut Cornflakes™ bar	72 ± 3	30	26	19
Cupcake, strawberry-iced, Squiggles	73 ± 3	38	26	19
Doughnut, wheat dough, deep-fried	75 ± 2	50	20	15
Fiber White™ bread	77 ± 2	30	15	11
French baguette bread with chocolate spread	72 ± 3	70	37	27
French bread, fermented with yeast	81 ± 2		30	16	13
Fruit and cinnamon bread	71 ± 3	30	16	11
Fruit and cinnamon bread	71 ± 2		30	16	11
Gluten Free Multigrain bread	79 ± 3	30	13	10
Gluten-free buckwheat bread, made with buckwheat meal & rice flour	72 ± 2	30	11	8
Gluten-free white bread, unsliced (gluten-free wheat starch)	71 ± 3	30	15	10
Golden Wheats™ breakfast cereal	71 ± 2	30	23	16
Granola Clusters breakfast cereal, Raisin & Almond, low fat, President's Choice® Blue Menu™	70 ± 4	30	22	15
Grapenuts™ breakfast cereal	75 ± 4	30	22	16

Food Name	GI	Serving (g)	Tot Carb (g)	GL
Honey Goldies™ wheat biscuits with additional ingredients	72 ± 4	30	21	15
Honey Rice Bubbles™ breakfast cereal	77 ± 3	30	27	20
Honey Smacks™ breakfast cereal	71 ± 4	30	23	16
Honey, Commercial Blend (28% fructose), NSW blend	72 ± 3	25	13	9
Instant oat cereal porridge prepared with water	83 ± 3	250	36	30
Instant oat porridge, cooked in microwave with water	82 ± 3	250	24	20
Japanese Wasabi & Honey Rice & Corn Crisps,	82 ± 3	50	39	32
Jelly beans, assorted colors (Allen's, Nestlé, Australia)	80 ± 4	30	28	22
Jelly beans, assorted colors (Savings, Grocery Holdings, Tooronga, Australia)	76 ± 3	30	28	21
Morning Coffee™ cookies	79 ± 4	25	19	15
Muesli	86 ± 4	30	21	18
Multigrain bread, with 5 g maragrine	80 ± 3	30	10	8
Pancakes, prepared from wheat flour	80 ± 3	80	20	16
Pikelets, Golden brand	85 ± 3	40	21	18
Pizza, plain baked dough, served with parmesan cheese and tomato sauce	80 ± 2	100	27	22
Potato, type not specified, boiled in salted water	76 ± 2	150	34	26
Potato, type not specified, peeled, boiled	85 ± 2	150	30	26
Pumpkin Soup, creamy, Heinz® Very Special™, with pumpkin, cream, potatoes	76 ± 2	250	18	14
Pumpkin, boiled in salted water	75 ± 2	80	4	3
Raspberry Fruit bar, fat-free, President's Choice® Blue Menu™ (Loblaw Brands Limited, Canada)	74 ± 2	40	31	23
Real Fruit Bars, strawberry (Uncle Toby's, Australia)	90 ± 3	30	26	23
Rice milk drink, low-fat, Australia's Own Natural™	92 ± 3	250	32	29
Rice Pops™, with 125 mL semi-skimmed milk	80 ± 4	30	25	20
Rice porridge	88 ± 3	150	15	13
Rockmelon/Cantaloupe, raw	70 ± 2	120	6	4
Special K™ breakfast cereal, made from rice	84 ± 4	30	23	20
Strawberry processed fruit bars, Real Fruit Bars	90 ± 2	30	26	23
Watermelon, raw	80 ± 2	120	6	5
Wheat based cereal biscuit, wheat biscuits (plain flaked wheat)	72 ± 4	30	20	14
Wheat-bites™ breakfast cereal	72 ± 3	30	25	18
White bread, wheat flour	78 ± 3	30	15	12
Wholemeal (whole wheat) bread	71 ± 2	30	12	9

NOTES

The information provided in this book is compiled from the most up-to-date sources in November 2019. The main source of the date is the United states Department of Agriculture.

Made in the USA
Las·Vegas, NV
10 January 2022

41015592R00152